Pulmonary Imaging

Pulmonary Imaging
Contributions to Key Clinical Questions

Edited by

Sujal R Desai MD FRCP FRCR

Consultant Radiologist
Department of Radiology
King's College Hospital
London
UK

Tomás Franquet MD PhD

Chief, Thoracic Radiology
Hospital de Sant Pau
Barcelona
Spain

Thomas E Hartman MD

Chief, Thoracic Radiology
Department of Radiology
Mayo Clinic
Rochester, MN
USA

Athol U Wells MD FRACP

Professor of Respiratory Medicine
Interstitial Lung Disease Unit
Royal Brompton Hospital
London
UK

informa
healthcare

First published in the United Kingdom in 2007 by Informa Healthcare, Telephone House, 69-77 Paul Street, London EC2A 4LQ. Informa Healthcare is a trading division of Informa UK Ltd. Registered Office: 37/41 Mortimer Street, London W1T 3JH. Registered in England and Wales number 1072954.

Tel: +44 (0)20 7017 5000
Fax: +44 (0)20 7017 6699
Website: www.informahealthcare.com

Although every effort has been made to ensure that all owners of copyright material have been acknowledged in this publication, we would be glad to acknowledge in subsequent reprints or editions any omissions brought to our attention.

Although every effort has been made to ensure that drug doses and other information are presented accurately in this publication, the ultimate responsibility rests with the prescribing physician. Neither the publishers nor the authors can be held responsible for errors or for any consequences arising from the use of information contained herein. For detailed prescribing information or instructions on the use of any product or procedure discussed herein, please consult the prescribing information or instructional material issued by the manufacturer.

A CIP record for this book is available from the British Library.
Library of Congress Cataloging-in-Publication Data

Data available on application

ISBN-10: 1 84214 324 7
ISBN-13: 978 1 84214 324 7

Distributed in North and South America by
Taylor & Francis
6000 Broken Sound Parkway, NW, (Suite 300)
Boca Raton, FL 33487, USA

Within Continental USA
Tel: 1 (800) 272 7737; Fax: 1 (800) 374 3401
Outside Continental USA
Tel: (561) 994 0555; Fax: (561) 361 6018
Email: orders@crcpress.com

Distributed in the rest of the world by
Thomson Publishing Services
Cheriton House
North Way
Andover, Hampshire SP10 5BE, UK
Tel: +44 (0)1264 332424
Email: tps.tandfsalesorder@thomson.com

Composition by Exeter Premedia Services Pvt Ltd, Chennai, India
Printed and bound in India by Replika Press Pvt Ltd

Dedications

To Mary and Emily for keeping me grounded and for sharing with me
the things that are more important than Radiology.
Thomas E Hartman

To my parents. For everything . . .
Sujal R Desai

I dedicate this to the late Dr Bill Douglas
Athol U Wells

To Salomé, Tomás, Pablo and Elisa Franquet
Tomás Franquet

Contents

Contributors

Alexander Bankier MD
Associate Professor of Radiology
University of Vienna
Chief of Thoracic Imaging Section
Medical University of Vienna
Vienna
Austria

Sujal R Desai MD FRCP FRCR
Consultant Radiologist
Department of Radiology
King's College Hospital
London
UK

Tomás Franquet MD PhD
Chief, Thoracic Radiology
Hospital de Sant Pau
Barcelona
Spain

Fergus V Gleeson FRCP FRCR
Consultant Radiologist
Churchill Hospital
Oxford
UK

Thomas E Hartman MD
Chief, Thoracic Radiology
Department of Radiology
Mayo Clinic
Rochester, MN
USA

David M Hansell MD FRCP FRCR
Professor of Thoracic Imaging
Department of Radiology
Royal Brompton Hospital
London
UK

John W Hildebrandt MD
Mayo Clinic College of Medicine
Rochester, MN
USA

Sanjay Kalra MD FRCP(UK)
Associate Professor
Mayo Clinic College of Medicine
Consultant, Division of Pulmonary and
Critical Care Medicine
Rochester, MN
USA

Joseph J Kavanagh MD
Division of Thoracic Imaging
Department of Radiology
Medical Univerisity of South Carolina
Charleston, SC
USA

YC Gary Lee PhD FCCP FRACP
Consultant Physician
Churchill Hospital
Oxford
UK

Douglas R Lake MD
Division of Thoracic Imaging
Department of Radiology
Medical University of South Carolina
Charleston, SC
USA

David L Levin MD PhD
Associate Professor of Radiology
Mayo Clinic College of Medicine
Department of Radiology
Mayo Clinic
Rochester, MN
USA

David E Midthun MD
Associate Professor of Medicine Consultant
Division of Pulmonary and Critical Care Medcine
Mayo Clinic College of Medicine
Rochester, MN
USA

Maureen Quigley MRCS FRCR
Radioloy Fellow
Royal Brompton Hospital
London
UK

Otis B Rickman DO
Division of Pulmonary and Critical Care Medicine
Mayo Clinic
Rochester, MN
USA

Jay H Ryu MD
Division of Pulmonary and Critical Care Medicine
Mayo Clinic
Rochester, MN
USA

U Joseph Schoepf MD
Division of Thoracic Imaging
Department of Radiology
Medical University of South Carolina
Charleston, SC
USA

Jacob Sellarés MD
Respiratory Physician
Pulmonology Department
Hospital Clinic
Barcelona
Spain

Leopold Stiebellehner MD
Associate Professor of Medicine
University of Barcelona
Pulmonology Department
Medical University of Vienna
Vienna
Austria

Stephen J Swenson MD
Department of Radiology
Mayo Clinic
Rochester
Minnesota, MN
USA

Anne-Marie Sykes MD
Department of Radiology
Mayo Clinic
Rochester, MN
USA

Antoni Torres MD
Associate Professor of Medicine
University of Barcelona
Head of Pulmonology Department
Hospital Clinic
Barcelona
Spain

Athol U Wells MD FRACP
Professor of Respiratory Medicine
Intersitial Lung Disease Unit
Royal Brompton Hospital
London
UK

Preface

Imaging tests have long been central to the practice of pulmonary medicine and surgery. Indeed, driven by an epidemic of tuberculosis and barely six months following the discovery of the x-ray, the American physician Francis H Williams saw the potential of radiologic tests when, using fluoroscopic screening, he was able to demonstrate non-invasively foci of pulmonary infection. Since those early days, there has been a steady revolution in imaging technology: for example, the advent of digital chest radiography sought to address some of the well-known constraints of conventional techniques. The development of computed tomography (CT) in the 1970s made it possible to view cross-sectional images of the body and, not long after that, high-resolution CT (HRCT) matured into a technique that is now seen as standard in the investigation of patients with diffuse interstitial lung disease. Most recently, multidetector CT machines, capable of imaging the whole thorax within a single breath hold, have become available and are having a significant impact.

Taken together, the advances in radiology have been of undoubted benefit. Certain radiologic techniques (for instance, HRCT in the diagnosis of bronchiectasis and CT pulmonary angiography for patients with suspected acute thromboembolism) have rendered more traditional tests (i.e. bronchography and conventional angiography) almost obsolete. However, it must be stressed that, in specific clinical scenarios, the enthusiasm for a particular radiologic test has sometimes leapt ahead of the evidence for its true utility. Thus, knowing which of the mulititude of radiologic tests is optimal to answer a specific clinical question is not always appreciated

Unlike other texts of imaging for clinicians, this book seeks not to teach the physician or surgeon about the radiologic signs of pulmonary disease but rather inform about the value of the various imaging tests in different clinical scenarios. Accordingly, each chapter has been written by a clinician and radiologist: the basic ethos is that the clinician identifies the common problem-areas and questions faced in a given field of pulmonology and that the radiologist attempts to critically define the role, if any, of the different imaging studies. It is our hope that this book will be valued not only by physicians and surgeons but also by Radiologist who regularly investigate and manage patients with pulmonary disease.

SUJAL R DESAI
TOMÁS FRANQUET
THOMAS E HARTMAN
ATHOL U WELLS

Color plates

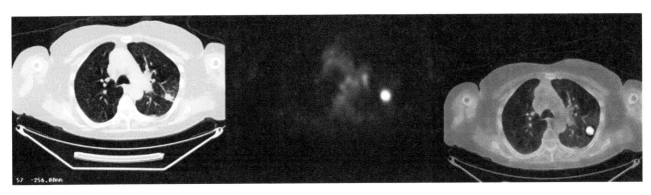

Figure 2.2
CT, PET, and fused PET/CT image of an 84-year-old woman with bronchogenic carcinoma. The left upper lobe nodule is shown to have increased uptake on the PET image which is confirmed on the fused PET/CT image.

(a)

(b)

(c)

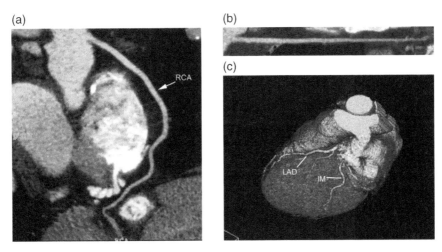

Figure 3.22
Normal coronary artery anatomy. (a) Two-dimensional multiplanar reconstruction of the right coronary artery (RCA) obtained at 16-row multidetector CT (MDCT); this technique is used to evaluate the entire coronary artery in one view. (b) Artery can also be seen in its long length and it can be displayed as a very straight line. (c) Three-dimensional volume-rendered reconstruction at MDCT coronary angiography. Left anterior oblique view showing left anterior descending coronary artery (LAD), and intermediate coronary artery branch (IM).

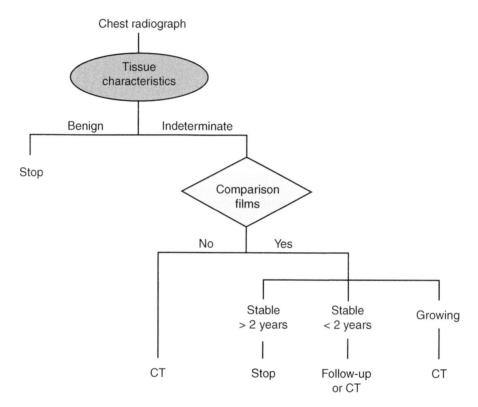

Figure 6.9
Decision algorithm for SPNs encountered on plain radiograph. Oval shaped branch point
represents decision made based on radiographic findings, whereas diamond shaped branch points represent decision made based
on clinical information.

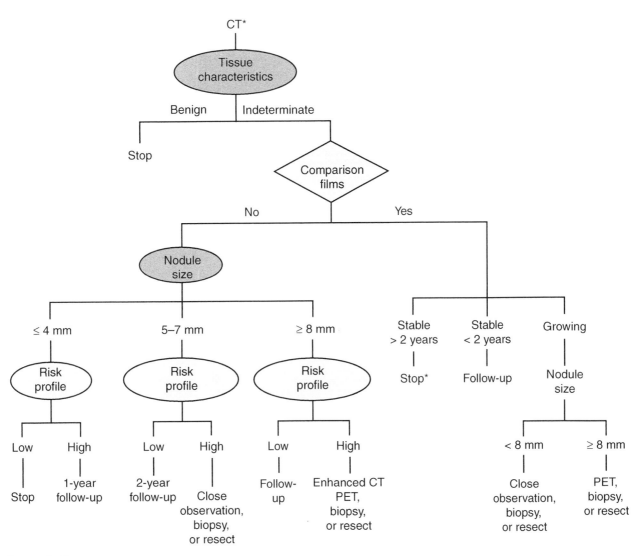

Figure 6.10

Decision algorithm for SPNs encountered on CT. *Ground glass partially solid nodules may require longer yearly follow-up to establish that they are begin. PET, positron emission tomography.

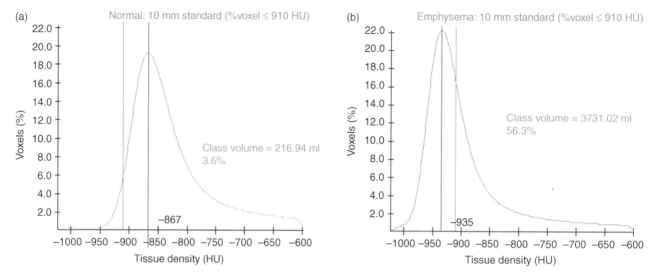

Figure 13.4

Quantitative evaluation of the lung parenchyma in a healthy subject (a) and a patient with emphysema (b). The histogram plots demonstrate the density distribution of voxels within the lung. In the healthy subject, the mean density for the lung is −867 HU and only 3.6% of all voxels have a density less than −910 HU. In the patient with emphysema, the mean lung density decreases to −935 HU and the percentage of lung voxels below −910 HU has increased to 56.3%.

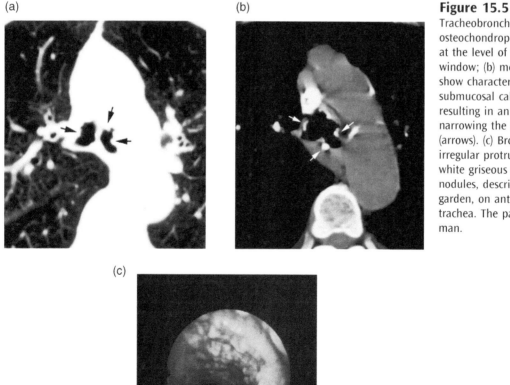

Figure 15.5

Tracheobronchopathia osteochondroplastica. Axial CT images at the level of the carina ((a) lung window; (b) mediastinal window) show characteristic appearance of submucosal calcified nodules, resulting in an irregular lumen narrowing the main bronchi lumen (arrows). (c) Bronchoscopic image shows irregular protrusions caused by multiple white griseous osteocartilaginous nodules, described as resembling a rock garden, on anterolateral wall of the trachea. The patient was a 67-year-old man.

(a)

(b)

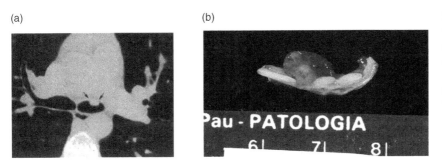

Figure 15.19
Mucoepidermoid carcinoma. (a) CT scan (2-mm collimation) at the level of the carina shows a well marginated nodule in left main bronchus. (b) Corresponding surgical specimen. The patient was a 18-year-old man with hemoptysis.

(a)

(b)

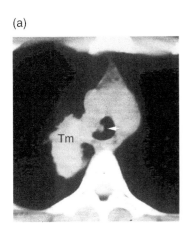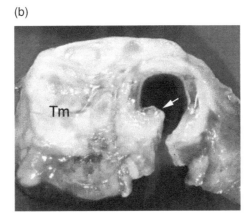

Figure 15.20
Bronchogenic carcinoma. (a) Non-enhanced CT scan (5-mm collimation) at the level of the aortic arch shows a right upper lobe lung cancer (Tm) invading the adjacent mediastinum and the lateral wall of the trachea (arrow). (b) Corresponding gross specimen obtained from autopsy confirms the mediastinal mass (Tm) and tracheal invasion (arrow).

(a)

(b)

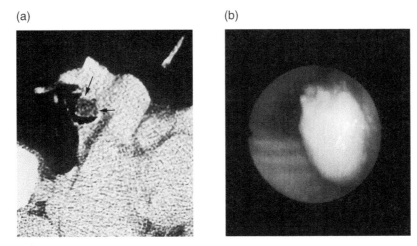

Figure 15.21
Intrabronchial lipoma. Mediastinal window CT scan (2.0-mm collimation) shows an endobronchial fatty mass (arrows) in the intermediate bronchus. (b) Fiberoptic bronchoscopy confirmed the lipomatous nature of the tumor. The patient was a 42-year-old man with persistent cough.

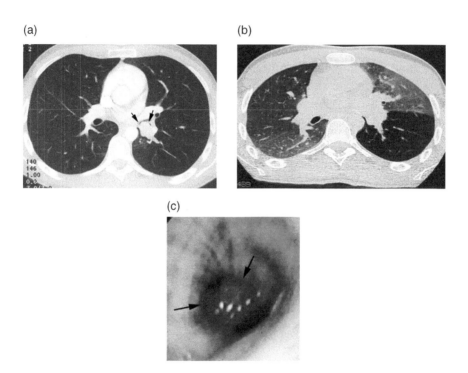

(a)

(b)

(c)

Figure 15.23

Bronchial carcinoid. (a) HRCT image (2.0-mm collimation) at the level of the intermediate bronchus shows a well defined, round, and partially endobronchial nodule (arrows) in the inferior bronchus of the left lower lobe. (b) Expiratory CT scan (lung windowing) shows overinflation and air trapping of the left lower lobe. (c) Photograph obtained during bronchoscopy shows a typical well defined 'reddy' nodule (arrows). The patient was a 18-year-old man with recurrent pneumonia and chronic cough.

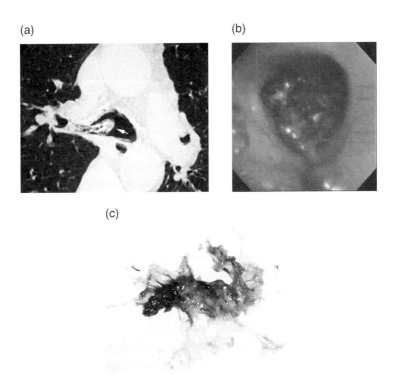

Figure 15.25
Mucus plug. (a) HRCT scan (2-mm collimation) at the level of the carina shows a 'tongue-like' material (arrow) filling the lumen of the main right bronchus and extending into the carina. Note the presence of tiny black lucencies (air bubbles) within the material. (b) Fiberoptic bronchoscopy demonstrated a tenacious mucous material that was subsequently removed. Note hematic content of mucus plug (c). The patient was a 55-year-old man with chronic bronchitis.

SECTION I: INTRODUCTION

Imaging in Pulmonary Medicine: A Chest Physician's Perspective

1

Imaging in pulmonary medicine: a chest physician's perspective

Athol U Wells

The accuracy of a diagnostic radiological test is generally quantified in the radiological literature as a statement of the sensitivity, specificity, overall accuracy, and the positive and negative predictive values of the test against a reference standard for diagnosis. However, for most new radiological procedures, there is a considerable time lag between the documentation of apparent diagnostic accuracy and the widespread adoption of a test in clinical practice. This phenomenon is a recurring theme in respiratory medicine, reflecting the inability of standard diagnostic statements to capture the true clinical utility of a test in routine management. In essence, the real contribution of radiological findings to the resolution of common clinical problems is seldom captured in the medical literature. In this introductory chapter, the inapplicability of keynote radiological series is reviewed. The investigation and management of diffuse lung disease is used as a basis for discussion as this difficult field amply illustrates the credibility gap between academic radiological studies and clinical practice.

Diagnostic radiological series necessarily examine a test such as high-resolution computed tomography (HRCT) without reference to pre-test probabilities. In the early landmark HRCT series in diffuse lung disease of the late 1980s, the accuracy of the test was evaluated against the histological diagnosis at surgical biopsy.[1-4] However, clinicians seeking to apply the findings in their day-to-day practice require a sense of the true value added by HRCT to routine diagnosis and management. In academic series, the HRCT findings are considered without reference to other information available to the clinician, with HRCT examined as though it provided the only data of diagnostic value. In reality, as in other respiratory subspecialties, there is a wealth of data available for diagnostic purposes in diffuse lung disease. A number of other tests have usually been performed before HRCT, including chest radiography, pulmonary function tests, and, often, serological tests to disclose underlying connective tissue disease or the presence of precipitins indicative of immunological reactivity

in patients with hypersensitivity pneumonia. Furthermore, a great deal of clinical information is woven into the act of diagnosis, including demographic data, the presence of likely causative factors, observed disease behavior (including the rapidity of previous decline and the degree of responsiveness to previous treatment), data on disease severity, and findings on clinical examination. In essence, HRCT can make only a partial contribution to diagnosis in diffuse lung disease. The use of HRCT to diagnose sarcoidosis illustrates the limitations of clinical series. In many cases, HRCT reveals virtually pathognomonic appearances but the diagnosis is often obvious from the clinical presentation and chest radiographic findings. Thus, many successful HRCT diagnoses in reported series, seeming to validate the utility of HRCT, make little if any real contribution to clinical diagnosis. Conversely, in other cases, in which HRCT is seen to fail, because the diagnosis of first choice is at odds with the histological diagnosis, HRCT information is diagnostically pivotal in distinguishing accurately between two likely diagnoses based on pre-test probabilities. In the entirety of the first 15 years, during which HRCT was increasingly applied in clinical practice, this aspect of HRCT was examined in only one series, in which increasing diagnostic accuracy against a histological diagnosis was seen when HRCT data were added to clinical and chest radiographic information.[5] The importance of this series, which can now be viewed as a decade ahead of its time, was not widely appreciated. Paradoxically, the real value and limitations of diagnostic HRCT in diffuse lung disease were widely appreciated by experienced clinicians and radiologists before their depiction in the radiological and respiratory literature.

In part, the problem arises from an understandable fixation with the validation of a new procedure against a reference standard. Reference standard tests are often cumbersome procedures which are undertaken in a selected minority of cases. This point is well illustrated by the use of HRCT to diagnose bronchiectasis. Prior to HRCT, bronchography was viewed as the 'gold standard' for diagnosis but was an unpleasant test for patients and was prone to significant interobserver variation.[6] HRCT was never validated definitively against bronchography but assumed a central role in the standard diagnosis of bronchiectasis, simply because it was widely found to provide useful information that was consistently compatible with clinical findings. In much the same way, ventilation/perfusion scanning and computed tomography (CT) evaluation largely supplanted pulmonary angiography in the detection of pulmonary embolism prior to formal validation. In diffuse lung disease, the perceived reference standard, a surgical lung biopsy, is often impracticable because of pulmonary disease severity, co-morbidity from other diseases, or advanced age. Furthermore, as a histological diagnosis it has lost its iconic diagnostic status,[7] there has been increasing focus on the considerable diagnostic variation between histopathologists[8] and the problem of 'sampling error' (in which a biopsy fails to capture the dominant histological process and may be diagnostically misleading).[9] It appears that the inherent clinical drawbacks of many diagnostic reference standards are not widely acknowledged until the advantages of a less invasive test become apparent. With time, the status of a reference standard test is subsumed as its role is re-evaluated.[10] In diffuse lung disease, optimal diagnosis is now widely acknowledged to be multidisciplinary with the construction of a final diagnosis from clinical, radiological, and histological information.[7,11] In a significant minority of patients, the histological diagnosis, made in isolation, is seen to be incorrect once clinical and radiological data have been considered. The demotion of a reference standard generally occurs after the true utility of an alternative test has been validated by clinical experience and, it appears, is seldom based upon prior landmark series. In other words, the value of a new test needs to be explored in clinical practice before academic radiological series are widely accepted.

Other inherent flaws in diagnostic radiological series are evident when studies of HRCT in diffuse lung disease are considered. In early series, evaluation was mostly confined to statements of the diagnostic sensitivity of HRCT against a final histological diagnosis. The relative prevalence of the key diseases contributing to differential diagnosis is seldom captured in referral center populations and, therefore, sensitivity and specificity statements are considered to be more reliable. However, in reality, the true value of a test lies in the positive and negative predictive values for the most frequently encountered diseases. In diffuse lung disease, the HRCT diagnosis of idiopathic pulmonary fibrosis (IPF), the most frequent, most aggressive disorder, is based upon knowledge of the high positive predictive value of typical HRCT appearances. However, the limitations of HRCT will only be understood if it is known that a large minority of patients with IPF have atypical HRCT findings: the exclusion of IPF cannot be based upon HRCT in isolation. This became anecdotally obvious to clinicians seeking to apply the radiological literature long before it was disclosed in clinical series, which were published after more than 10 years of HRCT usage.[12,13]

The artificial nature of studies performed in referral centers is problematic in other respects. Series are usually constructed by selecting key disorders from a hospital diagnostic codex, with appropriate care taken to ensure that a final diagnosis is secure. However, disorders that are seldom encountered in routine practice tend to be referred to specialist centers. Thus, in HRCT diagnostic series of diffuse lung disease, rare entities such as lymphangioleiomyomatosis and Langerhans' cell histiocytosis tend to be over-represented and evaluation is confined to the diffuse lung diseases without consideration of more frequently encountered disorders that may simulate diffuse lung disease. Diagnostic HRCT series in diffuse lung disease do not include patients with heart failure, metastatic malignancy (other than lymphangitis carcinomatosis), chronic infection, and bronchiectasis. However, as many clinicians have found to their cost, all these disorders may be overlooked once a diagnostic assumption of diffuse lung disease has been made. Radiologists who seek to apply HRCT series to routine diagnosis receive little or no guidance on the manifestations of these disorders and will often be biased towards a diagnosis of diffuse lung disease by the wording of a request form. The misdiagnosis of cancer as a benign disorder is a major source of stress for patients and clinicians, and this, almost certainly, occurs more often than is generally appreciated.

Misdiagnosis is less likely to occur at referral centers where radiologists tend to have a deeper knowledge of typical appearances of a relatively new diagnostic test and are more likely to alert the clinician that the diagnostic net needs to be cast more widely. The greater experience of radiologists participating in landmark series is a further problem when it comes to extrapolating the findings to routine practice. In diffuse lung disease, sporadic attempts have been made to examine the accuracy of less experienced observers[3,14] but the real problems experienced by radiologists who have not received preliminary training in the diagnostic use of a test cannot be overstated. In reality, this is well understood by most clinicians. The evolution of a test to routine clinical usage generally comes from partnerships between individual clinicians and radiologists, with informal audit of the accuracy of radiological diagnosis, based upon eventual final diagnoses and observed disease behavior. This process eventually leads to a second wave of radiological series, in which the limitations of a test are better understood, but which tend to document the real utility of the test well after it has assumed its true role in clinical practice. The confidence with which radiological observations are made is also pivotal to diagnosis but this aspect has also been difficult to quantify in routine practice, despite worthy attempts to do so in academic series.[1,2,5] A diffident HRCT diagnosis in diffuse lung disease, however accurate, cannot serve as a secure basis for prognosis or confident management. Once again, the experience of a radiologist in the use of the test is a key ingredient which cannot be easily factored into the diagnostic equation, based upon landmark series. Furthermore, although many patients have classical diagnostic findings, there are often overlapping features between disorders that complicate radiological diagnosis. This aspect is seldom disclosed in published series, in which photographic examples tend to be chosen to illustrate cases with typical appearances in which a diagnostic test is accurate.

The problems encountered in applying diagnostic series apply equally to other uses of a radiological test, including the staging of disease severity, the use of the test in monitoring, and the application of the test to prognosis. If anything, the problems are even greater than in diagnostic evaluation because these aspects tend to be less studied than diagnostic accuracy. In diffuse lung disease, HRCT findings and pulmonary function tests are usually considered together in reaching impressions about disease severity but no logical algorithm has been validated for the amalgamation of these tests. Similarly, HRCT is often used to monitor disease, on the supposition that it should be suited to this purpose because it is clearly a sensitive test, but this use of HRCT is wholly empirical with no overall consensus as to best practice. For all their flaws when it comes to clinical extrapolation, academic series do serve as a starting point from which the use of a test can evolve. However, clinicians have needs that are not always addressed in the medical literature. Prognostic evaluation is a key part of the assessment of diffuse lung disease. However, although the prognostic role of HRCT has been considered in IPF in several series,[15–17] the added value of HRCT in predicting the rapidity of progression in other diffuse lung disorders has not been formally considered. If clinicians are to make the best possible use of radiological data, there needs to be clear recognition of the lack of proof of radiological utility in many clinical scenarios. Radiological information may still be valuable when integrated with other information in a commonsensical fashion, but awareness of lack of validation needs to be kept constantly in mind. In diffuse lung disease, it is often possible to observe minor changes in disease extent on serial imaging but although this finding is sometimes useful when lung function trends are marginal, the greater importance of major functional change, validated in many clinical series, must not be forgotten.

The supposition that the superior sensitivity of a new radiological test is invariably advantageous does not stand up to close scrutiny. Low dose HRCT screening for lung cancer may seem to offer new opportunities for the earlier detection of malignant disease. However, the fact that most small nodules detected on screening HRCT are benign creates difficulties for clinicians, who must choose between active investigation, with a low probability of disclosing malignancy, and prolonged monitoring with attendant patient stress due to prolonged uncertainty. The widespread use of

CT pulmonary angiography has led to similar difficulties. Thrombi are sometimes isolated in small subsegmental vessels but their significance is wholly uncertain, with no data available on which to formulate a management strategy, be it non-intervention or anticoagulation. In connective tissue diseases, the sensitivity of HRCT is often advanced as a justification for routine HRCT screening, in order to detect early diffuse lung disease. It is now clear that in most connective tissue diseases, minor HRCT abnormalities are evident in the majority or a large minority of patients.[18–21] However, in many cases, limited abnormalities do not progress and the clinician has to deal with a new group of patients with subclinical disease in which there is ongoing uncertainty as to optimal management. Thus, the considerable sensitivity advantages of many radiological procedures may, at times, lead to difficult clinical dilemmas.

The unifying theme, when the radiological literature is extrapolated to clinical practice, is that clinical context is pivotal. For the most part, new radiological tests are applied to classical clinical problems, in which an established clinical approach is already in place: this applies equally to disease detection, diagnosis, prognostic evaluation, staging of severity, monitoring and the detection of complications. The value of radiological procedures lies in their ability to change clinical perception, when combined with pre-test clinical probabilities. However, this core role of radiological procedures is difficult to define for all the reasons discussed above, but depends upon informal validation in clinical practice. To appreciate the true utility of a radiological test, an iterative approach is needed, with consideration of the value added by radiological evaluation when key clinical problems are confronted. In this book, the difficulties encountered by clinicians in each respiratory subspecialty are enumerated, and contributions made by radiological tests to clinical problem solving are reviewed.

References

1. Mathieson JR, Mayo JR, Staples CA, Muller NL. Chronic diffuse infiltrative lung disease: comparison of diagnositic accuracy of CT and chest radiography. Radiology 1989; 171: 111–6.
2. Padley SPG, Hansell DM, Flower CDR, Jennings P. Comparative accuracy of high resolution computed tomography and chest radiography in the diagnosis of chronic diffuse infiltrative lung disease. Clin Radiol 1991; 44: 222–6.
3. Grenier P, Valeyre D, Cluzel P et al. Chronic diffuse infiltrative lung disease: diagnostic value of chest radiography and high-resolution CT. Radiology 1991; 178: 123–32.
4. Bergin CJ, Coblentz CL, Chiles C, Bell DY, Castellino RA. Chronic lung diseases: specific diagnosis by using CT. AJR Am J Roentgenol 1989; 152: 1183–8.
5. Grenier P, Chevret S, Beigelman C et al. Chronic diffuse infiltrative lung disease: determination of the diagnostic value of clinical data, chest radiography, and CT and Bayesian analysis. Radiology 1994; 191: 383–90.

6. Currie DC, Cooke JC, Morgan AD et al. Interpretation of bronchograms and chest radiographs in patients with chronic sputum production. Thorax 1987; 42: 278–84.

7. Wells AU. Histopathologic diagnosis in diffuse lung disease: an ailing gold standard. Am J Respir Crit Care Med 2004; 170: 828–9.

8. Nicholson AG, Addis BJ, Bharucha H et al. Inter-observer variation between pathologists in diffuse parenchymal lung disease. Thorax 2004; 59: 500–5.

9. Flaherty KR, Travis WD, Colby TV et al. Histologic variability in usual and nonspecific interstitial pneumonias. Am J Respir Crit Care Med 2001; 164: 1722–7.

10. Hansell DM, Wells AU. Towards complete and accurate reporting of studies of diagnostic accuracy: the STARD initiative [Editorial]. Clin Radiol 2003; 58: 573–4.

11. Flaherty KR, King TE Jr, Raghu G et al. Idiopathic interstitial pneumonia: what is the effect of a multidisciplinary approach to diagnosis? Am J Respir Crit Care Med 2004; 170: 904–10.

12. Raghu G, Mageto YN, Lockhart D et al. The accuracy of the clinical diagnosis of new-onset idiopathic pulmonary fibrosis and other interstitial lung disease. Chest 1999; 116: 1168–74.

13. Hunninghake GW, Zimmerman MB, Schwartz DA et al. Utility of a lung biopsy for the diagnosis of idiopathic pulmonary fibrosis. Am J Respir Crit Care Med 2001; 164: 193–6.

14. Nishimura K, Izumi T, Kitaichi M, Nagai S, Itoh H. The diagnostic accuracy of high-resolution computed tomography in diffuse infiltrative lung diseases. Chest 1993; 104: 1149–55.

15. Wells AU, Hansell DM, Rubens MB et al. The predictive value of appearances of thin-section computed tomography in fibrosing alveolitis. Am Rev Respir Dis 1993; 148: 1076–82.

16. Gay SE, Kazerooni EA, Toews GB et al. Idiopathic pulmonary fibrosis: predicting response to therapy and survival. Am J Respir Crit Care Med 1998; 157: 1063–72.

17. Flaherty KR, Thwaite EL, Kazerooni EA et al. Radiological versus histological diagnosis in UIP and NSIP: survival implications. Thorax 2003; 58: 143–8.

18. Fenlon HM, Doran M, Sant SM, Breatnach E. High resolution CT in systemic lupus erythematosus. AJR Am J Roentgenol 1996; 166: 301–7.

19. Schurawitzki H, Stiglbauer R, Graninger W et al. Interstitial lung disease in progressive systemic sclerosis: high resolution CT versus radiography. Radiology 1990; 176: 755–9.

20. Dawson JK, Fewins HE, Desmond J, Lynch MP, Graham DR. Fibrosing alveolitis in patients with rheumatoid arthritis as assessed by high resolution computed tomography, chest radiography, and pulmonary function tests. Thorax 2001; 56: 622–7.

21. Franquet T, Gimenez A, Monill JM et al. Primary Sjogren's syndrome and associated lung disease: CT findings in 50 patients. AJR Am J Roentgenol 1997; 169: 655–8.

SECTION II: KEY ASPECTS OF PULMONARY IMAGING

Basic Principles of Thoracic Imaging
Radiological Pulmonary Anatomy
Common Radiological Signs of Lung Disease

2

Basic principles of thoracic imaging

Thomas E Hartman

Introduction

The main role of imaging of the thorax is to establish the presence or absence of clinically suspected pulmonary pathology. Although there are a number of imaging modalities available, the primary modalities are the chest radiograph and chest computed tomography (CT). Other imaging modalities including positron emission tomography (PET) and PET/CT, magnetic resonance imaging (MRI), ultrasound, and angiography have roles to play in the evaluation of pulmonary diseases, but are typically complementary to the chest radiograph and chest CT. When evaluating parenchymal abnormalities, the pattern of the abnormality, the distribution and the chronicity of findings are the cornerstones upon which a workable differential diagnosis is built. Additional findings in the mediastinum, pleura, abdomen, or chest wall can be used to further refine the differential. Finally, correlating the imaging findings with available clinical information can help to focus the differential.

Radiography

The standard projections for radiographic evaluation of the chest are the posteroanterior (PA) and lateral projections with the patient standing. For patients who are unable to stand, an anteroposterior (AP) upright or supine projection can be obtained. While these are useful alternatives, they are typically less satisfactory because of inferior quality related to shorter focal film distance and greater magnification of the heart. This is important since the diagnostic accuracy of chest radiography is partially influenced by the quality of the images themselves.

Variables which can influence quality include patient positioning, respiration, exposure, and kilovoltage.[1] The X-ray beam must be centered properly with the patient's body aligned with the plane of the imaging device (not rotated).

Additionally, the scapulas should be rotated anteriorly so that they are projected away from the lungs. Imaging should be performed with respiration suspended at full inspiration. Exposure time should be as short as possible consistent with production of adequate contrast such that there is visualization of the intravertebral disk space in the thoracic spine and the lung markings behind the heart. A high kilovoltage technique (115–150 kVp) appropriate to the imaging device should be used for PA and lateral chest radiographs.

There are two main types of image devices for the production of PA and lateral chest images. Historically, these images have been produced on conventional screen film systems; however, more recently digital radiography systems have been employed in the production of these images. Film has several advantages including high sensitivity, good uniformity, and easy handling but it is limited by the small exposure range that provides diagnostic information and the inability of the images to be available to more than one individual at separate locations at any one time.[2,3]

Digital radiology has many advantages over conventional screen film systems including its wide exposure latitude.[2–6] The exposure latitude of digital radiography systems is 10–100 times greater than the best screen film system. As a result, the image quality is nearly independent of the X-ray exposure levels. The wider latitude of the digital system allows it to be used under a broader range of conditions and makes it especially attractive in bedside radiography where exposure can be difficult to control and can be highly variable. The other main advantage of a digitally acquired image is that the electronic images produced can be transmitted to any location and displayed at multiple sites simultaneously.

Computed tomography

CT is the other main imaging modality for the evaluation of pulmonary diseases. Traditionally, a CT image was a two-dimensional representation of a cross-sectional slice through a region of interest in the body. The third dimension of the CT image was the slice thickness which could range from 1 to 10 mm.

The CT image is composed of multiple picture elements which are called pixels. A pixel is a unit area defined by the number of pixel elements per image which typically is 512 × 512. The pixel area multiplied by the slice thickness defines the unit volume of tissue (voxel) sampled. The X-ray attenuation of the structures within a given voxel is averaged to produce the attenuation value of the pixel that is recorded to produce an image.

Slice thickness (collimation) has an influence on the images produced. Narrower collimation results in the ability to resolve smaller structures within the lung parenchyma. However, this comes at the cost of a noisier image since the narrower collimation results in fewer X-ray photons available to produce the image and the fewer the photons the greater the noise. Noisier images appear less smooth.

Another important consideration in production of CT images is the reconstruction algorithm that is applied to the reconstruction of the CT data to produce the image. In the evaluation of pulmonary pathology the two main algorithms used are the standard algorithm and the high spatial frequency reconstruction algorithm. The standard algorithm smooths the image and reduces visible image noise. This algorithm is preferred in the assessment of abnormalities of the mediastinum and chest wall. The high spatial frequency reconstruction algorithm increases spatial resolution which allows better depiction of parenchymal interfaces and better visualization of small vessels, airways, and subtle interstitial abnormalities.[7–9] However, this algorithm also increases image noise. The high spatial frequency reconstruction algorithm is typically used for assessment of the lung parenchyma in the setting of intersitial lung disease or bronchiectasis.[9–11]

Another important factor in the evaluation of CT images is the image display settings (window width and level). The window width and level is limited to 256 shades of gray on any particular image. However, there is a wider range of attenuation values within the structures of the thorax. These attenuation values are measured as Hounsfield units (HU) and range from −1000 HU for air in the trachea to approximately 700 HU for bones. With only 256 shades of gray, no single window setting can adequately display all of the information available on a CT scan. Therefore, several different variations on window width and level are necessary to adequately display the information on a CT of chest. The center CT attenuation value is called the window level and is chosen to correspond approximately to the mean attenuation value of the tissue being examined. This level allows the computer to assign a shade of gray to a certain number of CT values above and below the window level. The range of the CT numbers above and below the window level is called the window width. In practice to adequately display the lungs a window level of between −600 and −700 HU

and window width of 1000–1500 HU is typically used. For the best evaluation of the mediastinum, hila, and chest wall, a window level of 30–50 HU and a window width of 350–500 HU is typically used.[12]

Spiral and multidetector row computed tomography

The earliest CT scans of the chest were acquired axially, meaning that each individual image was produced by a single acquisition at that level followed by movement of the table with another acquisition at a specified level distinct from the first acquisition. In the late 1980s and early 1990s the development of spiral (helical) CT allowed continuous scanning while the patient moved through the CT gantry.[13] This continuous scanning allowed the data acquired to be manipulated to allow production of images of varying location and slice thicknesses.[14] During the late 1990s the single row detectors were replaced by scanners with multiple rows of detectors (multidetector row CT). The multiple rows of detectors allow acquisition of data from each of several detectors.[15] This resulted in improved temporal resolution, increased efficiency in X-ray tube use, decreased image noise, and improved spatial resolution in the z-axis. The improved temporal resolution allows the entire chest to be imaged with thin sections during a single breath hold. The increased efficiency in the X-ray tube use and decreased image noise can allow production of images with a lower dose to the patient. The increased spatial resolution in the z-axis allows production of multiplanar (sagittal and coronal) reconstructions (Figure 2.1) and three-dimensional reconstructions.

Magnetic resonance imaging

MRI does not rely on radiation to produce images but rather on the fact that when hydrogen nuclei are placed in a magnetic field and stimulated by radio waves of a particular sequence, they emit some of the absorbed energy in the form of radio signals. These signals can be used to create an image.[16] Hydrogen nuclei are used because of their abundance in the body. The greater number of hydrogen protons present the more intense the MR signal. Although several factors influence the energy emitted during MRI the most important are the relaxation times.

Relaxation time

The two relaxation times of interest in MRI are designated T1 and T2. T1 represents the time required for that portion

(a)   (b)

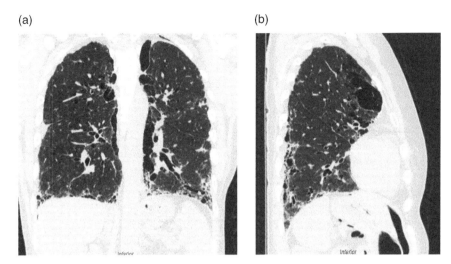

Figure 2.1

Sagittal and coronal reconstructed CT images of a 70-year-old man with idiopathic pulmonary fibrosis. (a) Coronal reconstruction at the level of the descending thoracic aorta shows peripheral and basilar honeycombing compatible with idiopathic pulmonary fibrosis. Emphysematous changes are seen in the upper lungs. (b) Sagittal reconstructed CT image shows posterior and basilar predominance of honeycombing and reticular fibrotic infiltrates compatible with idiopathic pulmonary fibrosis. Again noted are the emphysematous changes in the upper lungs.

of the net magnetization vector parallel to the external field to return to its initial value. The T1 relaxation time tends to be longer for fluids and shorter for fat. Processes that increase the fluid component of a tissue lengthen T1.[16] The T2 relaxation time is related to the exponential decay of the magnetization that is perpendicular to the external field. This relaxation time is the result of random molecular motion leading to signal dephasing. This signal dephasing is related to the local molecular environment with homogeneous local environments such as fluid having long T2 times while complex tissues such as muscle have short T2 times. An increase in fluid within tissues lengthens T2.[16]

Magnetic resonance imaging versus computed tomography

The advantages of MRI compared with CT include a lack of ionizing radiation; increased soft tissue contrast; the ability to directly image in coronal, sagittal, or oblique planes as well as the transverse plane; and intrinsic contrast in blood vessels as a result of flow phenomenon. The main disadvantage of MRI in the assessment of pulmonary diseases is the presence of physiological motion which severely degrades the image quality. MRI of the lungs is also hampered by the low signal to noise ratio of the lung parenchyma caused by the low proton density of the lungs and by the loss of signal caused by magnetic field inhomogeneity that is created by the difference in the diamagnetic susceptibilities between air and water. These limitations result in decreased resolution of MRI of the lung parenchyma when compared with CT and it is this loss of resolution which has prevented MRI from replacing CT as a primary imaging modality in the lungs.

MRI has advantages in the evaluation of the heart and great vessels as well as assessment of chest wall abnormalities. MRI is currently a complementary imaging modality for the assessment of mediastinal and hilar structures, and is used primarily as a problem solving technique in cases in which the CT findings are equivocal. However, because of its advantages related to vascular and chest wall structures, MRI is particularly helpful in assessment of mediastinal, chest wall, and vascular invasion by lung cancer. Although CT angiography is the current imaging modality of choice for evaluation of pulmonary emboli, MRI may soon challenge CT for the evaluation of the pulmonary arteries.

Nuclear medicine

The two primary radionuclide imaging techniques used in the evaluation of thoracic diseases are the ventilation perfusion (VQ) lung scan and a positron emission tomography (PET) scan utilizing 2-(fluorine-18)-fluoro-2-deoxy-D-glucose (FDG) scans. The PET scans can be acquired separately or in conjunction with a CT scan which can be used for better anatomic localization.

VQ scanning

VQ scanning consists of a ventilation scan and a perfusion scan. The most commonly used radiopharmaceuticals for ventilation images are xenon 133 and technetium 99m aerosols. The most common radiopharmaceuticals used for perfusion lung scanning are technetium 99m labeled human albumin microspheres and technetium 99m labeled macroaggregated albumin. While many conditions that affect the lung parenchyma and airways can cause decreased pulmonary arterial blood flow they will also often cause associated ventilation defects in the same lung region. These are typically referred to as matched defects. On the other hand, thromboembolic diseases characteristically cause perfusion defects in the setting of preserved ventilation. These mismatched defects, as they are referred to, are the basis for the VQ evaluation for pulmonary emboli. The VQ scan has been shown to be a safe non-invasive technique that has been widely used in the evaluation of patients with suspected thromboembolism.[17,18] However, it is rapidly being replaced by CT angiography of the pulmonary arteries which allows direct visualization of the pulmonary emboli.

Quantitative VQ scanning can be useful to determine lung function in patients who are scheduled to undergo pulmonary resection. Quantitative VQ scanning is used to predict postoperative function after lobectomy or pneumonectomy.[19] Estimating the predicted postoperative forced expiratory volume in 1 second (FEV1) is done by multiplying the preoperative value by the percentage of radionuclide activity in the lobes or lung that will remain after surgery. If the expected postoperative FEV1 is < 0.8 l or < 35% of predicted this will usually preclude lung resection.

Positron emission tomography

PET is an imaging technique that provides functional information as opposed to CT which typically provides anatomic information. Like CT, the images produced are tomographic images and similar to CT these tomographic images can be fused to form a three-dimensional representation of the area of interest.

PET is predicated on the idea that malignant cells have increased glucose transport and metabolism compared with benign cells.[20,21] The glucose analog FDG has mechanisms of uptake and phosphorylation that are similar to those of glucose. Once FDG is phosphorylated it is not metabolized further and remains in the cell. The amount of phosphorylated FDG within the cell is proportional to glucose uptake and metabolism, and can be assessed with PET.

The functional information provided by PET provides some distinct advantages related to CT. PET can play a role in the differentiation of benign from malignant pulmonary nodules, the identification of nodal metastases and the differentiation between parenchymal scarring and recurrent tumor in patients who have had previous therapy for carcinoma.[22–25] The main limitation of PET has been its low spatial resolution and lack of anatomic landmarks which limits the ability to localize lesions. This problem has been overcome with the introduction of scanners that allow the acquisition of CT images and PET images during the same session. These devices are referred to as PET/CT scanners and result in PET images that are co-registered (fused) with the CT images to allow the anatomic information from the CT to be displayed simultaneously with the metabolic or functional information from the PET scan (Figure 2.2). This type of imaging has been shown to be superior to either PET or CT alone for the assessment of primary tumors, mediastinal nodal involvement, and extrathoracic metastases.[26,27]

Ultrasonography

Ultrasonographic images are produced utilizing sound waves rather than ionizing radiation. The speed at which

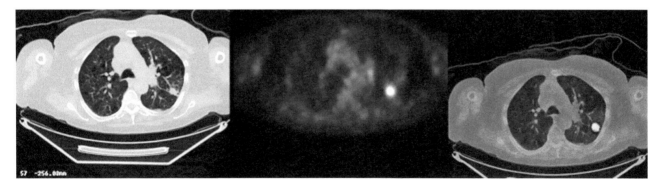

Figure 2.2
CT, PET, and fused PET/CT image of an 84-year-old woman with bronchogenic carcinoma. The left upper lobe nodule is shown to have increased uptake on the PET image which is confirmed on the fused PET/CT image.

sound waves are propagated through different tissues and the percentage of the sound waves that are reflected at tissue interfaces are utilized to produce an ultrasound image. Because air and bone reflect or absorb incoming sonic energy and do not transmit sound, the utility of ultrasound within the chest is limited to chest wall and mediastinal lesions, the heart, pleural and pericardial fluid collections, and to those pulmonary masses that abut the chest wall or mediastinum.

Another advantage ultrasound has relative to CT is that it is portable so bedside sonography can be performed eliminating the necessity of moving the patient to the radiology department for imaging. Ultrasound is particularly helpful in the evaluation of pleural fluid and can be helpful in differentiating transudates and exudates.[28,29] On ultrasound, exudative effusions typically contain septations and may often have echogenic as opposed to anechoic patterns. Because images are available in real-time, ultrasound can also be used to guide needle biopsy or catheter placement in pleural or mediastinal lesions or pulmonary lesions that are abutting the mediastinum, diaphragm, or chest wall.[30,31]

Angiography

Cut film angiography has largely been replaced by CT angiography or MR angiography as a diagnostic tool. It is still useful in the evaluation of pulmonary emboli in cases where the CT angiogram was technically inadequate or equivocal. Angiography also has a role in the diagnosis of arterial venous malformations[32] and for therapeutic planning.[33]

Conclusion

There are numerous modalities available for imaging suspected pulmonary pathology. The chest radiograph and CT are the primary imaging modalities, but there are other modalities that are particularly suited to specific disease processes. The subsequent chapters attempt to familiarize the reader with the appropriate modalities for specific clinical questions.

References

1. Müller N. Radiologic Diagnosis of Diseases of the Chest. Philadelphia: WB Saunders, 2001.
2. MacMahon H, Vyborny C. Technical advances in chest radiography. AJR Am J Roentgenol 1994; 163: 1049–59.
3. Ravin C, Chotas H. Chest radiography. Radiology 1997; 204: 593–600.
4. Wandtke J. Bedside chest radiography. Radiology 1994; 190: 1–10.
5. Schaefer C, Greene R, Llewellyn H et al. Interstitial lung disease: impact of postprocessing in digital storage phosphor imaging. Radiology 1991; 178: 733–8.
6. McAdams HP, Samei E, Dobbins J, Tourassi GD, Ravin CE. Recent advances in chest radiography. Radiology 2006; 241: 663–83.
7. Zwirewich C, Terriff B, Muller N. High-spatial-frequency (bone) algorithm improves quality of standard CT of the thorax. Am J Roentgenol 1989; 153: 1169–73.
8. Mayo J, Webb W, Gould R et al. High-resolution CT of the lungs: an optimal approach. Radiology 1987; 163: 507–10.
9. Müller N. Clinical value of high-resolution CT in chronic diffuse lung disease. Am J Roentgenol 1991; 157: 1163–70.
10. Leung A, Staples C, Muller N. Chronic diffuse infiltrative lung disease: comparison of diagnostic accuracy of high-resolution and conventional CT. Am J Roentgenol 1991; 157: 693–6.
11. McGuinness G, Naidich DP. Bronchiectasis: CT/clinical correlations. Semin Ultrasound CT MR 1995; 16: 395–419.
12. Webb W, Muller N, Naidich DP. High-resolution CT of the Lung. Philadelphia: Lippincott Williams & Wilkins, 2001.
13. Kalender W, Seissler W, Klotz E, Vock P. Spiral volumetric CT with single-breath-hold technique, continuous transport, and continuous scanner rotation. Radiology 1990; 176: 181–3.
14. Crawford CR, King KF. Computed tomography scanning with simultaneous patient translation. Medical Physics 1990; 17: 967–82.
15. Rydberg J, Buckwalter KA, Caldemeyer KS et al. Multisection CT: scanning techniques and clinical applications. Radiographics 2000; 20: 1787–1806.
16. Cutillo AG. Application of Magnetic Resonance to the Study of Lung. Armonk, NY: Futura Publishing Company, 1996.
17. Hull RD, Raskob GE, Ginsberg JS et al. A noninvasive strategy for the treatment of patients with suspected pulmonary embolism. Arch Intern Med 1994; 154: 289–97.
18. PIOPED Investigators. Value of the ventilation/perfusion scan in acute pulmonary embolism. Results of the prospective investigation of pulmonary embolism diagnosis (PIOPED). JAMA 1990; 263: 2753–9.
19. Ali MK, Mountain CF, Ewer MS, Johnston D, Haynie TP. Predicting loss of pulmonary function after pulmonary resection for bronchogenic carcinoma. Chest 1980; 77: 337–42.
20. Weber G. Enzymology of cancer cells: Part I. N Engl J Med 1977; 296: 486–92.
21. Weber G. Enzymology of cancer cells: Part II. N Engl J Med 1977; 296: 541–51.
22. Gupta N, Frank A, Dewan N et al. Solitary pulmonary nodules: detection of malignancy with PET with 2-[F- 18]-fluoro-2-deoxy-D-glucose. Radiology 1992; 184: 441–4.
23. Patz E Jr, Lowe V, Hoffman J et al. Focal pulmonary abnormalities: evaluation with F-18 fluorodeoxyglucose PET scanning. Radiology 1993; 188: 487–90.
24. Dwamena BA, Sonnad SS, Angobaldo JO, Wahl RL. Metastases from non-small cell lung cancer: mediastinal staging in the 1990s – meta-analytic comparison of PET and CT. Radiology 1999; 213: 530–6.
25. Marom EM, Erasmus JJ, Patz EF. Lung cancer and positron emission tomography with fluorodeoxyglucose. Lung Cancer 2000; 28: 187–202.

26. Lardinois D, Weder W, Hany TF et al. Staging of non-small-cell lung cancer with integrated positron-emission tomography and computed tomography. N Engl J Med 2003; 348: 2500–7.

27. Antoch G, Stattaus J, Nemat AT et al. Non-small cell lung cancer: dual-modality PET/CT in preoperative staging. Radiology 2003; 229: 526–33.

28. Hirsch J, Rogers J, Mack L. Real-time sonography of pleural opacities. Am J Roentgenol 1981; 136: 297–301.

29. Yang P, Luh K, Chang D et al. Value of sonography in determining the nature of pleural effusion: analysis of 320 cases. Am J Roentgenol 1992; 159: 29–33.

30. O'Moore P, Mueller P, Simeone J et al. Sonographic guidance in diagnostic and therapeutic interventions in the pleural space. Am J Roentgenol 1987; 149: 1–5.

31. Yang P. Ultrasound-guided transthoracic biopsy of peripheral lung, pleural, and chest wall lesions. J Thoracic Imaging 1997; 12: 272–84.

32. Dines DE, Seward JB, Bernatz PE. Pulmonary arteriovenous fistulas. Mayo Clin Proc 1983; 58: 176–81.

33. Puskas JD, Allen MS, Moncure AC et al. Pulmonary arterio-venous malformations: therapeutic options. Ann Thorac Surg 1993; 56: 253.

3

Radiological pulmonary anatomy

Tomás Franquet

The chest radiograph remains the screening procedure of choice in the thorax. However, the limitations of the chest radiograph in providing a definitive diagnosis are widely understood. Complicated chest radiographs, the lack of radiographic abnormalities in symptomatic patients, and the limitations of portable chest studies sometimes make the evaluation of conventional chest films difficult.

To date, it is well established that computed tomography (CT) is the most important imaging procedure in the evaluation of thoracic diseases. Compared with conventional radiographic techniques, CT provides a better spatial resolution, detects minor differences in radiographic contrast, and expands the ability of radiology to portray boundaries between different tissues.

Multidetector computed tomography (MDCT) is the latest technological breakthrough in CT scanners. It uses a multiple-row detector with narrow detector collimation in conjunction with a relatively rapid table translation to achieve faster scans with thinner slices than single detector CT.[1] With MDCT the performance of CT scanning has dramatically improved and machines can scan 16, 32, 64, and even more contiguous slices per rotation at subsecond times. MDCT scanners can provide continuous and/or overlapping high-resolution, near-isotropic thin sections throughout the lungs in a single breath hold. The provided additional information and its impact on clinical management has justified its use in the area of thoracic imaging.

The main disadvantages are that large amounts of data and images are created with the same amount of time and number of radiologists available for reporting[2] and there are potential increases in patient radiation dose.[3,4]

In combination with advanced image processing techniques including multiplanar reconstructions (MPRs), maximum intensity projections (MIPs), minimum intensity projections (MinIPs), external rendering with either three-dimensional (3D) shaded-surface displays (SSDs) or volumetric rendering, and internal rendering, or so-called virtual bronchoscopy (VB), CT has become a valuable tool for evaluating diseases affecting the airways. Moreover, MDCT is also extremely useful for cardiac imaging providing particular opportunities for quantitative assessment of coronary artery calcification, coronary CT angiography, assessment of ejection fraction, evaluation of ventricular wall motion, and evaluation of ventricular perfusion.[5] The value of MDCT for the evaluation of patients with chest pain presenting to the emergency department has also been recently discussed.[6]

A comprehensive understanding of the normal CT anatomy appearance can facilitate the detection and diagnosis of cardiothoracic diseases, as well as an awareness of the wide range of anatomic variants. Accurate interpretation of CT scans of the thorax requires high quality images and an accurate technique. In the chest, a wide range of attenuation values (CT numbers) are found depending on the physical density of the different tissues.

Anatomic computed tomography of mediastinum

The mediastinum is the part of the thoracic cavity between the lungs covered on each side by the mediastinal pleura. It is limited anteriorly by the sternum and chest wall, posteriorly by the spine and chest wall, and inferiorly by the diaphragm. It contains the thymus, the heart and its large blood vessels, the trachea, the esophagus, the bronchi, and lymph nodes.[7–9]

Anatomically, the mediastinum can be divided into anterior, middle, and posterior compartments. The anterior mediastinal compartment is bounded anteriorly by the sternum and posteriorly by the pericardium, aorta, and brachiocephalic vessels. This compartment contains the thymus gland, branches of internal mammary vessels, lymph nodes, the sternopericardial ligament, and fat. The middle mediastinal compartment lies between the anterior and posterior compartments and contains the ascending and transverse portions of the aorta, the superior and inferior vena cava, the brachiocephalic arteries and veins, the phrenic nerves and cephalad portion of the vagus nerves, the trachea and main bronchi, lymph nodes, and main pulmonary arteries and veins. The posterior mediastinal compartment is bounded anteriorly by the pericardium and the vertical part of the diaphragm, laterally by the mediastinal pleura, and posteriorly by bodies of the thoracic vertebrae. It contains the descending thoracic aorta, esophagus, thoracic duct, azygos and hemiazygos veins, autonomic nerves, lymph nodes, and fat.

On CT examination the anatomical boundaries of these compartments do not provide a clear-cut guide to disease and do not form any barriers to the spread of the disease.

The normal mediastinal structures always identified at CT are the heart and great vessels, airways, and esophagus.[8,10–14] Usually, these structures are surrounded by a considerable amount of fat that contains lymph nodes, nerves, and the thoracic duct. Use of intravenous contrast material helps the interpretation of CT scans of the mediastinum, facilitates the detection of vessel enlargement and abnormal vessels, and by enhancement can show highly vascular masses.[8,15,16]

A detailed mediastinal anatomy can be depicted using MDCT scanners. The vessels, heart, trachea, mediastinal pleura, and bony structures that border the mediastinum create real or potential spaces that can be visible with CT.[11,13] Normal mediastinal landmarks may be divided into lines, stripes, and interfaces.

Mediastinal spaces

Different 'mediastinal spaces' are well known and commonly used in the radiological literature. The retrosternal space lies immediately behind and to either side of the sternum, contains fat and connective tissue, and is variable in size among individuals. The mediastinum anterior to the great vessels, ascending aorta, and anterior aortic arch forms the prevascular space (Figure 3.1). This space is continuous with the retrosternal space and is bordered by the lungs laterally. Posteriorly it is limited by the ascending aorta and arch vessels. The prevascular space normally contains the left brachiocephalic vein, the thymus, and a variable amount of fat; lymph nodes are not normally seen in this space. The pretracheal space extends vertically from the thoracic inlet to the carina. It contains fat, connective tissue, and small lymph nodes (Figure 3.2). At lower levels, this space is bounded by the anterior convexity of the trachea, the medial wall of the azygos arch, the posteromedial wall of the superior vena cava, and the posterior wall of the ascending thoracic aorta. This space contains the innominate artery and the left common carotid and left subclavian arteries to the left.[13] The aortic–pulmonic window

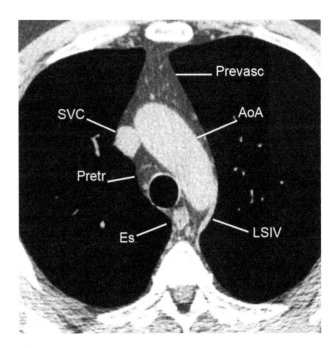

Figure 3.1
Normal prevascular and precarinal spaces. Non-enhanced CT at the level of the aortic arch (AoA) shows the prevascular space (Prevasc), bounded laterally by the lungs and containing fat. SVC, superior vena cava; LSIV, left superior intercostal vein; Es, esophagus; Pretr, pretracheal space.

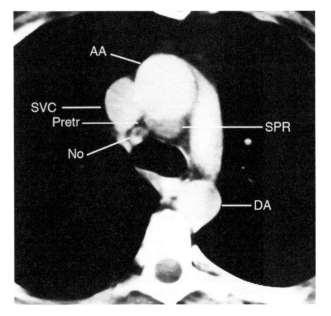

Figure 3.2
Normal superior pericardial recess and pretracheal space. Enhanced CT shows the superior pericardial recess (SPR) posterior to the ascending aorta (AA). The pretracheal space (Pretr) contains a normal lymph node with a visible fatty center (No). SVC, superior vena cava; DA, descending aorta.

is situated beneath the aortic arch and above the left pulmonary artery (Figure 3.3). This space is bounded medially by the lower trachea and esophagus, and laterally by the left lung. The aortic–pulmonic window contains lymph nodes, the ligamentum arteriosum, and the recurrent laryngeal nerve. The precarinal and subcarinal spaces extend inferiorly from the pretracheal space and is bounded by the right pulmonary artery, the mediastinal portion of the left superior pulmonary vein, the right and left main bronchi, and the esophagus (Figure 3.4). In its lower portion, the space is limited on the right by the intermediate bronchus and

inferiorly by the left atrium. In up to half of the population, the posterior tracheal wall can be outlined by lung that lies between the spine and the trachea (retrotracheal space)[17,18] (Figure 3.5). This space is best visualized on lateral chest images as a radiolucent triangular area bounded anteriorly by the trachea, posteriorly by the spine, inferiorly by the aortic arch, and superiorly by the thoracic inlet. Both lungs contribute to the radiolucency of the space; the right lung extends posterior to the trachea and outlines the tracheal wall, while the left lung extends above the transverse aorta and outlines the aortic arch.[17,18] The retrotracheal space is

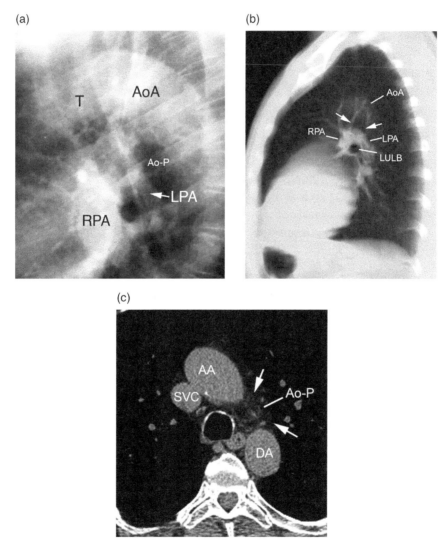

Figure 3.3

Normal anatomy at the level of the aortic–pulmonic window. (a) A detail view from a conventional lateral chest radiograph shows the aortic–pulmonic window (Ao-P) situated beneath the aortic arch (AoA) and above the left pulmonary artery (LPA). RPA, right pulmonary artery; T, trachea. (b) Sagittal multiplanar reconstruction (MPR), volume-rendered image through the left upper lobe bronchus (LULB) shows the aortic–pulmonic window (arrows). AoA, aortic arch; LPA, left pulmonary artery; RPA, right pulmonary artery. (c) Non-enhanced CT through the aortic–pulmonic window (Ao-P) shows the fatty component of this anatomic space (arrows). AA, ascending aorta; DA, descending aorta; SVC, superior vena cava.

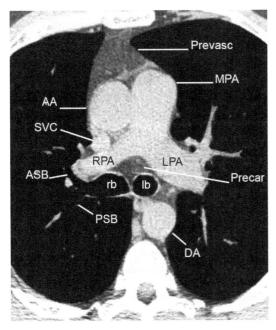

Figure 3.4
Normal precarinal space. Non-enhanced CT at the level of the carina shows the prevascular space (Prevasc), precarinal space (Precar), ascending aorta (AA), descending aorta (DA), superior vena cava (SVC), right pulmonary artery (RPA), left pulmonary artery (LPA), anterior segmental bronchus (ASB), and posterior segmental bronchus (PSB) of the right upper lobe. rb, right bronchus; lb, left bronchus.

triangular in shape and varies in size depending on the patient's age and body habitus. The size of the space is also affected by the degree of lung inflation. In patients with emphysema the size is typically larger and the upper margin of the space is extended and it may take on a trapezoidal shape. The retrocrural space is bounded by the diaphragmatic crura and the spine. It contains the descending aorta, the azygos and hemiazygos veins, intercostal arteries, splanchnic nerves, and variable amount of fat (Figure 3.6).

Mediastinal lines and interfaces

The posterior tracheal stripe is a vertically orientated line behind the tracheal air column that usually forms the anterior margin of the retrotracheal space[19–21] (see Figure 3.5). The line is produced by lung contacting the posterior wall of the trachea and is up to 2.5 mm in thickness. Occasionally a stripe up to 5.5 mm in thickness, the tracheoesophageal stripe, will form the anterior margin of the normal retrotracheal space.[19–21] The stripe is composed of the posterior wall of the tracheal and the anterior wall of the air-filled esophagus or, in some instances, the collapsed esophagus outlined by retroesophageal lung.[19–21]

The right paratracheal stripe is an important and sensitive indicator of disease on conventional chest radiographs. It comprises pleura, mediastinal fat, connective tissue, and

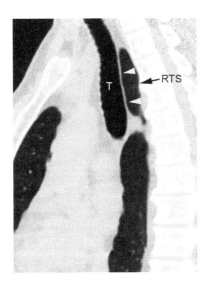

Figure 3.5
Retrotracheal space. Sagittal reformated image shows the radiolucent retrotracheal space (RTS) bounded anteriorly by the trachea (T) and posteriorly by the spine. The posterior tracheal stripe is a vertically orientated line behind the tracheal air column (arrowheads) that usually forms the anterior margin of the retrotracheal space (RTS). Inferiorly the retrotracheal space is limited by the aortic arch (not shown).

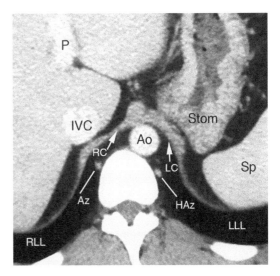

Figure 3.6
Normal CT anatomy of the retrocrural spaces. Enhanced CT showing normal retrocrural spaces posterior to the diaphragmatic crura (arrows). RC, right crura; LC, left crura; RLL, right lower lobe; LLL, left lower lobe; Az, azygos vein; HAz, hemiazygos vein; Ao, aorta; IVC, inferior vena cava; P, portal vein; Stom, stomach; Sp, spleen.

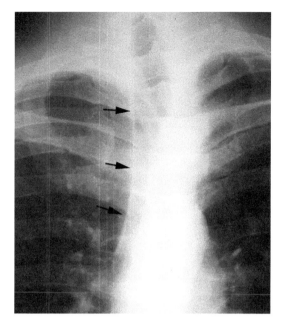

Figure 3.7

Right paratracheal stripe. A detail view from a conventional posteroanterior chest radiograph shows a linear zone of contact between the right upper lobe and the right tracheal wall forming the right paratracheal stripe (arrows).

the wall of the trachea (Figure 3.7). Abnormal thickening of the stripe can be caused by tracheal, mediastinal, and pleural disease. CT can easily show the cause of a thickened right paratracheal stripe.

Junctional lines consist of four sheets of pleura (two layers of visceral pleura covering both lungs and two layers of mediastinal pleura) representing regions of contact between both lungs in the mediastinum.

The term anterior junction (prevascular space) represents a mediastinal area that lies anterior to the pulmonary artery, the ascending aorta, and the three major branches of the aortic arch. When the two lungs approximate each other closely enough, the so-called anterior junction line describes a region of contact between the anterior portions of the right and left lungs posterior to the sternum (Figure 3.8). The term posterior junction describes the mediastinal space posterior to the trachea and the heart where the two lungs lie close to each other. Similarly, the posterior junction line represents a linear region of contact between the posterior portions of both lungs in the superior mediastinum, behind the esophagus, and anterior to the upper thoracic vertebral bodies (Figure 3.9).

(a)

(b)

(c)

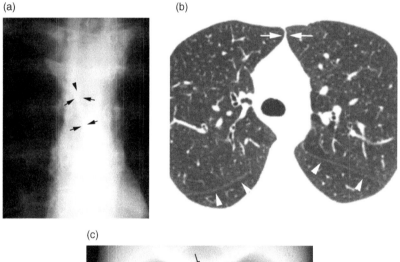

Figure 3.8

Anterior junction line. (a) A detail view from a conventional posteroanterior chest radiograph shows the anterior junction line (arrows) extending from the right to the left caudally from the level of the thoracic arch. Note the presence of a V-shaped shadow (arrowhead) representing the anterior mediastinal triangle. (b) CT at the level of the aortic arch shows the anterior junction line, a linear region of contact between the anterior portions of both lungs, posterior to sternum (arrows). Major fissures are also seen (arrowheads). (c) Coronal multiplanar reconstruction (MPR), volume-rendered image shows the anterior junction line (white arrows). The anterior mediastinal triangle (black arrow) is clearly demonstrated.

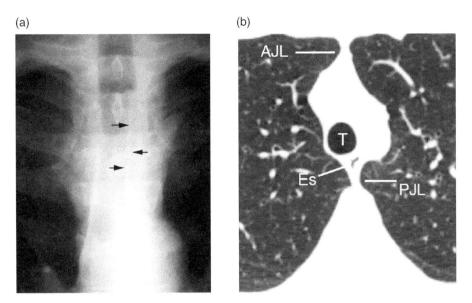

(a)   (b)

Figure 3.9
Posterior junction line. (a) A detail view from a conventional posteroanterior chest radiograph shows the posterior junction line (arrows) projecting through the air column of the trachea; it may be straight or slightly convex to the left. (b) CT shows the posterior junction line (PJL) behind the esophagus (Es) and anterior to the upper thoracic vertebral bodies. The anterior junction line (AJL) is also seen. T, trachea.

Anatomic computed tomography of pulmonary airways

Anatomic CT of trachea

The trachea is a cartilaginous and fibromuscular midline tubular structure, 16–20 cm in length and slightly deviated to the right at the level of the aortic arch, that extends from the inferior aspect of the cricoid cartilage to the carina where it divides into the left and right main bronchi. In cross section, there is a marked variability in the appearance of the trachea, which may appear rounded, oval, or horseshoe shaped.[22–24] The 16–22 cartilaginous 'rings' that contain the trachea are horseshoe shaped and posteriorly incomplete. Calcification of the cartilage rings is a common CT finding. The posterior tracheal wall is a thin fibromuscular membrane termed posterior tracheal membrane. A flat posterior membrane is seen in 25% of normal individuals; a pear-shape or square appearance can also be observed.[23–25] Cross-sectional diameters and areas have been documented by CT; the mean transverse diameter is 15.2 mm (SD 1.4) for women and 18.2 mm (SD 1.2) for men.[25]

Anatomic CT of bronchi (main and intrapulmonary)

The trachea divides into right and left main bronchi at the carina. On CT, anatomic features of the hila can be depicted by examining a series of axial scans. When no intravenous contrast agent is administered the anatomy of bronchi is best assessed on the lung windows. Using MDCT scanners the anatomy of central airways is easily demonstrated and acquired CT data can be used to produce high quality MPRs, 3D reconstructions, and virtual bronchoscopy[26–29] (Figure 3.10).

The pulmonary hila are complex anatomic areas formed by pulmonary arteries and veins, bronchi, surrounding connective tissue, and lymph nodes. Normal CT hilar anatomy can be conveniently described by examining a series of scans obtained at different anatomic levels: level I (supracarinal trachea), level II (carina/right upper lobe bronchus), level III (proximal intermediate bronchus/left upper lobe bronchus), level IV (distal intermediate bronchus/lingular bronchus), level V (middle lobe bronchus), and level VI (basilar lower lobe bronchi/inferior pulmonary veins) (Figure 3.11).

The right main bronchus is about 2.2 cm long whereas the left main bronchus is about 5 cm in length. The right main bronchus divides into an upper lobe bronchus and an intermediate bronchus. The right upper lobe bronchus divides into three segmental bronchi that are usually visible on CT. The intermediate bronchus is 4 cm long and its posterior wall is visible on CT scans outlined by the right lower lobe. The middle lobe bronchus arises from the right antero-lateral wall of the intermediate bronchus, at the same level as the right lower superior segment, and divides into the medial and lateral segments. Beyond the origin of the right lower superior segment, the right basal trunk divides into medial, anterior, lateral, and posterior basal segments.

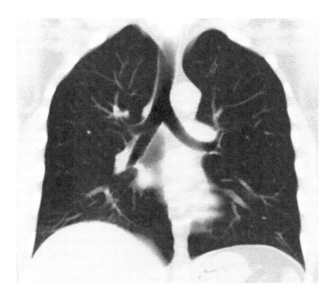

Figure 3.10
Normal CT anatomy of the tracheobronchial tree. Coronal multiplanar reconstruction (MPR) volume-rendered image through the carina shows a normal tracheobronchial tree. This image was reconstructed using five contiguous 1-mm sections obtained from a 16-detector CT scanner using 1-mm collimators.

The main left bronchus divides directly into upper and lower lobe bronchi. The upper lobe bronchus gives off a lingular bronchus and a short common trunk before dividing into anterior and apicoposterior segments. The lingular bronchus bifurcates into superior and inferior segmental bronchi. As on the right, the first branch of the left lower lobe is the left lower superior segment; the anteromedial, lateral, and posterior basal segments arise distal to the superior segmental bronchus.

On CT, appearance of bronchi depends on their orientation. Bronchi oriented horizontally in the scan plane are seen along their axes and appear as tubular structures. These bronchi are the right and left upper lobe bronchi, the anterior segmental bronchi of the upper lobes, the middle lobe bronchus, and the superior segmental bronchi of the lower lobes. Bronchi which have a vertical orientation are seen in cross section and appear as circular shadows. These bronchi are the apical segmental bronchus of the right upper lobe, the apicoposterior segmental bronchus of the left upper lobe, the bronchus intermedius, the lower lobe bronchi, and the basal segmental bronchi. Bronchi oriented obliquely to the scan plane appear as elliptical structures on CT. These are the lingular bronchi, the superior and inferior segmental lingular bronchi, and the medial and lateral segmental bronchial branches of the right middle lobe.

The lung contains over 300 000 branching airways. Ten generations of bronchi divide in a generally dichotomous manner, decreasing in diameter from 12.2 mm centrally to 1.3 mm peripherally. Bronchioles, both membranous and respiratory, are airways that lack cartilage. The smallest normal airways that can be visualized on CT scan are 1.5–2 mm in diameter. The membranous bronchiole proximal to a respiratory bronchiole is called the terminal bronchiole. Terminal bronchioles measure about 0.6 mm in diameter whereas respiratory bronchioles measure about 0.4 mm. Normal centrilobular bronchioles are not identified by HRCT scanning because their wall thickness (300 μm) is less than the maximum scanner resolution. It is the presence of bronchiolar wall thickening or plugging of the lumen ('tree-in-bud') that renders small airways visible in the lung periphery. Using 1–3-mm thick sections, Napel et al.[30] described a new reconstruction technique for rapidly computing a series of overlapping MIPs or MinIPs obtained with use of a sliding thin-slab of lung while retaining a normal axial orientation. This resulted in acquisition of reconstructions with high contrast resolution that allowed improved visualization of peripheral blood vessels (MIP) or bronchi (MinIP)[30] (Figure 3.12).

Anatomic computed tomography of aorta, great veins, and pulmonary arteries

Aortic arch and supraaortic vessels

In the upper part of the supraaortic mediastinum the esophagus, usually collapsed and flattened, lies posterior to the trachea.

The thoracic aorta is divided into the ascending aorta, the aortic arch, and the descending aorta. At the level of the superior mediastinum the proximal part of the aortic arch gives rise to three arterial branches: the brachiocephalic artery (innominate artery), left common carotid artery, and left subclavian artery. These vessels are usually seen behind the right and left brachiocephalic veins. The left brachiocephalic vein has a horizontal course and crosses the anterior mediastinum from left to right to joint the right brachiocephalic vein to form the superior vena cava (Figure 3.13).

The distal part of the aortic arch, between the origin of the left subclavian artery and the ligamentum arteriosum, is known as aortic isthmus. The ascending aortic diameter is approximately 3 cm and a diameter greater than 4 cm is considered abnormal. The diameter of the descending aorta, distal to the ligamentum arteriosum, is almost constant and some degree of dilatation and tortuosity may develop with increasing age.

Great veins

The brachiocephalic veins are the most anterior and lateral mediastinal vessels. The left brachiocephalic vein is 6 cm

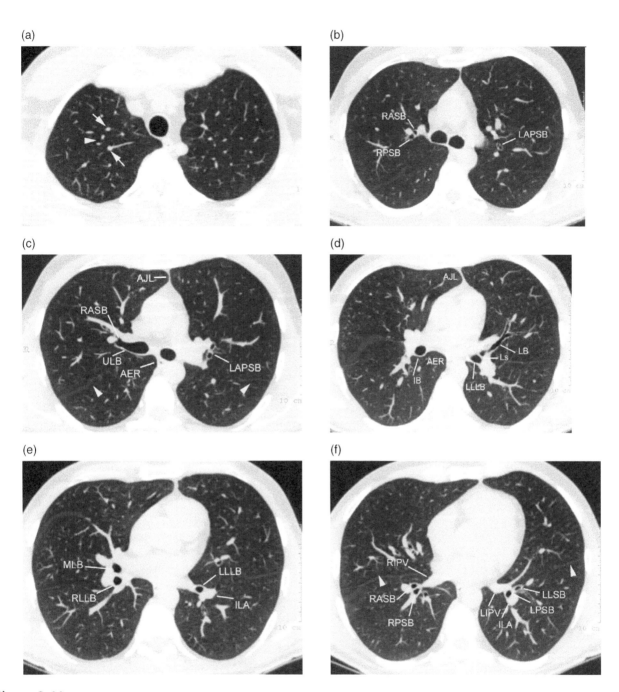

Figure 3.11

Normal bronchial CT anatomy. (a) CT scan at the level of the supracarinal trachea shows the right apical bronchus and artery (arrowhead) and veins (arrows). (b) CT scan at the level of the tracheal carina right anterior segmental bronchus (RASB), right posterior segmental bronchus (RPSB), and left apicoposterior segmental bronchus (LAPSB) of the upper lobe. (c) CT scan slightly below level shown in (b) shows right upper lobe bronchus (ULB); right anterior segmental bronchus (RASB), and left apicoposterior segmental bronchus (LAPSB) of the upper lobe. (d) CT scan at the level of the intermediate bronchus (IB) shows the lingular bronchus (LB) and the left lower lobe bronchus (LLLB). Note the presence of the lingular spur (Ls) separating the lingular bronchus (LB) from the left lower lobe bronchus (LLLB). (e) Slightly more caudal CT scan shows the middle lobe bronchus (MLB), the right lower lobe bronchus (RLLB), and the left lower lobe bronchus (LLLB); the left interlobar artery (ILA) is also seen. (f) CT scan at the level in which the inferior pulmonary veins join the left atrium shows the right inferior pulmonary vein (RIPV), left inferior pulmonary vein (LIPV), right anterior segmental bronchus (RASB), and right posterior segmental bronchus (RPSB) of the right lower lobe; left lateral segmental bronchus (LLSB) and left posterior segmental bronchus (LPSB) of the left lower lobe; the left interlobar artery is also visible (ILA). Arrowheads, major fissures; AJL, anterior junction line; AER, azygo-esophageal recess.

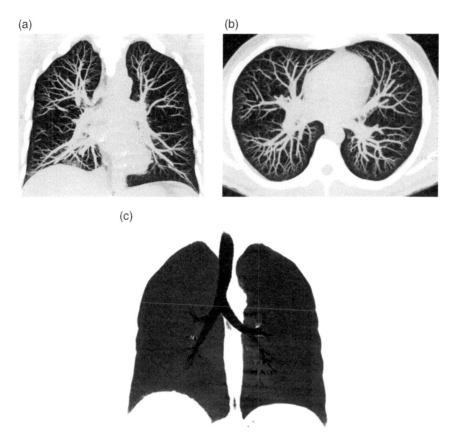

(a) (b)

(c)

Figure 3.12

Multiplanar image reconstruction. (a) Coronal and (b) axial multiplanar reconstructions (MPR), maximum intensity projection images (MIP) show a normal pulmonary vasculature. MIP enhance visualization of the pulmonary vessels. (c) Coronal MPR, minimum intensity projection image (MinIP) shows a normal visualization of the tracheobronchial tree. Images were reconstructed using five contiguous 1-mm sections obtained from a 16-detector CT scanner using 1-mm collimators.

long and crosses horizontally the mediastinum to the right-sided superior vena cava; the right brachiocephalic vein is 2.5 cm long, lies anterolateral to the trachea, and has a nearly vertical course throughout its length.

The superior vena cava forms the upper right border of the mediastinum. On CT, the superior vena cava is visible anterior and to the right of the trachea, has an oval or round configuration, and drains into the right atrium. It is located in front of the trachea and separated from it by the pretracheal space. Its lower portion is located within the pericardium and lies anterior to the right main bronchus.[31,32] A left superior vena cava resulting from failure of obliteration of the left common cardinal vein during fetal development can be identified in 0.3% of healthy individuals. At unenhanced CT, a left superior vena cava may be confused with lymphadenopathy.

The anterior portion of the aortic arc lies in front of the trachea and is closely related to the anteromedial aspect of the superior vena cava, the medial portion lies just to the left of the trachea and the posterior portion lies just lateral to the esophagus (Figure 3.14).

One centimeter below the aortic arch, the only consistent vascular structure to the right of the intrathoracic trachea is the arch of the azygos vein. The azygos vein enters the thorax through the aortic hiatus in the diaphragm, and passes along the right side of the vertebral column to the fourth thoracic vertebra, where it arches forward over the root of the right lung, and ends in the superior vena cava, just before that vessel pierces the pericardium.[31–34] The azygos and hemiazygos veins are routinely identifiable at CT.[35]

Pulmonary arteries and veins

The main pulmonary artery is a short, wide vessel, about 5 cm in length and 3 cm in diameter, arising from the base of the right ventricle. It extends obliquely upward and backward, passing at first in front and then to the left of the ascending aorta, as far as the under surface of the aortic arch, where it divides into right and left branches of nearly equal size (Figure 3.15). The right pulmonary artery divides within the mediastinum into upper and lower divisional

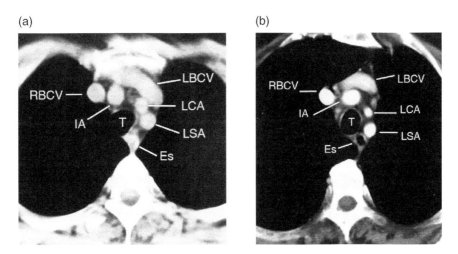

Figure 3.13
Normal CT anatomy at the level of supraaortic mediastinum. (a) Unenhanced CT shows the left brachiocephalic vein (LBCV), right brachiocephalic vein (RBCV), innominate artery (IA), left carotid artery (LCA), left subclavian artery (LSA), trachea (T), and esophagus (Es). (b) Contrast-enhanced CT at the same level shows left brachiocephalic vein (LBCV), right brachiocephalic vein (RBCV), innominate artery (IA), left carotid artery (LCA), left subclavian artery (LSA), trachea (T), and esophagus (Es).

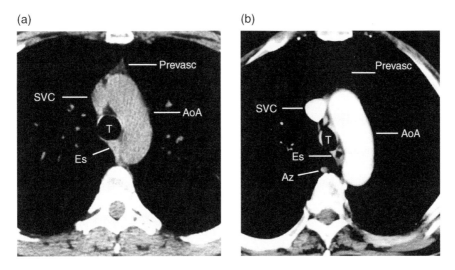

Figure 3.14
Normal CT anatomy at the level of aortic arch. (a) Unenhanced CT shows the prevascular space (Prevasc), superior vena cava (SVC), aortic arch (AoA), trachea (T), and esophagus (Es). (b) Contrast-enhanced CT at the same level shows the prevascular space (Prevasc), superior vena cava (SVC), aortic arch (AoA), azygos vein (Az), trachea (T), and esophagus (Es).

arteries. The upper division of the right pulmonary artery (anterior trunk) is immediately in front of the right main bronchus. The apical, anterior, and posterior branches of the anterior trunk accompany their respective bronchi. The lower division of the right pulmonary artery (interlobar artery) is anterolateral to the intermediate bronchus and gives branches to the right middle lobe and to the superior and basal segments of the right lower lobe. The left pulmonary artery does not divide into distinct upper and lower divisions. Different upper lobe arterial branches arise from the superior and lateral surfaces of the main trunk. The left pulmonary artery passes over the left main bronchus and turns rapidly caudad as the descending left pulmonary artery. An anterior branch to the lingular segment of the left upper lobe and a posterior branch to the superior segment of the left lower lobe are the first two major branches of the descending left pulmonary artery. The descending left pulmonary artery divides with the basal segmental bronchi of the left lower lobe.

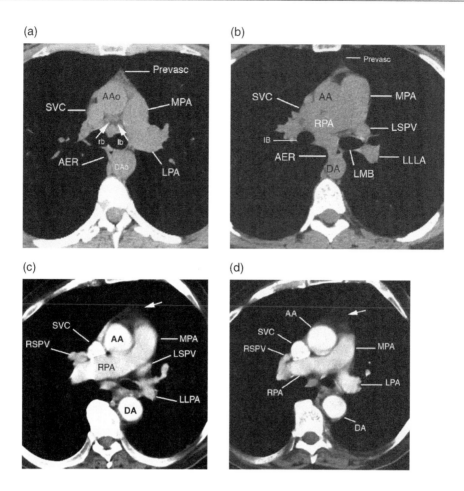

Figure 3.15

Normal CT anatomy of the pulmonary arteries. (a) Unenhanced CT shows the prevascular space (Prevasc), superior vena cava (SVC), ascending aorta (AAo), descending aorta (DAo), main pulmonary artery (MPA), left pulmonary artery (LPA), azygo-esophageal recess (AER), right bronchus (rb), and left bronchus (lb). The superior pericardial recess (arrows) is seen posterior to the ascending aorta (AAo). The anterior reflection of the superior pericardial recess (arrowhead) is also visible in the groove between the ascending aorta (AAo) and main pulmonary artery (MPA). (b) Unenhanced CT scan slightly below level shown in (a) shows the prevascular space (Prevasc), superior vena cava (SVC), main pulmonary artery (MPA), right pulmonary artery (RPA), ascending aorta (AA), descending aorta (DA), left superior pulmonary vein (LSPV), left lower lobe artery (LLLA), azygo-esophageal recess (AER), intermediate bronchus (IB), and left main bronchus (LMB). (c) Contrast-enhanced CT at the level of the pulmonary arteries shows the prevascular space (arrow), superior vena cava (SVC), ascending aorta (AA), descending aorta (DA), major pulmonary artery (MPA), right pulmonary artery (RPA), right superior pulmonary vein (RSPV), left superior pulmonary vein (LSPV), and left lower lobe pulmonary artery (LLPA). (d) Contrast-enhanced CT at a slightly lower level than (c) shows the prevascular space (arrow), superior vena cava (SVC), ascending aorta (AA), descending aorta (DA), major pulmonary artery (MPA), right pulmonary artery (RPA), left pulmonary artery (LPA), and right superior pulmonary vein (RSPV).

The pulmonary veins return the arterialized blood from the lungs to the left atrium of the heart. They are four in number, two from each lung, and lack valves. At the root of the lung, the superior pulmonary vein lies in front of and a little below the pulmonary artery; the inferior pulmonary vein is situated at the lowest part of the hilus of the lung and on a plane posterior to the upper vein. Behind the pulmonary artery is the bronchus. The right pulmonary veins pass behind the right atrium and superior vena cava; the left in front of the descending thoracic aorta.

Anatomic computed tomography of thoracic lymph nodes

CT is the primary non-invasive technique for the diagnostic evaluation of thoracic lymph nodes. Lymph nodes are usually oval in cross section with low attenuation centers or fatty hila. Although there is a significant variation in the number and locations of lymph nodes within the mediastinum, lymph nodes are considered normal if they are less than 10 mm in short axis diameter.[36,37] Lymph nodes with a short axis diameter greater than 2 cm usually indicate pathology. The different regional nodal stations have been numbered by the American Thoracic Society (ATS) and are routinely used in the staging of lung cancer.[38] CT can determine the exact location of pathological node groups in order to determine the best means of biopsy. Whereas subcarinal nodes are easily approached by bronchoscopic transbronchial needle aspiration, right paratracheal lymphadenopathy can be approached by either mediastinoscopy or transbronchial needle aspiration.

Anatomic computed tomography of the lung parenchyma

Lung density

Attenuation (density) on a CT scan is expressed in terms of Hounsfield units (HU); under normal circumstances water is 0 HU and air is −1000 HU. CT scans of the lung are usually obtained during maintained full inspiration. Normally, the attenuation of lung parenchyma is determined by its relative proportions of blood, gas, extravascular fluid, and pulmonary tissue.[39] The normal lung parenchyma has a fairly homogeneous attenuation that is slightly greater than that of air. As lung gas volume is reduced, lung attenuation increases. A significant increase in the attenuation of the lung parenchyma is seen on expiratory scans.[40] Attenuation values are variable and influenced by the pulmonary volume and different parameters such as kilovoltage, patient size, and the particular region of the lung being assessed.[41]

The appearance of CT images on the monitor or film (hard copy) depends on the display parameters used (window level and window width) and is limited to 256 shades of gray. For clinical practice a window level of −600 to −700 HU and a window width of 1000–1500 HU are recommended. Window levels of 30–50 HU and window widths of 350–500 HU are the recommended parameters to evaluate mediastinum, hila, and pleura.

Secondary pulmonary lobule

The secondary pulmonary lobule is a fundamental unit of lung structure defined as the smallest portion of the lung that is surrounded by connective tissue septa.[42] An understanding of lobular anatomy is essential to the interpretation of thin-section CT of the lung.[43–45] The most typical secondary pulmonary lobules are recognized in the outermost part of the lung, where each lobule is bounded by the visceral pleura, interlobular septa, and pulmonary veins (Figure 3.16). The secondary lobule of the lung is separated incompletely by the interlobular septa from adjacent lobules.[42,45]

Structures in the centrilobular region include terminal and proximal respiratory bronchioles, accompanying pulmonary arteries, interstitial tissue enveloping these bronchovascular structures and immediately adjacent alveolar ducts, sacs, and alveoli.[46] The smallest pulmonary arteries and accompanying bronchioles are situated in the centrilobular area but bronchioles cannot be seen in normal conditions because they are no more than 1 mm in diameter and their walls are less than 0.1 mm thick.[43,46] Lambert canal connects airspace to bronchioles. The number of terminal bronchioles included in one lobule varies from three

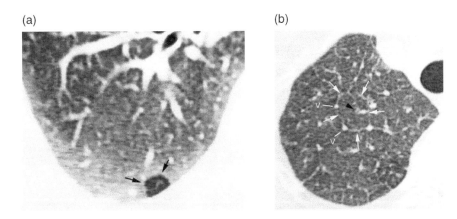

(a) (b)

Figure 3.16
Secondary pulmonary lobule. (a) Close up view of a CT scan (5-mm collimation) shows physiological air-trapping in a peripheral secondary pulmonary lobule (arrows). (b) High-resolution CT scan (2-mm collimation) shows smooth septal thickening (arrows) in a patient with pulmonary edema; thickened septa outline the polygonal shape of the secondary pulmonary lobule; the interlobular septa contain pulmonary venules (V). Bronchovascular structures are seen in a centrilobular location (arrowhead).

to approximately 30, depending upon the size of the lobule. The marginal structures of the lobule (interlobular septa) contain pulmonary venules and lymphatics.[45]

Anatomic computed tomography of pleura

The pleural space is bounded by two serosal membranes: the visceral and parietal pleurae.[47] While visceral pleura covers the lungs, the surfaces of mediastinum, chest wall, and diaphragm are lined by parietal pleura. The combined thickness of visceral and parietal pleural layers is approximately 0.2 mm. Using HRCT a 1–2-mm thick line of soft tissue density, representing the combined thickness of the visceral pleura, normal pleural fluid, parietal pleura, endothoracic fascia, and innermost intercostal muscle, is seen in the intercostal space between the lung and chest wall. The pleura and endothoracic fascia are too thin to be seen over the inner aspect of the ribs and they are not visualized unless pathologically thickened.

Interlobar and accessory fissures

On CT the pleura may be identified when it forms an interlobar fissure.[48] The normal fissures include a major or oblique fissure that runs obliquely through each lung and separates the upper and lower lobes (Figure 3.17) and a minor or horizontal fissure that runs horizontally through the right lung and separates the right upper and middle lobes.[49] Depending on the section thickness, interlobar fissures manifest as lucent bands, lines, and dense bands. On thick section scans (10 mm collimation) they appear as lucent bands that are devoid of vessels. On thin section CT scans (1–2-mm collimation) the fissures will usually appear as thin lines or dense bands. With advanced image processing techniques, including MPRs and MIPs, fissures are accurately identified as dense thin lines.

Fissures may or may not be complete, and incomplete fissures allow collateral air drift or spread of disease from one lobe to the other.[50,51] Fissures are incomplete on 12–75% of CT scans and are more commonly seen on the right lung, especially between the upper and lower lobes.

Accessory fissures can be identified in approximately 20% of conventional CT scans; they are seen with higher frequency on MDCT.[51,52] The most common is the azygos fissure, created by downward invagination of the azygos vein through the apical portion of the right upper lobe.[53] On CT scan azygos fissure is manifested by a curvilinear shadow that extends obliquely across the upper portion of the right upper lobe (Figure 3.18). The fissure can be identified in approximately 20% of CT examinations.[54,55] Because the vein runs outside the parietal pleura, four pleural layers (two parietal and two visceral) form the fissure.[33,34] Other accessory fissures are the inferior accessory

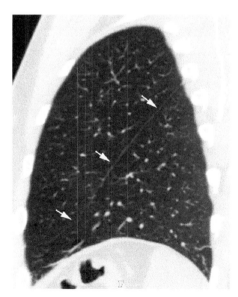

Figure 3.17
Left major fissure. Sagittal reconstruction from a high-resolution multidetector CT shows a well-defined thin line (arrows) across the left lung.

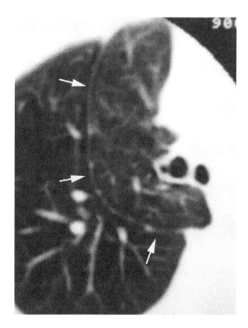

Figure 3.18
Azygos fissure. CT scan through the upper thorax shows a curvilinear line (arrows) across the right upper lobe that ends at the superior vena cava. Lung tissue is seen between the azygos vein and the trachea.

fissure, the superior accessory fissure, and the left minor fissure; the latter, analogous to the right minor fissure, separates the lingula from the left upper lobe.

Inferior pulmonary ligament

The pulmonary ligaments are reflections of a double layer of mediastinal parietal pleura that tethers the medial aspect of the lower lobes to the adjacent mediastinum and diaphragm.[56] They contain small systemic vessels and several lymph nodes, and contribute to the fixation of the lung to the mediastinum. Pulmonary ligaments extent from just below the inferior margins of the pulmonary hila inferiorly to the diaphragm posteriorly[56,57] (Figure 3.19).

Although it is anatomically extraparenchymal, the pulmonary ligament is contiguous laterally with a cleavage plane in the parenchyma of the lower lobe (intersegmental septum) which separates the medial from the posterior basal segments.[58] Intersegmental septa are bounded at the mediastinum by the base of the pulmonary ligament and laterally by a vein.[56,57]

The left pulmonary ligament is related closely to the esophagus and is bordered posteriorly by the descending aorta. The right pulmonary ligament is shorter than the left and can be situated anywhere along an arch extending from the inferior vena cava to the azygous vein.

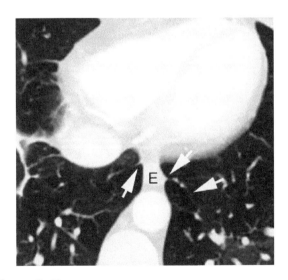

Figure 3.19
Inferior pulmonary ligaments. CT scan through the lower lungs shows bilateral well defined thin lines (arrows) showing small peaks on the mediastinal surface. Note that the left inferior pulmonary ligament is closely related to the esophagus (E).

Anatomic computed tomography of heart and pericardium

Cross-sectional cardiac anatomy can be studied by CT.[59] Contrast-enhanced electrocardiogram (ECG)-gated multi-detector CT provides high contrast and spatial resolution for imaging the thoracic organs.[60] The right atrium and right ventricle form the right lateral border of the heart. The right ventricle contains anterior and posterior papillary muscles, and its wall is typically more trabeculate and thinner than the left ventricular wall. The left ventricle also contains papillary muscles. The left atrium is the most superior and posterior chamber of the heart. The interatrial septum is thin and may be difficult to identify on CT scans. On CT, papillary muscles can be seen in both axial and coronal reformatted images (Figure 3.20). Knowledge of the location of these structures helps the radiologist to avoid a misdiagnosis of lymphadenopathy or other mediastinal processes.

The pericardium, like the pleura, is a two-layered stiff membrane lined by mesothelial cells that envelops the heart and the origin of the great vessels. It is divided into two distinct layers, the visceral and parietal pericardium, that become contiguous at the attachment of great vessels and forms a space that surrounds the heart (pericardial space). This space normally contains a small amount of serous fluid (20–25 ml) for lubrication during cardiac motion.

The pericardium can be identified at cross-sectional imaging when it is outlined by mediastinal and subepicardial fat or when it contains fluid or is thickened.[61] On CT the normal pericardium appears as a thin line measuring 1–2 mm in thickness (Figure 3.21). The normal 'potential' capacity of the pericardial space is approximately 300 ml. Whereas rapid accumulation of pericardial fluid greater than this amount impairs cardiac function, larger pericardial effusions may be physiologically adjusted for when accumulation occurs slowly.

Several pericardial recesses are demonstrated with cross-sectional imaging. On CT, these recesses can be recognized as areas of water attenuation around the great vessels.[62,63] The pericardial recesses can be categorized on the basis of whether they arise from the pericardial cavity proper, the transverse sinus, or the oblique sinus. The transverse sinus lies posterior to the ascending aorta and main pulmonary artery, just above the left atrium. The oblique sinus is the posterior extension of the pericardium and lies posterior to the left atrium and anterior to the esophagus. The transverse sinus lies superior and anterior to the oblique sinus. However, the transverse and oblique sinuses do not communicate at this level and are separated by two pericardial reflections.[61,63]

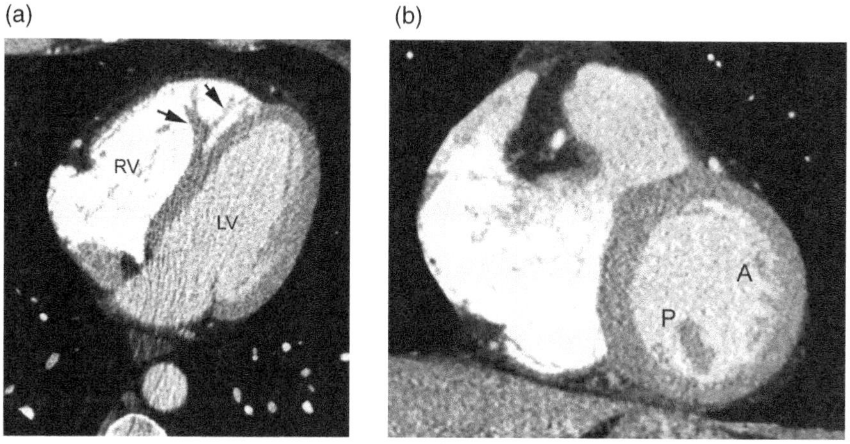

(a)

(b)

Figure 3.20

Normal ventricular anatomy. (a) Image obtained at 16-row multidetector CT. The right ventricle (RV), left ventricle (LV), and anterior papillary muscle (arrows) are shown. (b) Reformatted image of the left ventricle from CT data shows a modified short-axis view of the anterior (A) and posterior (P) papillary muscles.

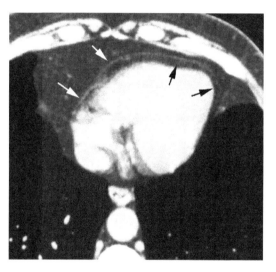

Figure 3.21

Normal pericardium. At CT the pericardium is seen as a thin, curvilinear soft-tissue density line (arrows) outlined by mediastinal and epicardial fat.

Anatomic computed tomography of the diaphragm

The diaphragm is a dome-shaped musculotendinous structure, approximately 5 mm thick, which separates the thoracic and abdominal cavities and performs most of the physiological work of inspiration. It has two distinct anatomic parts: a central tendinous portion and a peripheral muscular portion. There are three major openings to permit the passage of structures between the thorax and abdomen: the aortic hiatus, the esophageal hiatus, and the inferior vena cava foramen. The diaphragm is covered by pleura on its thoracic side and by peritoneum on its abdominal side.

The diaphragm is sometimes difficult to evaluate in the axial plane. MDCT has enhanced the capabilities of CT in imaging the diaphragm and has replaced conventional or slice-by-slice CT acquisition[64] (Figure 3.23). Sagittal and coronal reformatted images are of particular importance in the evaluation of the peridiaphragmatic area.[64] On CT, the anterior diaphragm most often appears as a relatively smooth or slightly undulating soft-tissue curve, concave posteriorly and continuous across the midline with the lateral diaphragmatic arcs.[65] An understanding of the normal anatomy of the anterior diaphragmatic attachments is valuable in assessing a variety of anterior paradiaphragmatic air collections.[66]

Diaphragmatic crura are tendinous structures that arise inferiorly from the anterior surfaces of the upper lumbar vertebral bodies and intervening disks. The right crus is larger and longer than the left. They appear as discrete oval

MDCT has also proved especially valuable in the evaluation of coronary artery anatomy and vessel patency. This technique also allows the 3D simultaneous imaging of additional vascular structures such as coronary veins, pulmonary arteries, aorta, and other thoracic arterial and venous structures[5] (Figure 3.22).

(a)

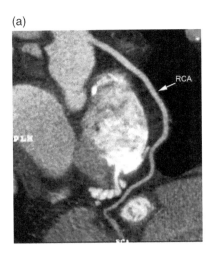

(b)

(c)

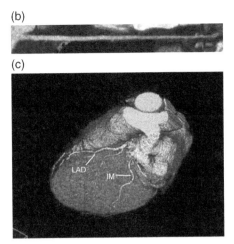

Figure 3.22

Normal coronary artery anatomy.
(a) Two-dimensional multiplanar reconstruction of the right coronary artery (RCA) obtained at 16-row multidetector CT (MDCT); this technique is used to evaluate the entire coronary artery in one view. (b) Artery can also be seen in its long length and it can be displayed as a very straight line.
(c) Three-dimensional volume-rendered reconstruction at MDCT coronary angiography. Left anterior oblique view showing left anterior descending coronary artery (LAD), and intermediate coronary artery branch (IM).

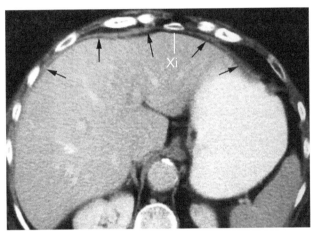

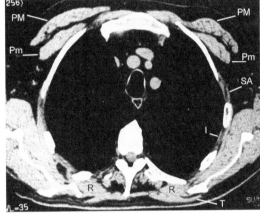

Figure 3.23

Normal diaphragm. A CT scan at the lower level of the xiphoid (Xi) demonstrates a well defined anterior portion of the diaphragm (arrows). The diaphragm is well visualized in the areas where it is outlined by lung, peritoneal, or retroperitoneal fat.

Figure 3.24

CT of the chest wall muscles. CT scan at the superior thorax demonstrates normal chest wall muscles. PM, pectoralis major; Pm, pectoralis minor; T, trapezius; R, romboideus; SA, serratus anterior; I, intercostal muscles.

or round structures that join anterior to the aorta to form the aortic hiatus. The diaphragmatic crura can be mistaken for enlarged lymph nodes or masses.

Anatomic computed tomography of the chest wall

The chest wall consists of the thoracic skeleton and its associated musculature and the soft tissues including the skin and subcutaneous fat. Chest wall musculature is easily visualized on CT because of the presence of fat separating the various muscle groups (Figure 3.24). The bony thorax includes components of the axial skeleton (vertebral bodies, ribs, and sternum) and appendicular skeleton (clavicles and scapula). The ribs are elastic arches of bone, which form a large part of the thoracic skeleton. They are twelve

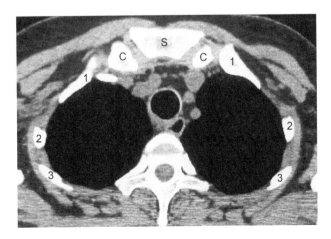

Figure 3.25

CT of chest wall bony structures. A CT scan at the level of the thoracic inlet shows the right and left clavicles (C), and the first (1), second (2), and third (3) ribs; the upper part of the sternum (S) is also seen.

in number on each side; however, this number may be increased by the development of a cervical or lumbar rib. Because of their oblique orientation, only a portion of any given rib is seen in a single CT section (Figure 3.25). The first rib is the most curved and usually the shortest of all the ribs. In some patients, a bony spur projects inferiorly from the undersurface of the first rib at its junction with the sternal manubrium. This protuberance may simulate a pulmonary nodule on CT (Figure 3.26). The typical location of this density should suggest its true nature.[67] Another common CT finding is the visualization of a normal 'vacuum

phenomenon' with visible gas within the sternoclavicular joint space.[68]

The body of the sternum is clearly identified in cross-sectional imaging with a narrower and more rectangular shape than the manubrium. In the parasterna-internal mammary zone, the internal mammary artery, one or two internal mammary veins, and the internal mammary lymph node run parallel to the lateral border of the sternum.[69]

The role of CT in the diagnosis of chest wall diseases has dramatically improved since the introduction of multidetector CT (MDCT). The complex anatomy of the chest wall is particularly well suited to multiplanar and 3D volume-rendering imaging.

(a)

(b)

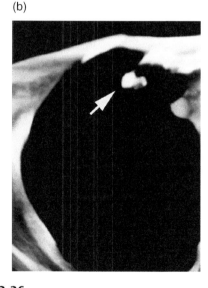

Figure 3.26
CT of the costomanubrial junction. (a) Lung window CT scan at the level of the superior thorax shows an anterior focal nodular opacity (arrow). (b) Mediastinal window demonstrates that the nodule corresponds to the articulation of the first rib and the sternal manubrium (arrow).

References

1. Kalender WA, Seissler W, Klotz E, Vock P. Spiral volumetric CT with single-breath-hold technique, continuous transport, and continuous scanner rotation. Radiology 1990; 176: 181–3.

2. Rubin GD. Data explosion: the challenge of multidetector-row CT. Eur J Radiol 2000; 36: 74–80.

3. Majos A, Tybor K, Stefanczyk L, Gorj B. Cortical mapping by functional magnetic resonance imaging in patients with brain tumors. Eur Radiol 2005; 15: 1148–58.

4. Brix G, Nagel HD, Stamm G et al. Radiation exposure in multi-slice versus single-slice spiral CT: results of a nationwide survey. Eur Radiol 2003; 13: 1979–91.

5. de Roos A, Kroft LJ, Bax JJ, Lamb HJ, Geleijns J. Cardiac applications of multislice computed tomography. Br J Radiol 2006; 79: 9–16.

6. White CS, Kuo D, Kelemen M et al. Chest pain evaluation in the emergency department: can MDCT provide a comprehensive evaluation? AJR Am J Roentgenol 2005; 185: 533–40.

7. Hyson EA, Ravin CE. Radiographic features of mediastinal anatomy. Chest 1979; 75: 609–13.

8. Proto AV. Mediastinal anatomy: emphasis on conventional images with anatomic and computed tomographic correlations. J Thorac Imaging 1987; 2: 1–48.

9. Chukwuemeka A, Currie L, Ellis H. CT anatomy of the mediastinal structures at the level of the manubriosternal angle. Clin Anat 1997; 10: 405–8.

10. Goldwin RL, Heitzman ER, Proto AV. Computed tomography of the mediastinum. Normal anatomy and indications for the use of CT. Radiology 1977; 124: 235–41.

11. Heitzman ER, Goldwin RL, Proto AV. Radiologic analysis of the mediastinum utilizing computed tomography. Radiol Clin North Am 1977; 15: 309–29.

12. Kondo T, Arita H, Ohta Y, Yamabayashi H. Role of the mediastinum as a part of the chest wall: analyzed by computed tomography. Respiration 1989; 56: 116–26.

13. Schnyder PA, Gamsu G. CT of the pretracheal retrocaval space. AJR Am J Roentgenol 1981; 136: 303–8.

14. Vock P, Owens A. Computed tomography of the normal and pathological thoracic inlet. Eur J Radiol 1982; 2: 187–93.

15. Diagnostic problems in the mediastinum. J Thorac Imaging 1987; 2: 1–100.

16. Heitzman ER. Fleischner Lecture. Computed tomography of the thorax: current perspectives. AJR Am J Roentgenol 1981; 136: 2–12.

17. Raider L. The retrotracheal triangle. Chest 1973; 63: 835–8.

18. Raider L, Landry BA, Brogdon BG. The retrotracheal triangle. Radiographics 1990; 10: 1055–79.

19. Proto AV, Speckman JM. The left lateral radiograph of the chest. Part 1. Med Radiogr Photogr 1979; 55: 29–74.

20. Proto AV, Speckman JM. The left lateral radiograph of the chest. Med Radiogr Photogr 1980; 56: 38–64.

21. Franquet T, Erasmus JJ, Gimenez A, Rossi S, Prats R. The retrotracheal space: normal anatomic and pathologic appearances. Radiographics 2002; 22 Spec No: S231–46.

22. Gamsu G, Webb WR. Computed tomography of the trachea: normal and abnormal. AJR Am J Roentgenol 1982; 139: 321–6.

23. Gamsu G, Webb WR. Computed tomography of the trachea and mainstem bronchi. Semin Roentgenol 1983; 18: 51–60.

24. Breatnach E, Abbott GC, Fraser RG. Dimensions of the normal human trachea. AJR Am J Roentgenol 1984; 142: 903–6.

25. Stern EJ, Graham CM, Webb WR, Gamsu G. Normal trachea during forced expiration: dynamic CT measurements. Radiology 1993; 187: 27–31.

26. Boiselle PM, Ernst A. Recent advances in central airway imaging. Chest 2002; 121: 1651–60.

27. De Wever W, Vandecaveye V, Lanciotti S, Verschakelen JA. Multidetector CT-generated virtual bronchoscopy: an illustrated review of the potential clinical indications. Eur Respir J 2004; 23: 776–82.

28. Eberle B, Weiler N, Vogel N, Kauczor HU, Heinrichs W. Computed tomography-based tracheobronchial image reconstruction allows selection of the individually appropriate double-lumen tube size. J Cardiothorac Vasc Anesth 1999; 13: 532–7.

29. Boiselle PM, Lee KS, Ernst A. Multidetector CT of the central airways. J Thorac Imaging 2005; 20: 186–95.

30. Napel S, Rubin GD, Jeffrey RB, Jr. STS-MIP: a new reconstruction technique for CT of the chest. J Comput Assist Tomogr 1993; 17: 832–8.

31. Chasen MH, Charnsangavej C. Venous chest anatomy: clinical implications. Eur J Radiol 1998; 27: 2–14.

32. Godwin JD, Chen JT. Thoracic venous anatomy. AJR Am J Roentgenol 1986; 147: 674–84.

33. Heitzman ER, Scrivani JV, Martino J, Moro J. The azygos vein and its pleural reflections. I. Normal roentgen anatomy. Radiology 1971; 101: 249–58.

34. Heitzman ER, Scrivani JV, Martino J, Moro J. The azygos vein and its pleural reflections. II. Applications in the radiological diagnosis of mediastinal abnormality. Radiology 1971; 101: 259–66.

35. Lawler LP, Fishman EK. Thoracic venous anatomy multidetector row CT evaluation. Radiol Clin North Am 2003; 41: 545–60.

36. Genereux GP, Howie JL. Normal mediastinal lymph node size and number: CT and anatomic study. AJR Am J Roentgenol 1984; 142: 1095–100.

37. Glazer GM, Gross BH, Quint LE et al. Normal mediastinal lymph nodes: number and size according to American Thoracic Society mapping. AJR Am J Roentgenol 1985; 144: 261–5.

38. Mountain CF, Dresler CM. Regional lymph node classification for lung cancer staging. Chest 1997; 111: 1718–23.

39. Rosenblum LJ, Mauceri RA, Wellenstein DE et al. Density patterns in the normal lung as determined by computed tomography. Radiology 1980; 137: 409–16.

40. Webb WR, Stern EJ, Kanth N, Gamsu G. Dynamic pulmonary CT: findings in healthy adult men. Radiology 1993; 186: 117–24.

41. Verschakelen JA, Van fraeyenhoven L, Laureys G, Demedts M, Baert AL. Differences in CT density between dependent and nondependent portions of the lung: influence of lung volume. AJR Am J Roentgenol 1993; 161: 713–7.

42. Reid L. The secondary lobule in the adult human lung, with special reference to its appearance in bronchograms. Thorax 1958; 13: 110–5.

43. Webb WR. Thin-section CT of the secondary pulmonary lobule: anatomy and the image – the 2004 Fleischner lecture. Radiology 2006; 239: 322–38.

44. Bergin C, Roggli V, Coblentz C, Chiles C. The secondary pulmonary lobule: normal and abnormal CT appearances. AJR Am J Roentgenol 1988; 151: 21–5.

45. Heitzman ER, Markarian B, Berger I, Dailey E. The secondary pulmonary lobule: a practical concept for interpretation of chest radiographs. I. Roentgen anatomy of the normal secondary pulmonary lobule. Radiology 1969; 93: 507–12.

46. Murata K, Itoh H, Todo G et al. Centrilobular lesions of the lung: demonstration by high-resolution CT and pathologic correlation. Radiology 1986; 161: 641–5.

47. Kuhlman JE, Singha NK. Complex disease of the pleural space: radiographic and CT evaluation. Radiographics 1997; 17: 63–79.

48. Hayashi K, Aziz A, Ashizawa K et al. Radiographic and CT appearances of the major fissures. Radiographics 2001; 21: 861–74.

49. Raasch BN, Carsky EW, Lane EJ, O'Callaghan JP, Heitzman ER. Radiographic anatomy of the interlobar fissures: a study of 100 specimens. AJR Am J Roentgenol 1982; 138: 1043–9.

50. Dandy WE, Jr. Incomplete pulmonary interlobar fissure sign. Radiology 1978; 128: 21–5.

51. Godwin JD, Tarver RD. Accessory fissures of the lung. AJR Am J Roentgenol 1985; 144: 39–47.

52. Otsuji H, Uchida H, Maeda M et al. Incomplete interlobar fissures: bronchovascular analysis with CT. Radiology 1993; 187: 541–6.

53. Felson B. The azygos lobe: its variation in health and disease. Semin Roentgenol 1989; 24: 56–66.

54. Berkmen T, Berkmen YM, Austin JH. Accessory fissures of the upper lobe of the left lung: CT and plain film appearance. AJR Am J Roentgenol 1994; 162: 1287–93.

55. Caceres J, Mata JM, Alegret X, Palmer J, Franquet T. Increased density of the azygos lobe on frontal chest radiographs simulating disease: CT findings in seven patients. AJR Am J Roentgenol 1993; 160: 245–8.

56. Rabinowitz JG, Cohen BA, Mendelson DS. Symposium on Nonpulmonary Aspects in Chest Radiology. The pulmonary ligament. Radiol Clin North Am 1984; 22: 659–72.

57. Rost RC, Jr., Proto AV. Inferior pulmonary ligament: computed tomographic appearance. Radiology 1983; 148: 479–83.

58. Berkmen YM, Drossman SR, Marboe CC. Intersegmental (intersublobar) septum of the lower lobe in relation to the

pulmonary ligament: anatomic, histologic, and CT correlations. Radiology 1992; 185: 389–93.

59. Guthaner DF, Wexler L, Harell G. CT demonstration of cardiac structures. AJR Am J Roentgenol 1979; 133: 75–81.

60. Boxt LM. CT anatomy of the heart. Int J Cardiovasc Imaging 2005; 21: 13–27.

61. Broderick LS, Brooks GN, Kuhlman JE. Anatomic pitfalls of the heart and pericardium. Radiographics 2005; 25: 441–53.

62. Levy-Ravetch M, Auh YH, Rubenstein WA, Whalen JP, Kazam E. CT of the pericardial recesses. AJR Am J Roentgenol 1985; 144: 707–14.

63. Kodama F, Fultz PJ, Wandtke JC. Comparing thin-section and thick-section CT of pericardial sinuses and recesses. AJR Am J Roentgenol 2003; 181: 1101–8.

64. Brink JA, Heiken JP, Semenkovich J et al. Abnormalities of the diaphragm and adjacent structures: findings on multiplanar spiral CT scans. AJR Am J Roentgenol 1994; 163: 307–10.

65. Gale ME. Anterior diaphragm: variations in the CT appearance. Radiology 1986; 161: 635–9.

66. Kleinman PK, Raptopoulos V. The anterior diaphragmatic attachments: an anatomic and radiologic study with clinical correlates. Radiology 1985; 155: 289–93.

67. Paling MR, Dwyer A. The first rib as the cause of a "pulmonary nodule" on chest computed tomography. J Comput Assist Tomogr 1980; 4: 847–8.

68. Destouet JM, Gilula LA, Murphy WA, Sagel SS. Computed tomography of the sternoclavicular joint and sternum. Radiology 1981; 138: 123–8.

69. Kuhlman JE, Bouchardy L, Fishman EK, Zerhouni EA. CT and MR imaging evaluation of chest wall disorders. Radiographics 1994; 14: 571–95.

4

Common radiological signs of lung disease

Sujal R Desai

Introduction

The plain chest radiograph and, now increasingly, computed tomography (CT) are indispensible tools in the investigation of patients with suspected lung disease. The chest radiograph has long enjoyed an enduring role in radiology and remains one of the most commonly requested radiological tests. Not only is the radiation dose associated with plain radiography acceptably low, but also the technique is relatively simple and not infrequently provides the first clue to the presence of pulmonary disease. Furthermore, in patients with an established diagnosis of lung disease and where the physician needs to monitor progress or the effects of treatment, serial chest radiography is certainly easier to justify than repeated CT examinations.

Despite the acknowledged benefits, conventional chest radiography has limitations. In contrast to CT, the chest radiograph is constrained by problems of anatomical superimposition, poorer contrast resolution, and issues of observer disagreement. All of these factors have the potential to hinder plain radiographic interpretation. The corollary, which is particularly true in the context of diffuse interstitial lung diseases, is that CT is not only more sensitive and specific but also significantly more accurate in diagnosis.[1,2] However, the disadvantages of CT must always be borne in mind. The obvious and important drawback is the significantly increased exposure to ionizing radiation. In this regard, because of the interslice spacing and the facility to use low dose protocols (which do not significantly hinder image quality)[3] the radiation burden may be kept to a minimum with high-resolution CT.

In this chapter, the more common radiological signs (which physicians regularly encounter in radiologists' reports) and their pathological/diagnostic significance are discussed. Because they are the 'work-horse' radiological tests in the vast majority of patients with suspected lung disease, this chapter deals exclusively with plain radiographic and CT signs of disease.

Basic principles of radiological interpretation

When interpreting radiological images it is good practice for the observer to first determine the dominant radiological pattern or combination of signs, instead of making instant (and frequently erroneous) judgments about pathology. Most physcians will be all too familiar, for instance, with the radiological report which begins with the statement that 'there is an interstitial pattern in the lower zones'. Leaping towards a pathological diagnosis before a careful assessment of the radiological signs is best avoided. In this regard, it must be appreciated by the reader that the range of possible radiological patterns, which reflect the multitude of possible lung pathologies, is relatively narrow. A good illustration is the pattern of ground-glass opacification which may be caused by diseases that predominantly involve the air spaces, the interstitium or, indeed, both.[4,5] Even with the apparently non-contentious term 'consolidation' some caution is warranted, not least because of the variable meaning of the term when used by pathologists (who refer to the presence of an exudative process) and radiologists (who tend to apply the term more loosely, to indicate any pathological process within the air spaces). Suffice to say that infection is not the sole cause of consolidation in the lungs; intra-alveolar hemorrhage, eosinophilic lung disease, and some malignancies (to name but a few) can all give rise to a pattern of air space filling on chest radiography or CT.

Although the spectrum of histopathological responses to lung injury, is relatively narrow, it is a sobering thought that, even when there is unequivocal diffuse lung disease on the chest radiograph, careful analysis of the radiographic pattern alone will seldom allow a histospecific diagnosis to be reached;[6] the distinction between a reticular and a nodular pattern on a chest radiograph is not always easy[7] and does not usually allow the differential diagnosis to be refined.

Surprisingly, the situation is not significantly improved with experienced radiologists, since the correct diagnosis is included in only half the cases.[8] However, notwithstanding this, plain chest radiography and CT should be analyzed in terms of the basic radiographic patterns. Thus, only the standard terms such as nodular, reticular, ground-glass opacification, and consolidation should be used. Only when the observer has decided on the nature of the radiological pattern or patterns, should judgments be made about the likely pathological process. In the sections which follow, the common radiological patterns and their likely pathological correlates are considered.

Common radiological patterns of lung disease

In routine practice, the radiologist generally only has to deal with a handful of radiological signs. In this chapter, the following CT patterns of consolidation, ground-glass opacification, reticular pattern, nodular pattern, mosaic attenuation, and the tree-in-bud pattern will be discussed. The interested reader, requiring detailed information on radiological signs, is referred to a number of excellent reference texts and articles.[4,9–11]

Consolidation

Consolidation refers to an area of increased parenchymal opacification which obscures the margins of both vessels and the walls of airways. The reader should contrast this with the definition of ground-glass opacification given below[4] (Figure 4.1). Put simply, consolidation is seen when *any* disease process fills the alveoli and alveolar ducts and, thus, consolidation must be regarded as a non-specific radiological sign. Air spaces diseases are reasonably common and the approach to diagnosis is potentially mind boggling (Table 4.1). When interpreting the pattern of consolidation, the observer should be mindful of a few important facts. First, contrary to the belief of many junior radiologists, consolidation is not synonymous with infection! Second, interpretation of the radiological findings is seldom fruitful without due consideration of the available clinical data. Third, an appreciation of the distribution of radiographic abnormalities (i.e. upper zones versus lower, central versus peripheral) may be of diagnostic value and, finally, where available, a review of serial radiological studies is crucial.

Clearly, a knowledge of the clinical background is crucial. For instance, when there is a history of pyrexia and a productive cough in a patient known to be immunosuppressed, it is entirely reasonable for the radiologist to conclude that widespread consolidation on chest radiography is due to an opportunistic chest infection (Figure 4.2). In contrast, the same radiological sign in someone known to

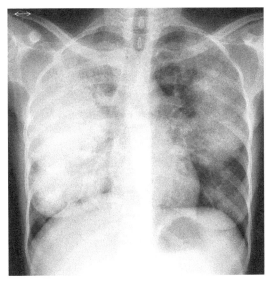

Figure 4.1
Consolidation on a chest radiograph in a patient with multidrug-resistant tuberculosis. There is dense bilateral opacification and an air bronchogram is clearly visible on the right.

Table 4.1 Miscellaneous causes of consolidation on chest radiography and computed tomography

- Infection
- Intra-alveolar hemorrhage
- Infarction
- Organizing pneumonia
    cryptogenic
    secondary (e.g. drug reaction, connective tissue disease)
- Eosinophilic pneumonias
- Malignancy
    adenocarcinoma/bronchioloalveolar cell carcinoma
    primary pulmonary lymphoma
    metastases
- Sarcoidosis

have presented with massive hemoptysis should suggest the possibility of intra-alveolar hemorrhage. The distribution of air space opacities on the plain radiograph might also be a helpful differentiating feature. In cryptogenic organizing pneumonia, areas of consolidation tend to be most pronounced in the periphery and the lower zones,[12] whereas in patients with chronic eosinophilic pneumonia, the changes have a predilection for the upper zones and characteristically are parallel to the chest wall.[13] A review of serial radiographs, to ascertain disease progression or regression, should also be part of the radiologist's routine. Relatively rapid changes (occurring over a period of hours or, at most, a few days as opposed to weeks) are more in keeping with pulmonary edema or hemorrhage, whereas gradual improvement over a week or so is suggestive of infective consolidation (Figure 4.3). Opacities that are transient and migratory, perhaps associated with constitutional disturbance, should prompt the radiologist to suggest a diagnosis of an eosinophilic lung disease (Figure 4.4).

CT is frequently requested in patients with airspace disease and may, just occasionally, reveal features hitherto masked on chest radiography: an example is the discovery

of a small focus of cavitation and perhaps an associated tree-in-bud infiltrate on CT which may prompt the radiologist to consider a mycobacterial infection rather than one of the myriad other causes of consolidation. However, apart from a few select cases, the salutary point is that even with CT the observer might only be able to limit the list of diagnostic possibilities and, in general, the advantages of CT over plain radiography in the diagnosis of air space diseases have yet to be proven.[14]

Ground-glass opacification

Ground-glass opacification is an important and common radiological sign. On plain radiographs, there is veil-like increased density that obscures the vascular markings. In contrast, because of the better density resolution, when there is ground-glass opacification on CT bronchovascular markings remain visible despite the increased attenuation (Figure 4.5).[4] As with consolidation, the demonstration of ground-glass opacification (regardless of whether this is on chest radiography or CT) indicates that air has been displaced from the lungs. However, unlike consolidation, the finding of ground-glass opacification does not always imply that the pathology is in the air spaces. Predominant interstitial lung diseases and a combination of interstitial and air space pathology can also result in a pattern of ground-glass opacification (Figure 4.6). Thus, in patients with diffuse interstitial lung disease, the notion (implied in some CT reports) that ground-glass opacification always depicts a 'reversible alveolitis' is too simplistic. Indeed, the presence of dilated segmental or subsegmental airways (so-called traction bronchiectasis) within regions of ground-glass opacification, indicates that there is established fibrosis which is below the resolution limits of CT (Figure 4.7).

The causes of ground-glass opacification are legion (Table 4.2) and it is important to appreciate that this radiological pattern is non-specific. The most frequent causes of ground-glass opacification in clinical practice include

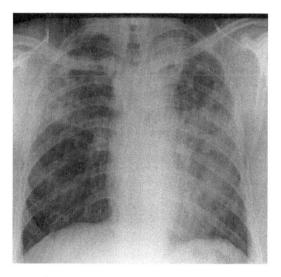

Figure 4.2
Chest radiograph in a patient with human immunodeficiency virus infection and acquired immunodeficiency syndrome presenting with pyrexia and a productive cough. There is widespread bilateral consolidation (which obscures vascular markings) more pronounced in the left lung. The diagnosis of *Pneumocystis jiroveci* pneumonia was confirmed following bronchoalveolar lavage.

(a)

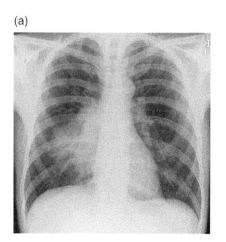

(b)

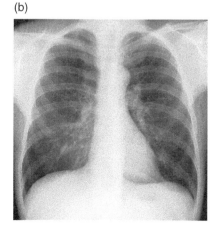

Figure 4.3
Serial chest radiographs taken in a patient with the classical symptoms and clinical signs of pneumonia. (a) There is dense consolidation in the right lower lobe which obscures vessel markings. (b) A repeat radiograph performed 10 days later and following antibiotics shows resolution of pneumonia.

(a)   (b)

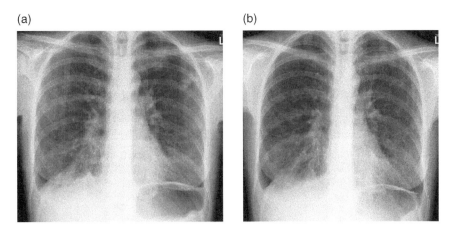

Figure 4.4
Chest radiographs in a patient with asthma, elevated peripheral eosinophil level, and pulmonary infiltrates. (a) Chest radiograph at presentation demonstrates ill-defined foci of opacification in the left upper zone. (b) The second radiograph (performed 5 days later and on no treatment) demonstrates significant resolution of the left upper lobe opacities.

(a)   (b)

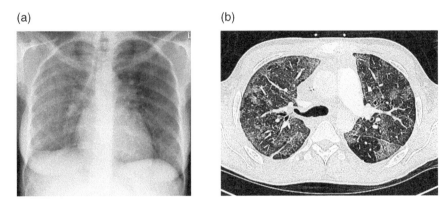

Figure 4.5
Ground-glass opacification on chest radiography and CT. (a) Chest radiograph in a patient with *Pneumocystis jiroveci* pneumonia. There is a subtle but definite increase in parenchymal attenuation in the right lung which renders vessels invisible. (b) CT in another patient with *Pneumocystis jiroveci* pneumonia. Despite the increase in parenchymal density bronchial walls and vessels are easily seen.

pulmonary edema (typically due to fluid overload or heart failure), infection (such as pneumonia due to *Pneumocystis jiroveci* (formerly *Pneumocystis carinii*), inflammatory lung diseases (for instance, subacute extrinsic allergic alveolitis), and intra-alveolar hemorrhage. As with the pattern of consolidation, it is important that the pattern of ground-glass opacification is considered in concert with the clinical data and, where available, a review of serial radiological findings.

Reticular pattern (reticulation)

The presence of fine, intermediate thickness or coarse criss-crossing lines on a chest radiograph or CT is termed a reticular pattern (Figure 4.8). On plain chest radiographs, because of the effects of superimposition, there is often the impression of an associated nodular element and most physicians will have come across the phrase 'reticulonodular pattern' in radiologists' reports. In patients with fibrotic lung disease there may be associated honeycomb destruction of

the lung but it is perhaps fair to state that this is more easily recognized at CT than plain chest radiography. The importance of the reticular or reticulonodular pattern is that it generally indicates significant interstitial lung disease. However, it must be emphasized that although fibrotic lung diseases are probably the best known cause of a reticular pattern, the radiological differential diagnosis must consider other potential causes of this sign. In this regard, pathological processes that primarily involve the lymphatics (the most familiar example of which is lymphangitis carcinomatosa) or pulmonary venous circulation (typically in patients with pulmonary edema) will lead to thickening of the interlobular septa and hence a reticular pattern. In addition, a distinction should be made between a linear pattern (defined as any linear opacity, measuring up to 3 mm in thickness, that is not an interlobular septum or bronchovascular bundle)[4] and reticulation. Linear opacities due to subsegmental atelectasis and irregular bands of parenchymal distortion sometimes seen in association with

(a)

(b)

(c)

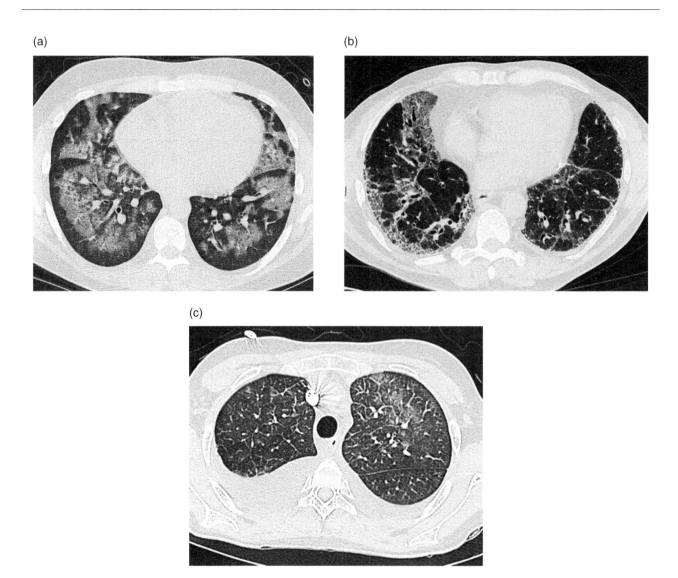

Figure 4.6
Triptych of images demonstrating different categories of causes of ground-glass opacification on CT. (a) Predominant air space disease due to acute intra-alveolar hemorrhage; (b) predominant interstitial (fibrotic) lung disease; and (c) mixed interstitial and airspace filling due to pulmonary edema.

exudative pleural effusions are a relatively frequent finding on chest radiography and CT. Some of the causes of a reticular pattern most commonly encountered in clinical practice are given in Table 4.3.

When evaluating the chest radiograph it is worth focusing on the distribution of abnormality for it is known that different disease processes have a predilection for different lung zones. Thus, despite the long list of possible causes of a reticular pattern, knowing that diseases such as asbestosis and idiopathic pulmonary fibrosis have a propensity to involve the lower zones, whereas sarcoidosis and certain pneumoconioses generally cause fibrosis in the upper zones is helpful (Figure 4.9). In addition to the distribution of a reticular pattern, noting the presence of ancillary radiological findings may be of value in refining what might

otherwise be a long (and ultimately, unhelpful) list of differential diagnoses. Thus, in a patient with a lower zone reticular pattern, the presence of associated pleural thickening makes the diagnosis of idiopathic pulmonary fibrosis less likely. Similarly, the demonstration of so-called Kerley B lines in the lower zones (particularly if this is unilateral and associated with ipsilateral hilar lymph node enlargement) should prompt the radiologist to at least consider lymphangitis carcinomatosa in the differential diagnosis.

Nodular pattern

Nodules are a common finding on radiological examination. A nodule has been defined as any rounded and usually well marginated opacity which measures no more than 3 cm in

(a)

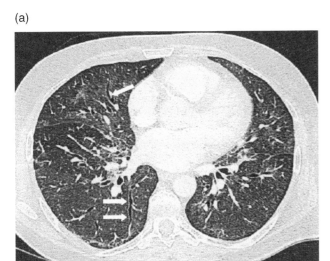

(b)

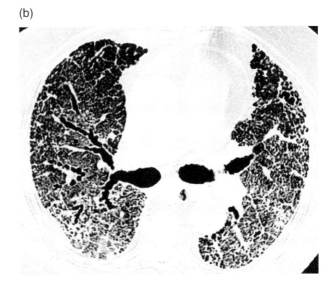

Figure 4.7

Ground-glass opacification reflecting intrapulmonary fibrosis in two patients. (a) CT through the midzone in a patient with resolving Pneumocystis jiroveci pneumonia. There is subtle ground-glass attenuation in which there are dilated segmental and subsegmental airways (arrows). (b) CT at the level of the carina in acute interstitial pneumonia. There is a fine reticular pattern and widespread ground-glass opacification. However, in addition, there is gross dilatation of airways (particularly in the right lung) indicating established interstitial fibrosis. Image courtesy of Professor Jud W Gurney, University of Nebraska Medical Center, Nebraska, USA.

Table 4.2 Causes of ground-glass opacification

Common
- Infection (bacterial, fungal, viral)
  edema (cardiogenic or non-cardiogenic)

Less frequent
- Intra-alveolar haemorrhage
- Interstitial pneumonias
  non-specific interstitial pneumonia
  respiratory bronchiolitis/respiratory
    bronchiolitis-interstitial lung disease
  lymphocytic interstitial pneumonia
  desquamative interstitial pneumonia
  cryptogenic organizing pneumonia
  acute interstitial pneumonia
- Other diffuse interstitial lung disease
  eosinophilic lung diseases
  sarcoidosis
  subacute extrinsic allergic alveolitis
  alveolar proteinosis
- Miscellaneous
  bronchioloalveolar cell carcinoma
  radiation pneumonitis
  'spurious' (lungs imaged at less than total
    lung capacity)

---

diameter.[4] The subject of the solitary pulmonary nodule is deserving of a separate volume in itself and will not be discussed further. However, a pattern of multiple nodules is a reasonably frequent finding and, depending to a certain extent on whether a chest radiograph or CT is being reviewed, radiologists will attempt to characterize nodules based on their margin (smooth versus irregular), distribution (upper versus lower zone, perilymphatic, centrilobular, or random), and the presence or absence of cavitation.

As with other radiological signs, the finding of multiple pulmonary nodules is non-specific. However, there are examples of scenarios in which the observer might make a reasonable stab at a diagnosis. Thus, in the context of a patient with a known extrathoracic malignancy, the finding of multiple well-defined spherical nodules in the periphery of the lungs is highly suspicious for metastatic disease. Multiple small nodules in a peribronchovascular or subpleural distribution are typical of sarcoidosis, whereas numerous small nodules of ground-glass attenuation, in a centrilobular distribution, are seen in patients with subacute extrinsic allergic alveolitis and also respiratory bronchiolitis.

Mosaic attenuation pattern

The term mosaic attenuation pattern (still referred to as mosaic oligemia or mosaic perfusion by some) implies that there are admixed regions of variable parenchymal attenuation. Put simply, there are patchy 'black' and 'white' areas of lung (Figure 4.10). In essence, mosaic attenuation is a CT sign of disease; the inferior contrast resolution means that this sign is not depicted on conventional chest radiographs. The categories of causes of the mosaic pattern are conveniently considered in three broad groups: infiltrative

(a) 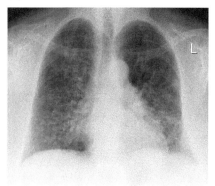   (b)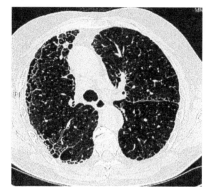

Figure 4.8
Reticular pattern on (a) chest radiography in a patient with chronic extrinsic allergic alveolitis (hypersensitivity pneumonitis) and (b) CT in idiopathic pulmonary fibrosis where there is a coarse reticular pattern with honeycombing predominantly in the subpleural lung on the right.

Table 4.3 Causes of reticular or reticulo-nodular pattern

Fibrosing lung diseases
- Mid- and upper zone distribution
    tuberculosis
    sarcoidosis
    chronic extrinsic allergic alveolitis
    ankylosing spondylitis
    pneumoconioses
    berylliosis
    Marfan's syndrome
    radiation fibrosis
- Mid- and lower zone distribution
    Idiopathic pulmonary fibrosis/cyptogenic
    fibrosing alveolitis
    asbestosis
    chronic extrinsic allergic alveolitis
    connective tissue disease related fibrosis
        rheumatoid arthritis
        systemic sclerosis
        dermatomyositis
        systemic lupus erythematosus
Diffuse interstitial lung diseases
    Langerhans' cell histiocytosis
    lymphangioleiomyomatosis
    tuberose sclerosis
    neurofibromatosis
    lymphocytic interstitial pneumonia
    idiopathic pulmonary hemorrhage
Miscellaneous causes
    lymphangitis carcinomatosa and other causes
        of malignant infiltration
    infection (viral, mycoplasma)
    paraseptal emphysema
    veno-occlusive disease
    alveolar proteinosis
    lipoid pneumonia
    bronchioloalveolar carcinoma
    Niemann–Pick disease

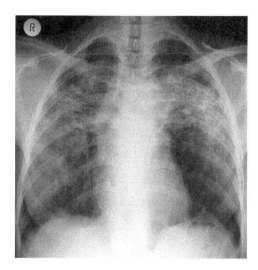

Figure 4. 9
Coarse symmetrical reticular pattern in the upper zones, the characteristic chest radiographic distibution of fibrosis in sarcoidosis.

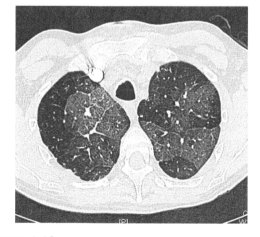

Figure 4.10
Mosaic attenuation pattern on CT. There is heterogeneity of lung parenchymal density in this patient with small airways disease in the context of primary ciliary dyskinesia.

lung disease, small airways disease (specifically, constrictive obliterative bronchiolitis), and occlusive vascular disease. It should be mentioned that although the exact etiology of lung infiltration or constrictive obliterative bronchiolitis might not be identified, the principal challenge for the radiologist is to determine the category (infiltrative, small airways, or vascular) of disease in individual patients.

When faced with a mosaic attenuation pattern, the radiologist will first decide whether regions of low or high attenuation are abnormal. In this regard, the vessels are the key (Figure 4.11). Where there is no obvious disparity in the number and/or caliber of vessels between regions of low and high attenuation, it can be assumed that the areas of black lung represents regions of 'sparing' and that the primary pathology is pulmonary infiltration. Conversely, any reduction in the number and/or caliber of vessels in regions of low density generally excludes infiltrative disease and the radiologist will then look for certain ancillary features that point towards either small airways disease or occlusive vascular pathology. Bronchial dilatation and air trapping on images taken at end-expiration should suggest a diagnosis of obliterative bronchiolitis. In contrast, dilatation of the main pulmonary trunk in relation to the diameter of the ascending aorta,[15] pericardial effusions or thickening,[16] and laminated filling defects in the pulmonary arteries on contrast-enhanced CT are the associated findings in chronic thromboembolic disease. The diagnostic pathway described above appears reasonably straightforward and is useful in many cases. However, in practice, it must be stressed that the division into infiltrative, small airways, and vascular disease is sometimes difficult, not least because of the tendency for radiologists (including experienced observers) to misclassify the last category.[17]

Tree-in-bud pattern

Because the walls of bronchioles cannot be resolved, normal peripheral airways (unlike branches of the homologous pulmonary arteries), are not seen at CT. However, the presence of exudate in the lumen and the surrounding peribronchiolar inflammation can render these small airways visible. At CT there are centrilobular nodules of soft-tissue attenuation. Depending on the orientation of the airway with respect to the plane of section, some will demonstrate clear branching or have a 'V'- or 'Y-shaped' configuration (Figure 4.12). As with mosaic attenuation, the tree-in-bud pattern is essentially a CT sign: although an abnormality might be seen it is unlikely that the branching nature of this pattern would be appreciated on plain radiographs.

The most common cause of this pattern is infection. In this group mycobacterial disease (both tuberculous and non-tuberculous), viral (cytomegalovirus, respiratory syncytial virus), and, occasionally, fungal (*Aspergillus* and *Candida* species) infection are the widely documented causes of this

(a) (b)

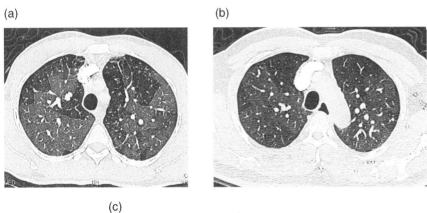

(c)

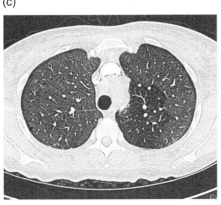

Figure 4.11
Mosaic attenuation pattern due to (a) constrictive obliterative bronchiolitis in a patient with bronchiectasis, (b) chronic thromboembolic disease, and (c) pulmonary edema. Note that in obliterative bronchiolitis, and vascular disease there is a reduction in the number/caliber of pulmonary vessels in regions of 'black' lung. This is not the case in the patient with pulmonary edema.

(a)

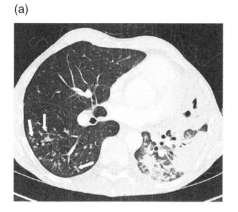

(b)

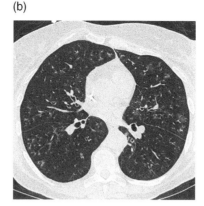

Figure 4.12
Two examples of a tree-in-bud pattern. (a) Localized tree-in-bud infiltrate (arrows) in the right lower lobe in a patient with smear-positive tuberculosis. Extensive cavitating consolidation is present in the left lung. (b) Widespread tree-in-bud pattern in a patient with presumed infection following allogeneic bone marrow transplantation.

CT pattern.[18–20] Sometimes the tree-in-bud pattern will be an ancillary finding in patients with more proximal (large) airway disease. Thus, in bronchiectasis, for instance, plugging of the peripheral small airways will give rise to a tree-in-bud infiltrate. Less frequent causes of this sign include aspiration, toxic fume inhalation, and the bronchiolitis associated with certain connective tissue diseases (notably rheumatoid arthritis and Sjögren's syndrome). Rarely, the tree-in-bud pattern will be a manifestation of (malignant) vascular pathology as opposed to small airways disease. On occasion, tumor microemboli incite intense intimal cellular proliferation and, ulitmately, occlusion of small arteries and arterioles.[21] This phenomenon, which leads to a 'vascular' tree-in-bud pattern, has been termed thrombotic microangiopathy.

Conclusions

The correct interpretation of radiological studies is dependent on not only a knowledge of the common patterns but also an understanding of the possible relationships between these signs and different pathological processes. Before making judgments about the nature of the pathological process it is good practice to first decide which pattern or combination of patterns predominates. Only then should statements about the pathology (e.g. air space disease, pulmonary fibrosis) be made. Finally, the observer must also remember that many of the common radiological signs such as consolidation and ground-glass opacification are non-specific and accurate diagnosis requires that the imaging features are considered together with the available clinical data.

References

1. Epler GR, McLoud TC, Gaensler EA, Mikus JP, Carrington CB. Normal chest roentgenograms in chronic diffuse infiltrative lung disease. N Engl J Med 1978; 298: 934–9.

2. Mathieson JR, Mayo JR, Staples CA, Müller NL. Chronic diffuse infiltrative lung disease: comparison of diagnostic accuracy of CT and chest radiography. Radiology 1989; 171: 111–6.

3. Zwirewich CV, Mayo JR, Müller NL. Low-dose high-resolution CT of lung parenchyma. Radiology 1991; 180: 413–7.

4. Austin JHM, Müller NL, Friedman PJ et al. Glossary of terms for computed tomography of the lungs: recommendations of the nomenclature committee of the Fleischner society. Radiology 1996; 200: 327–31.

5. Collins J, Stern EJ. Ground-glass opacity at CT: the ABCs. AJR Am J Roentgenol 1997; 169: 355–67.

6. Felson B. A new look at pattern recognition of diffuse pulmonary disease. AJR Am J Roentgenol 1979; 133: 183–9.

7. Carstairs LS. The interpretation of shadows in a restricted area of lung field on the chest radiograph. Pro R Soc Med 1961; 54: 978–80.

8. McLoud TC, Carrington CB, Gaensler EA. Diffuse infiltrative lung disease: a new scheme for description. Radiology 1983; 149: 353–63.

9. Webb WR, Müller NL, Naidich DP. High-resolution computed tomography findings of lung disease. In: Webb WR, Müller NL, Naidich DP, eds. High-resolution CT of the Lung, 3rd edn. Philadelphia: Lippincott Williams & Wilkins, 2001; 71–192.

10. Hansell DM, Armstrong P, Lynch DA et al. Basic patterns in lung disease. In: Hansell DM, Armstrong P, Lynch DA, McAdams HP, editors. Imaging of Diseases of the Lung. 4th edn. Philadelphia: Elsevier Mosby; 2005; 69–141.

11. Hansell DM, Armstrong P, Lynch DA et al. Basic HRCT patterns of lung disease. In: Hansell DM, Armstrong P, Lynch DA, McAdams HP, editors. Imaging of Diseases of the Chest. 4th edn. Philadelphia: Elsevier Mosby; 2005; 143–81.

12. Haddock JAA, Hansell DM. The radiology and terminology of cryptogenic organizing pneumonia. Br J Radiol 1992; 65: 674–80.

13. Gaensler EA, Carrington CB. Peripheral opacities in chronic eosinophilic pneumonia: the photographic negative of pulmonary oedema. AJR Am J Roentgenol 1977; 128: 1–13.

14. Johkoh T, Ikezoe J, Kohno N et al. Usefulness of high-resolution CT for differential diagnosis of multi-focal pulmonary consolidation. Radiat Med 1996; 14(3): 139–46.

15. Ng CS, Wells AU, Padley SP. A CT sign of chronic pulmonary arterial hypertension: the ratio of main pulmonary artery to aortic diameter. J Thorac Imaging 1999; 14: 270–8.

16. Baque-Juston MC, Wells AU, Hansell DM. Pericardial thickening or effusion in patients with pulmonary artery hypertension: a CT study. AJR Am J Roentgenol 1999; 172: 361–4.

17. Worthy SA, Müller NL, Hartman TE et al. Mosaic attenuation pattern on thin-section CT of the lung: differentiation among infiltrative lung, airway, and vascular diseases as a cause. Radiology 1997; 205: 465–70.

18. Rossi SE, Franquet T, Volpacchio M, Gimenez A, Aguilar G. Tree-in-bud pattern at thin-section CT of the lungs: radiologic-pathologic overview. Radiographics 2005; 25: 789–801.

19. Franquet T, Müller NL, Lee KS, Oikonomou A, Flint JD. Pulmonary candidiasis after hematopoietic stem cell transplantation: thin-section CT findings. Radiology 2005 Jul 1; 236: 332–7.

20. Jeong YJ, Lee KS, Koh WJ et al. Nontuberculous mycobacterial pulmonary infection in immunocompetent patients: comparison of thin-section CT and histopathologic findings. Radiology 2004 Jun 1; 231(3): 880–6.

21. Franquet T, Gimenez A, Prats R, Rodriguez-Arias JM, Rodriguez C. Thrombotic microangiopathy of pulmonary tumors: a vascular cause of tree-in-bud pattern on CT. AJR Am J Roentgenol 2002 Oct 1; 179: 897–9.

SECTION III: CONTRIBUTIONS OF IMAGING TESTS IN SPECIFIC CLINICAL SETTINGS

Lung Cancer
The Solitary Pulmonary Nodule
Interstitial Lung Diseases
Connective Tissue Disorders
Immunologic Diseases (other than asthma)
Pulmonary Thromboembolic Disease
Pleural Sepsis
Pulmonary Sepsis
Chronic Obstructive Pulmonary Disease
Hemoptysis
Cough

5

Lung cancer

Otis B Rickman and Stephen J Swensen

Introduction

According to recent estimates there were 172 570 new cases and 163 510 deaths from lung cancer in 2005 and these accounted for 28% of deaths from cancer in the United States.[1] When identified early, non-small cell lung carcinoma is routinely resected with survival rates of 40–85%.[2] Unfortunately, most lung cancers present at an advanced stage resulting in a dismal overall 5-year survival of 15%.[3] Chest radiography was the first imaging technique to advance the diagnosis and staging of lung cancer and still plays a role.[4] However, plain chest radiography and tomography have largely been supplanted by newer imaging techniques such as computed tomography (CT) or positron emission tomography (PET). CT scanning is currently the cornerstone imaging study for diagnosis and staging of lung cancer. Since its introduction in 1973 and widespread deployment in the 1980s it has become the indispensable technology for work-up of lung cancer. Many national organizations including the American College of Chest Physicians and American Thoracic Society[5] list CT prominently in their respective lung cancer guidelines. In general a chest CT is obtained in all patients with known or suspected lung cancer to help characterize the nodule, determine best biopsy or surgical approach, and assess the locoregional extent. Fluorodeoxyglucose (FDG)-PET is a newer modality that is rapidly evolving into the cornerstone imaging technique in the diagnosis and staging of lung cancer. In this chapter we identify some of the clinical questions that arise during diagnosis and staging of lung cancer, and explore the role of imaging in answering those questions.

Should patients at high risk for lung cancer be screened with low dose spiral computed tomography?

Currently there is insufficient evidence to support widespread screening for lung cancer with low dose spiral CT (LDCT). However, in recent years there have been several trials that have demonstrated that LDCT can detect lung cancer at an early stage.[6–9] For example, Swensen et al.[6] recently published their 5-year experience with LDCT. In a prospective study they found 3356 uncalcified lung nodules in 1118 (74%) participants. Sixty-eight lung cancers were diagnosed in 66 participants. Twenty-eight cases of non-small cell cancers were detected on annual screening examinations after the initial prevalence scan, of which 17 (61%) were stage I tumors. Diameters of cancers detected on screening CT were 5–50 mm (mean 14.4 mm; median 10.0 mm). Lung cancer mortality rate for the incidence portion of trial was 1.6 per 1000 person-years and there was no stage shift demonstrated. Other trials have reported similar findings.[7,10,11] It should be noted that these single arm prospective studies are confounded by lead time, length time, and over diagnosis bias. Only a randomized trial with a true control arm will be able to determine whether there is a mortality benefit conferred by screening with LDCT. A large randomized study (National Lung Screening Trial) is currently underway in the United States that hopes to provide conclusive evidence for or against screening for lung cancer with LDCT.[12]

How long and often should a patient with an incidental pulmonary nodule be followed?

An incidental pulmonary nodule is defined as a nodule detected on a scan obtained for reasons other than cancer detection. The standard of care in the recent past has been to follow every nodule until it shows growth, disappears, calcifies, or remains stable for a period of 2 years. Ost et al.[13] recommended serial CT scans at 3, 6, 12, 18, and 24 months for all nodules that had a low likelihood of malignancy regardless of size. The 2003 American College of Chest Physicians (ACCP) guidelines[14] had similar recommendations of 3, 6, 12, and 24 month follow-up scans. These guidelines remain appropriate for indeterminate nodules larger than 1 cm. However, in recent years there has been an explosion of new information regarding solitary pulmonary nodules obtained from the many LDCT studies being undertaken for early detection of lung cancer. The Fleischner Society (an international group of thoracic radiologists, pulmonologists, thoracic surgeons, and pulmonary pathologists) reviewed the literature and based on the data regarding nodule size, growth rate, and relative risk of malignancy have promoted new guidelines for management of incidental small pulmonary nodules.[15] For patients at low risk of cancer with a nodule ≤ 4 mm no follow-up is needed; with a 4–6 mm nodule a CT should be obtained at 12 months and if no change is observed no further follow-up is needed; for a nodule > 6–8 mm the first CT should be at 6–12 months and then again at 18–24 months; a nodule > 8 mm should be followed at 3, 9, and 24 months or have CT enhancement study, PET, or biopsy. In high risk patients (those at risk for lung cancer, e.g.

smokers, prior lung cancer, etc.) with a ≤ 4 mm nodule, CT should be obtained at 12 months, if no change is observed then no further follow-up is required; with a 4–6 mm nodule follow-up is the same as low risk patients with a > 6–8 mm nodule; for those with > 6–8 mm nodule CT should be obtained at 3–6 months, 9–12 months, and 24 months if unchanged; for a nodule > 8 mm recommendations are the same as for low risk patients.

What technique should be used for evaluation of a patient with a solitary pulmonary nodule?

The diagnostic work-up of pulmonary nodules is complex. Patient and radiological risk factors should guide the work-up. Patient risk factors for malignancy include advancing age, smoking history, and prior malignancy.[16] Radiological risk factors include size, spiculated margins, and approximate doubling time.[16] For low risk patients with a small nodule (≤ 8 mm) a conservative approach as noted in the previous discussion of how long to follow nodules would apply. For high risk patients with a high risk nodule that is a surgical candidate no further diagnostic work-up is needed and a staging work-up should be started in anticipation of excisional biopsy and potential lobectomy if malignancy is confirmed. For intermediate risk patients with an indeterminate nodule further diagnostic work-up is required. Many options are available, however, the focus of this chapter is on the role of CT and PET. Thin section imaging can show features of benignity (benign calcification, fat, etc.) (Figure 5.1) or malignancy (semisolid ground-glass

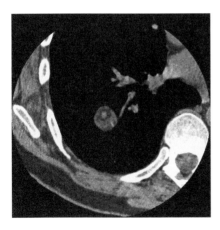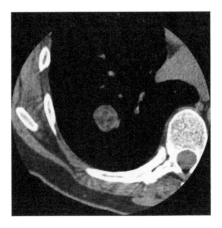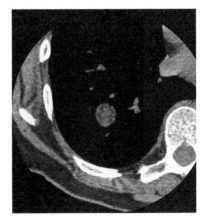

Figure 5.1
Thin section CT demonstrating a nodule with a smooth border and fat density. This is a hamartoma.

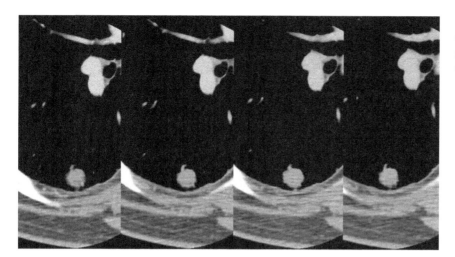

Figure 5.2
CT enhancement of pulmonary nodule showing baseline image and no enhancement on serial 1-minute images.

opacity or spiculation).[17] If the nodule is still indeterminate after initial thin section CT, dynamic contrast enhancement of the nodule can be helpful. CT enhancement study is a non-invasive method for evaluating lung nodules (Figure 5.2). If a nodule enhances less than 15 HU after radiocontrast injection, it is strongly predictive of benignity (sensitivity 98%, specificity 58%).[18]

^{18}F-FDG-PET provides complementary information on the metabolic activity of a nodule that cannot be obtained by CT or plain chest radiograph (Figure 5.3). Generally the sensitivity and specificity of PET for pulmonary nodules larger than 1 cm is quoted to be around 90%.[19] Critics cite cost of PET as a deterrent to its routine use in the evaluation of pulmonary nodules. However, PET has been shown to be at least as cost effective as traditional evaluation. An Italian study[20] compared conventional work-up of a solitary pulmonary nodule with CT, fine-needle aspiration, and thoracoscopic biopsy to a strategy that included ^{18}F-FDG-PET. This study demonstrated a cost reduction of approximately $60 per patient when PET was part of work-up.

In general small pulmonary nodules less than 1 cm in size and ground-glass opacities cannot be evaluated accurately by PET. Nomori et al.[21] found that all of the malignant nodules less than 1 cm in size were PET negative and the sensitivity and specificity for nodules with ground-glass opacities images were 10 and 20%, respectively, which was significantly lower than 90 and 71% for solid nodules ($P < 0.001$). Lindell et al.[22] demonstrated in a post hoc analysis of a spiral CT lung cancer screening study that PET was falsely negative in 32% of the non-small cell lung carcinomas detected on screening CT. The high false negative rate was attributed to the small size of the cancer and the high prevalence of bronchioloalveolar cell carcinoma. Because the spatial resolution of the current PET scanners is 7–8 mm, use of FDG-PET for nodules less than 1 cm should await further technological refinements.

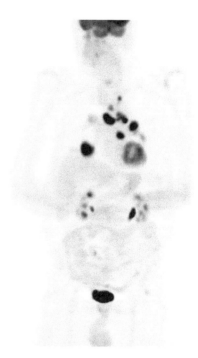

Figure 5.3
Whole body FDG-PET demonstrating activity in the primary right lower lobe mass. In this case PET re-staged the patient up to IIIB and unresectable based on the contralateral hilar lymphadenopathy. The contralateral disease was confirmed by bronchoscopic needle aspiration.

What is the diagnostic yield of computed tomography guided transthoracic needle aspiration for lung nodules?

The recent ACCP guidelines state 'It is the procedure of choice for confirming the diagnosis of lung cancer in patients in whom it is indicated (i.e., patients for whom preoperative therapy is planned or surgery is not feasible).'[23] In the recent ACCP guidelines, data on 11 279 patients were pooled.[23] The overall sensitivity and specificity of transthoracic needle aspiration (TTNA) for diagnosing peripheral lung cancers were 0.90 and 0.97, respectively. The false positive rate is only 0.01–0.02, indicating that a diagnosis of cancer made by TTNA is reliable. However, the false negative rate is high (0.20–0.30). Therefore, a negative biopsy does not rule out cancer. There is a trend toward a lower diagnostic yield for lesions less than 2 cm in size, however, this difference is not statistically significant.[24] It is generally accepted that the technical lower limit in size for successful biopsy is about 8 mm.

If imaging shows mediastinal lymph nodes to be abnormal, is further staging work-up necessary?

Lung cancer staging is based on the tumor, node, metastases (TNM) system. Stage of cancer is intimately associated with prognosis and survival. Accurate staging is extremely important for establishing treatment regimens. In non-small cell lung cancer, lymph node involvement in the mediastinum generally precludes primary resection of the lung cancer. Hence, accurate staging of the mediastinum is crucial. CT has been the standard non-invasive method for mediastinal staging. It is generally accepted that the criterion for abnormality is a lymph node ≥ 1 cm in short-axis diameter. In a recent review Toloza et al.[25] found the pooled sensitivity of CT scanning to be 0.57 (95% confidence interval (CI) 0.49–0.66), and the pooled specificity was 0.82 (95% CI 0.77–0.86). The overall positive predictive value and negative predictive value of CT scanning were 0.56 (0.26–0.84) and 0.83 (0.63–0.93), respectively. Thus, neither the positive predictive value nor negative predictive value are high enough to prove or refute disease, respectively. Magnetic resonance imaging (MRI) has no advantages over CT for detecting nodal involvement.[26] Other methods such as PET or endobronchial ultrasound (EBUS) are more sensitive and specific.[25] However, the sensitivity and specificity of PET is only approximately 90% (see section on role of PET for staging non-small cell lung cancer). It is therefore inappropriate to rely solely on imaging for staging the mediastinum and ultimate determination of the resectability of a lung cancer. CT remains an important tool in staging the mediastinum especially since it is used to guide more invasive staging modalities such as transbronchial needle aspiration or mediastinoscopy.

What is the role of positron emission tomography for staging non-small cell lung cancer?

PET was developed as a research tool for brain function and cardiac metabolism studies. PET has evolved into an important metabolic imaging technique for staging non-small cell lung cancer. The most frequently used tracer in PET is FDG. The basis for using FDG for in vivo cancer imaging is that there is a higher rate of glucose metabolism in cancer cells compared with non-malignant tissue.

In a recent review, PET had a sensitivity of 89% (range 67–100%), specificity of 92% (range 79–100%), and accuracy of 90% (range 78–100%). For CT, the corresponding figures were 65% (range 20–86%), 80% (range 43–90%), and 75% (range 52–79%), respectively.[27] However, it should be noted that CT is complementary to PET in evaluating lymph node status. PET/CT has high negative predictive value for mediastinal lymph node metastases. The sensitivity, specificity, and accuracy of PET/CT are 93%, 95%, and 94%, respectively. This is advantageous in the approach to patients with non-small cell lung cancer, because invasive mediastinal procedures are probably not necessary for patients with negative findings on PET/CT.[28]

PET is also useful for evaluation of metastatic disease. PET is reported to change the conventional staging in 27–62% of patients. Re-staging upwards is more frequent than re-staging downwards, mainly because of detection of unexpected distant lesions.[29] This results in a change in patient management in 25–41% of patients. In a recent randomized trial of potentially operable non-small cell lung cancer patients, it was reported that the preoperative addition of PET to a standard staging algorithm prevented unnecessary surgery in one out of five patients.[30]

Although the specificity of PET is high, false positive results do occur in reactive lymph nodes due to infectious or inflammatory conditions. Because FDG uptake is not always indicative of malignancy, and surgery is the only chance of cure for most patients with non-small-cell lung cancer, PET findings that would preclude surgical treatment need to be verified by biopsy.

What is the role of imaging in assessing the locoregional extent of lung cancer?

Thoracic CT has historically been very poor at assessing chest wall and mediastinal invasion.[31,32] Findings that are considered diagnostic of unresectable disease are gross invasion of the mediastinum with encasement and distortion of the vascular structures of the mediastinum, or bony destruction of a vertebral body. It should be noted that more subtle involvement is difficult to ascertain, e.g. tumor adjacent to mediastinum. Glazer et al.[31] found in a retrospective study that 82% of tumors deemed indeterminate for mediastinal invasion by CT were in fact resectable. They then developed a set of criteria predicting resectability: contact of ≤ 3 cm with mediastinum, less than 90 degrees of contact with aorta, and mediastinal fat between mass and mediastinal structures. After applying these criteria 97% of tumors were resectable. Therefore, unless there is encasement of mediastinal structures or vertebral body involvement by tumor, findings of invasion on CT should not preclude a patient from potentially curable surgery.

The presence of chest wall invasion does not eliminate surgical therapy as a treatment choice. However, it does adversely affect prognosis.[33] CT criteria used for predicting chest wall invasion include pleural thickening adjacent to the tumor, encroachment on or increased density of the extrapleural fat, asymmetry of the extrapleural soft tissues adjacent to the tumor, apparent mass invading the chest wall, and rib destruction.[34] Of these criteria only clear invasion with rib destruction is unequivocal evidence of invasion. In a study by Pennes et al.[32] it was found that the sensitivity of CT was 38%, specificity was 40%, and accuracy was 39% for evaluation of invasion of chest wall if equivocal/indeterminate CT results were counted as radiological errors.

Many experts believe that MRI is superior to CT for detection of chest wall or mediastinal invasion due to the higher resolution and anatomic detail provided by MRI. However, differentiating between adjacency, adherency, and invasion is difficult at best with both techniques. The only sign that confidently excludes invasion is motion or sliding between mass and adjacent structure. Brightness of fat on T1 imaging and ability to see vascular wall are the characteristics of MRI that give it the resolution and anatomic detail advantages over CT.[35] When the mediastinal or extrapleural fat line is disrupted this is predictive of invasion. MRI is also thought to be more accurate than CT in determining the extent of involvement of chest wall, subclavian vessels, brachial plexus, and vertebral column by superior sulcus tumors.[26]

Concurrent with advances in CT technology such as thin section multiplanar reformatted images from multidetector-row CT, the performance of CT has improved in detecting both chest wall and mediastinal invasion over conventional CT techniques.[36] Multidetector CT capable of multi-planar reformatting may eventually provide the level of anatomic detail currently provided by MRI to reliably detect subtle locally invasive disease.

Conclusion

A chest CT should be obtained in all operable patients with known or suspected lung cancer to help characterize the nodule, determine best biopsy or surgical approach, and to assess the locoregional extent. PET scanning should be obtained in all patients prior to planned surgical resection to more accurately stage patients and to avoid futile thoracotomy. PET findings that would preclude surgical resection should be confirmed with biopsy. MRI is superior to CT in determining the local extent of cancer in relation to the mediastinum and chest wall. However, the presence of chest wall invasion does not eliminate surgical therapy as a treatment choice.

References

1. Jemal A, Murray T, Ward E et al. Cancer statistics, 2005. CA Cancer J Clin 2005; 55: 10–30.
2. Naruke T, Tsuchiya R, Kondo H et al. Implications of staging in lung cancer. Chest 1997; 112 (4 Suppl): 242S–8S.
3. Ries L, Eisner M, Kosary C et al. SEER Cancer Statistics Review, 1975–2000. Bethesda, MD: National Cancer Institute, 2003.
4. Bondi G, Leites V. Malignant neoplastic disease discovered in chest x-ray surveys. N Engl J Med 1952; 247: 506–12.
5. Pretreatment evaluation of non-small-cell lung cancer. The American Thoracic Society and The European Respiratory Society. Am J Respir Crit Care Med 1997; 156: 320–32.
6. Swensen SJ, Jett JR, Hartman TE et al. CT Screening for lung cancer: five-year prospective experience. Radiology 2005; 235: 259–65.
7. MacRedmond R, Logan PM, Lee M et al. Screening for lung cancer using low dose CT scanning. Thorax 2004; 59: 237–41.
8. Kaneko M, Kusumoto M, Kobayashi T et al. Computed tomography screening for lung carcinoma in Japan. Cancer 2000; 89 (11 Suppl): 2485–8.
9. Sone S, Takashima S, Li F et al. Mass screening for lung cancer with mobile spiral computed tomography scanner. Lancet 1998; 351: 1242–5.
10. McWilliams A, Mayo J, MacDonald S et al. Lung cancer screening: a different paradigm. Am J Respir Crit Care Med 2003; 168: 1167–73.
11. Henschke CI, Yankelevitz DF, Libby D et al. Computed tomography screening for lung cancer. Clin Chest Med 2002; 23: 49–57, viii.
12. Moore SM, Gierada DS, Clark KW et al. Image quality assurance in the prostate, lung, colorectal, and ovarian cancer screening trial network of the National Lung Screening Trial. J Digit Imaging 2005; 18: 242–50.
13. Ost D, Fein AM, Feinsilver SH. Clinical practice. The solitary pulmonary nodule. N Engl J Med 2003; 348: 2535–42.
14. Tan BB, Flaherty KR, Kazerooni EA et al. The solitary pulmonary nodule. Chest 2003; 123: 89S–96.
15. MacMahon H, Austin JH, Gamsu G et al. Guidelines for management of small pulmonary nodules detected on CT

scans: a statement from the Fleischner Society. Radiology 2005; 237: 395–400.

16. Swensen SJ, Silverstein MD, Ilstrup DM et al. The probability of malignancy in solitary pulmonary nodules. Application to small radiologically indeterminate nodules. Arch Intern Med 1997; 157: 849–55.

17. Li F, Sone S, Abe H et al. Malignant versus benign nodules at CT screening for lung cancer: comparison of thin-section CT findings. Radiology 2004; 233: 793–8.

18. Swensen SJ, Viggiano RW, Midthun DE et al. Lung nodule enhancement at CT: multicenter study. Radiology 2000; 214: 73–80.

19. Lowe VJ, Fletcher JW, Gobar L et al. Prospective investigation of positron emission tomography in lung nodules. J Clin Oncol 1998; 16: 1075–84.

20. Gugiatti A, Grimaldi A, Rossetti C et al. Economic analyses on the use of positron emission tomography for the work-up of solitary pulmonary nodules and for staging patients with non-small-cell lung cancer in Italy. Q J Nucl Med Mol Imaging 2004; 48: 49–61.

21. Nomori H, Watanabe K, Ohtsuka T et al. Evaluation of F-18 fluorodeoxyglucose (FDG) PET scanning for pulmonary nodules less than 3 cm in diameter, with special reference to the CT images. Lung Cancer 2004; 45: 19–27.

22. Lindell RM, Hartman TE, Swensen SJ et al. Lung cancer screening experience: a retrospective review of PET in 22 non-small cell lung carcinomas detected on screening chest CT in a high-risk population. AJR Am J Roentgenol 2005; 185: 126–31.

23. Rivera MP, Detterbeck F, Mehta AC. Diagnosis of lung cancer: the guidelines. Chest 2003; 123: 129S–36.

24. Laurent F, Latrabe V, Vergier B et al. CT-guided transthoracic needle biopsy of pulmonary nodules smaller than 20 mm: results with an automated 20-gauge coaxial cutting needle. Clin Radiol 2000; 55: 281–7.

25. Toloza EM, Harpole L, McCrory DC. Noninvasive staging of non-small cell lung cancer: a review of the current evidence. Chest 2003; 123: 137S–46.

26. Grover FL. The role of CT and MRI in staging of the mediastinum. Chest 1994; 106 (6 Suppl): 391S–6S.

27. Vansteenkiste JF, Stroobants SG. The role of positron emission tomography with 18F-fluoro-2-deoxy-D-glucose in respiratory oncology. Eur Respir J 2001; 17: 802–20.

28. Vansteenkiste JF, Stroobants SG, De Leyn PR et al. Lymph node staging in non-small-cell lung cancer with FDG-PET scan: a prospective study on 690 lymph node stations from 68 patients. J Clin Oncol 1998; 16: 2142–9.

29. Pieterman RM, van Putten JW, Meuzelaar JJ et al. Preoperative staging of non-small-cell lung cancer with positron-emission tomography. N Engl J Med 2000; 343: 254–61.

30. van Tinteren H, Hoekstra OS, Smit EF et al. Effectiveness of positron emission tomography in the preoperative assessment of patients with suspected non-small-cell lung cancer: the PLUS multicentre randomised trial. Lancet 2002; 359: 1388–93.

31. Glazer H, Kaiser L, Anderson D et al. Indeterminate mediastinal invasion in bronchogenic carcinoma: CT evaluation. Radiology 1989; 173: 37–42.

32. Pennes DR, Glazer GM, Wimbish KJ et al. Chest wall invasion by lung cancer: limitations of CT evaluation. AJR Am J Roentgenol 1985; 144: 507–11.

33. Allen M, Mathisen D, Grillo H et al. Bronchogenic carcinoma with chest wall invasion. Ann Thorac Surg 1991; 51: 948–51.

34. Verschakelen JA, Bogaert J, De Wever W. Computed tomography in staging for lung cancer. Eur Respir J 2002; 19 (35 Suppl): 40S–8.

35. Schaefer-Prokop C, Prokop M. New imaging techniques in the treatment guidelines for lung cancer. Eur Respir J 2002; 19 (35 Suppl): 71S–83.

36. Higashino T, Ohno Y, Takenaka D et al. Thin-section multiplanar reformats from multidetector-row CT data: utility for assessment of regional tumor extent in non-small cell lung cancer. Eur J Radiol 2005; 56: 48–55.

6

The solitary pulmonary nodule

John W Hildebrandt and David E Midthun

Introduction

The management of a solitary pulmonary nodule (SPN) is one of the more common diagnostic problems arising from findings on chest radiograph or computed tomography (CT). In the past, it has been estimated that approximately 150 000 SPNs are detected in the US each year or in approximately one out of every 500 chest X-rays.[1,2] With the increasing use of multidetector row CT to evaluate a variety of conditions and the preliminary results from use of CT for screening for lung cancer, the number of SPNs detected will be far greater. The vast majority of detected nodules will be benign. In the single arm prospective study of CT screening reported by Swensen et al.[3] 51% of the participants had one or more non-calcified nodules detected on the baseline scan, and 98% of these were benign. Efficiently identifying which nodules are benign will avoid additional radiation exposure, considerable expense from performing unnecessary examinations, and limit unnecessary interventions. This chapter presents an algorithm to categorize nodules into benign versus indeterminate category and to guide appropriate work-up based on radiographic and clinical information. Our discussion starts with the defining of a SPN and continues with a review of the radiographic and clinical characteristics which are most pertinent to the evaluation of SPNs.

What is a pulmonary nodule?

The definition of a SPN is a fairly well circumscribed, round density in the lung parenchyma that is 3 cm or less in diameter (keeping in line with TI tumor size designation). The nodule should not significantly alter the surrounding tissue to the adjacent lung parenchyma, pleura, or mediastinum and not be associated with adenopathy. Lesions greater than 3 cm are considered to be a lung mass and have a high likelihood of malignancy. Lesions that are commonly mistaken for SPNs on chest radiographs include vascular opacities, focal bone densities, skin lesions, summation artifacts, and nipple shadows.

What features are helpful in determining the management of solitary pulmonary nodes?

The crux of the evaluation of patients with a pulmonary nodule is to intervene promptly in those with a malignant nodule and avoid invasive pursuits in those with benign nodules. Clinical history, physical examination, and radiographic features play vital roles in the management of SPNs.

Clinical considerations

Clinical considerations can be used to suggest a benign cause for the nodule. For example, a 3-cm opacity in a patient with fever and purulent sputum may represent a rounded area of pneumonia. A patient with a family history of fatal epistaxis and lip telangiectasias may have an arteriovenous malformation as the cause for the nodule seen on chest radiograph. Similarly, a patient with seropositive rheumatoid arthritis and subcutaneous nodules may have one or more rheumatoid nodules in the lung. Clinicians need to be alert to the clues in the history and examination that may indicate the cause of the pulmonary nodule.

Risk for lung cancer is most strongly associated with smoking history. Cancer risk increases with the duration of smoking, tar content, and early age at initiation of smoking. Exposure to passive smoke or radon and a family history of lung cancer are also helpful to assess the patient's 'relative risk' of lung cancer. A prior history of malignancy can be a helpful clue that the identified nodule may be a metastasis. Common sources of metastatic nodules to the lung include breast, thyroid, head and neck, renal, and colorectal cancers.

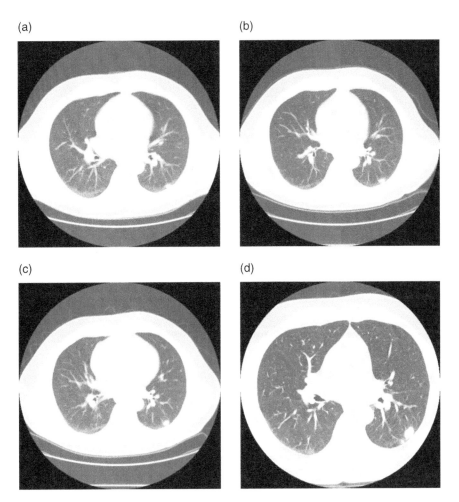

(a)   (b)

(c)   (d)

Figure 6.1
Left lower lobe nodule in a 67-year-old male. (a) Initial scan, (b) 6-month follow-up, (c) 18-month follow-up, and (d) 24-month follow-up. Serial studies demonstrate slow interval growth over a 2-year period. Transthoracic needle aspiration yielded bronchogenic adenocarcinoma. Surgical resection revealed stage IV adenocarcinoma.

Radiographic considerations

There are many radiographic features that are helpful in determining whether a nodule is likely to be benign or malignant. The majority of SPNs are benign and understanding which radiographic features reliably exclude malignancy is of great clinical utility. Nodules that remain indeterminate after radiological evaluation require assessment of clinical features and other less specific radiographic findings to determine the likelihood of malignancy.

What are the imaging findings that can reliably predict benignity?

Stability

A solid SPN with lack of growth for 2 years or longer can safely be considered benign. This is based on the premise

that most lung malignancies have a doubling time of between 1 and 18 months with an average time between 4.2 and 7.3 months.[4] The 'doubling' of a lesion refers to the volume of a nodule and not simply its diameter. However, the measurement recorded and compared is the average diameter of a lesion (average of width plus length). Based on the volume relationship of a sphere, $4/3\pi r^3$, a 25% increase in diameter correlates to an approximate doubling of a lesion's volume. For example, a SPN that grows from 4 to 5 mm has essentially doubled in volume. Due to the fact that small differences in diameter measurement reflect significant volumetric change, care in measurement is important. One needs to be aware of the fact that differences in slice selection may falsely indicate a change and this can be particularly problematic for a nodule of only a few millimeters in size. Because small increments of growth may not be appreciated in comparing subsequent examinations, it is usually a wise practice to compare the 2-year follow-up examination with that when the lesion was first discovered (Figure 6.1).

Nodule growth increases the likelihood that a nodule is malignant. Malignant nodules may grow in an irregular

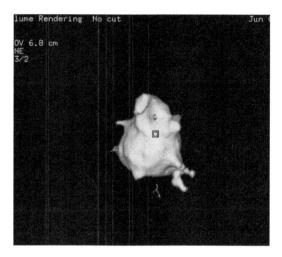

Figure 6.2
Three-dimensional volumetric imaging demonstrates oblong shape and irregular surface with spiculation of a bronchogenic adenocarcinoma.

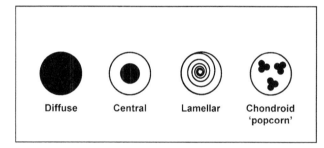

Figure 6.3
Benign calcification patterns in nodules. Courtesy of the Mayo Clinic Foundation, Rochester, MN with permission.

fashion or not uniformly in all dimensions (Figure 6.2). Volumetric measurements of nodules, utilizing CT measurement tools, are currently being investigated.[5,6] This will probably lead to more accurate measurements and shorten the time intervals between studies that can reliably detect changes in volume. A tissue diagnosis should be obtained in nodules which demonstrate a growth rate with a doubling time of between 1 and 18 months. Nodules which demonstrate no interval growth for a time period of less than 2 years need continued follow-up. Nodules discovered on chest X-rays in which there are no prior radiographs should be further evaluated by thin sliced unenhanced CT.

Attenuation

The tissue features in a nodule that rule out malignancy include benign calcification pattern or presence of fat. Benign calcification patterns include diffuse, solid, laminar, and chondroid (popcorn) as demonstrated in Figure 6.3. Eccentric or stippled calcification patterns can be associated

with malignant or benign lesions and thus are considered indeterminate. The one exception to a solid calcification nodule representing a benign lesion is pulmonary metastases from an osteosarcoma and chondrosarcoma. Thus, calcified nodules cannot be considered benign in patients who have a history of these types of sarcomas. Fat within a nodule, whether central or eccentric, is consistent with a hamartoma (Figure 6.4).

Although the presence of calcification can sometimes be diagnosed on chest radiographs, CT is better at demonstration of both calcification and/or fat within the nodule. Thin section (1–3 mm slice width) CT is more likely to recognize these features than standard collimation (5–7 mm). False interpretation of calcium can occur in the CT evaluation of pulmonary nodules if images are only obtained after the use of intravenous contrast. Contrast can lead to enhancement of a malignant lesion which can increase the attenuation of the lesion giving it the appearance that is uniformly calcified. False interpretation of the absence of calcification can occur when evaluating a pulmonary nodule the diameter of which is smaller than the slice thickness. This can lead to volume averaging of solid calcification with aerated lung parenchyma giving the appearance of a non-calcified nodule (Figure 6.5). For these reasons it is important that evaluation of a SPN is included in the indication for the study to ensure non-contrast images are obtained and that thin slices are obtained through the SPN of interest. An additional reason for performing the initial scan without contrast is to allow for the opportunity to perform a nodule enhancement CT study at the time of the initial scan.

How can additional imaging characteristics aid in the management of solitary pulmonary nodules?

There are additional radiographic features such as size, margin characteristics, nodule attenuation, and satellite nodules that are not specific but are helpful in determining the likelihood of malignancy.

Size

The larger the pulmonary nodule, the more likely it is to be malignant. Nodules 3 cm or larger, that lack a benign calcification pattern or fat on CT, are more than 90% likely to be malignant. Data from CT screening studies have shown that nodules smaller than 7 mm have a less than 1% chance of malignancy, 8–20 mm have an approximately 20% chance of malignancy, and those larger than 20 mm have a 50% chance of malignancy.[7] Based on these data, in 2005, the Fleischner Society (an international organization of pulmonologists, pulmonary pathologists, thoracic surgeons and thoracic radiologists) published a set of practical guidelines for the management of small SPNs detected incidentally on CT examinations.[8]

Patients are divided into either a high or low risk category. High risk factors include history of smoking, lung cancer in first-degree relatives, and exposure to asbestos, radon, or uranium. Low risk profile consists of absence or minimal history of smoking and other previously mentioned risk factors. Nodules discovered in patients with suspected or known malignancy or with unexplained fever do not fit into either high or low risk profile as they may require immediate intervention or shorter term follow-up. Additionally, SPNs found incidentally in young patients are overwhelmingly benign.[9] Thus, the follow-up guidelines set up by the Fleischner Society do not apply to patients younger than 35 years of age, those presenting with unknown fever, or those diagnosed with or suspected of having a malignancy.

According to the Fleischner criteria, for patients with a nodule 4 mm or smaller, a 1-year follow-up study is recommended to document stability in patients with a high risk profile, while no follow-up examination is recommended in patients with a low risk profile. Nodules 5 mm or larger require a 2-year follow-up for both high and low risk profiles. Management options for nodules less than 8 mm in diameter are mostly limited to follow-up examinations and surgical resection. In patients with a nodule 8 mm and larger further evaluation should be considered which could include nodule-enhancement CT, positron emission tomography (PET) scan, or biopsy.

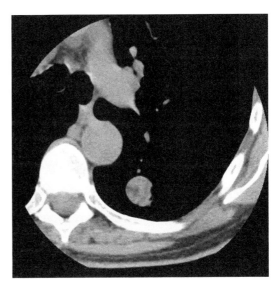

Figure 6.4
Thin slice CT through a nodule in the left lower lobe of a 65-year-old woman shows areas of fat within the nodule that allow the diagnosis of a hamartoma.

glass, or contain air bronchograms have an increased likelihood of malignancy compared with that of a completely solid nodule. Approximately 34% of ground-glass (non-solid) nodules are malignant.[12] and 40–50% of partially solid nodules are malignant.[12,13] Air bronchograms are present in approximately 30% of malignant nodules, while only 6% are associated with benign nodules.[14]

Margins

The more spiculated or lobular the margin of a SPN, the more likely it is to be malignant. Spiculated nodules have a 90% predicted value for malignancy.[10] Thus, spiculated nodules should be more aggressively worked up with biopsy if they are of sufficient size or with resection if they are too small for biopsy but demonstrate interval growth over 6–12 months. However, 21% of malignant nodules have smooth borders.[11] Therefore, a smooth margin does not indicate that a lesion is benign.

Attenuation

As previously noted, the presence of fat or benign calcification pattern essentially excludes malignancy. However, there are other attenuation patterns that may be encountered that are less specific with regard to malignancy, but can be stratified regarding relative risk. Nodules that are ground glass in attenuation, part solid and part ground

Cavitation

The presence of cavitation in and of itself is not a good predictor of whether a lesion is benign or malignant. Thin smooth walled cavities are more likely to be benign, while nodules containing irregular and thicker walls are more likely to be malignant. For example, approximately 92% of nodules with a greatest wall thickness between 1 and 4 mm are benign, while 95% with greatest wall thickness larger than 15 mm are malignant.[15] However, other lesions such as a lung abscess or Wegener's granulomatosis can present as a thick, irregular cavitary lesion, and thus cavitation alone cannot be used to determine whether the lesion is malignant.

Satellite nodules

Multiple small nodules surrounding a larger dominant nodule are referred to as satellite nodules. A dominant

(a)   (b)

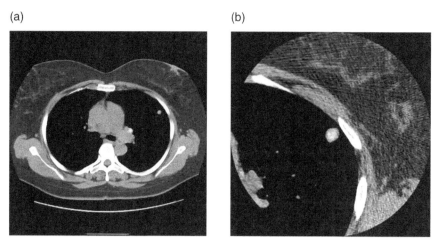

Figure 6.5
(a) Standard CT image at the level of the carina in a 55-year-old woman shows an indeterminate nodule in the left upper lobe laterally. (b) Thin slice CT through the nodule shows calcification diagnostic of a granuloma.

nodule with associated satellite nodules is likely to be benign with a positive predictive value of 90% (Figure 6.6).[10] Frequently, CT will reveal satellite nodules in a patient thought to have a solitary nodule on chest radiograph.

What additional imaging is helpful in managing a solitary pulmonary nodule?

PET or nodule-enhancement CT imaging should be performed on those lesions which are 8 mm or more in diameter, have a moderate degree of risk of malignancy, and have no comparison studies to demonstrate stability over time.

Nodule-enhancement CT

A nodule-enhancement CT study evaluates the increase in density of a nodule after intravenous contrast administration. The study is based on the premise that malignant nodules have an increased blood supply compared with benign lung nodules, resulting in a substantially greater enhancement of malignant nodules. Following the initial non-contrast examination, thin slice images are obtained through the center of the nodule at 1 minute intervals for 4 minutes following intravenous contrast administration (Figure 6.7). The peak level of enhancement is subtracted from the precontrast density measurement. Less than a 15 HU increase in density is consistent with a benign nodule. The absence of significant nodule enhancement is a strong

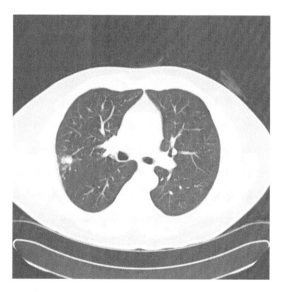

Figure 6.6
CT image at the level of the bronchus intermedius shows a dominant nodule in the right upper lobe laterally with surrounding tiny (satellite) nodules. This was stable for more than 2 years and was classified as benign.

predictor of benignity. Studies have shown that the sensitivity and negative predictive value of a nodule-enhancement CT are both greater than 95%.[16,17] The value of a nodule-enhanced CT study is that it is readily available (can be performed at the time of initial CT investigation), is less expensive than 2-fluorine-18-fluoro-2-deoxy-D-glucose (FDG)-PET scan, and a negative result can alleviate

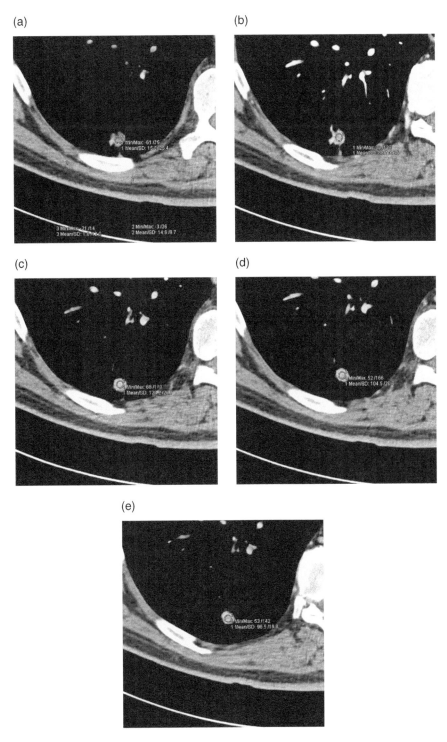

Figure 6.7

CT nodule enhancement of a lesion in the right lower lobe. Precontrast image compared with four other images obtained at 1 minute intervals demonstrates avid contrast enhancement (112 HU) consistent with a high likelihood of malignancy. Surgical resection revealed a diagnosis of adenocarcinoma. (a) Precontrast density 15.6 HU; (b) 1 min postcontrast 88.7 HU; (c) 2 min postcontrast 128 HU; (d) 3 min postcontrast 105 HU; (d) 4 min postcontrast 96.5 HU.

the need for biopsy or PET scan. In high risk patients, a negative nodule-enhancement CT study should be followed up with serial CT imaging to document stability. In low risk patients, generally no additional follow-up is needed. The disadvantage of this study is that inflammatory conditions such as histoplasmosis, sarcoidosis, foreign body (FB) reaction to talc, or necrotizing granulomas can have increased vascularity leading to a false positive result. Because of this, nodule enhancement CT studies have a low specificity which results in a large number of benign lesions having a positive result. For this reason, a positive result should be followed by a FDG-PET scan or biopsy which have a higher specificity and positive predictive value. Limitations of nodule-enhancement CT examination are that nodules must be 8 mm or larger and not contain calcification, air bronchogram, or fat attenuation material. The nodule must also not be in areas of substantial imaging artifact from cardiac motion or beam hardening from adjacent bone. When used for its strong negative predictive value, nodule-enhanced CT study is a valuable tool in the work-up of indeterminate solitary pulmonary nodules.

Positron emission tomography

FDG-PET imaging works on the premise that malignant nodules have a higher glucose metabolism relative to benign nodules and thus have an increased uptake of glucose or a glucose analog. PET imaging uses a radionuclide glucose analog 2-fluorine-18-fluoro-2-deoxy-D-glucose (FDG). There is usually a significant difference in the accumulation of radionuclide between malignant and benign lesions with substantially more uptake in malignant lesions. The sensitivity, specificity, positive predictive value, and negative predictive value have recently been shown to be as high as 96, 76, 86, and 93%, respectively.[17] False positive PET results can occur in focal infectious or inflammatory lesions such as tuberculosis, histoplasmosis, sarcoidosis, FB reaction to

talc, and caseating granulomas (Figure 6.8). False negative results can occur in malignancies with low metabolic rates such as carcinoid and bronchioloalveolar carcinomas. Therefore, nodules with a negative FDG-PET result should be observed with serial CT examinations.

In addition to having good sensitivity and specificity, FDG-PET imaging has the advantage of being able to detect distant and mediastinal lymph node metastases and leads to more accurate tumor staging. Similar to nodule enhancement CT, a limitation of FDG-PET imaging is that it requires a nodules to be 8 mm or larger in diameter due to its limited spatial resolution. The cost of FDG-PET imaging is also higher than that of nodule-enhancement CT, and FDG-PET is not as widely available as CT. FDG-PET imaging is best utilized in nodules of 8 mm or larger either as the initial work-up or for nodules that had a positive nodule-enhancement CT examination. It may also be utilized following a positive biopsy result in order to assess for mediastinal lymph nodes involvement or distant metastases. Integrated PET/CT simultaneously combines the metabolic and anatomic information, and has been shown to provide greater accuracy in tumor evaluation and staging than either CT or PET alone.[18]

What are the roles for bronchoscopy and transthoracic needle aspiration in the management of solitary pulmonary nodules?

Pursuit of biopsy is usually reserved for nodules 8 mm in diameter or larger depending on location. Biopsy may be appropriate for newly detected nodules that have a high likelihood for malignancy or have a positive result on PET

(a)   (b)

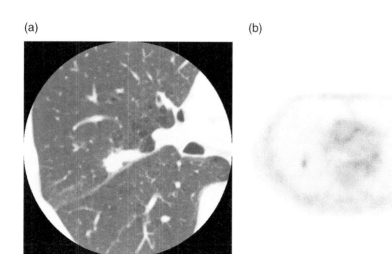

Figure 6.8
(a) Right upper lobe mildly spiculated oblong shaped nodule in a 67-year-old male with a 55 pack year history of smoking. (b) FDG/PET scan demonstrates isolated hypermetabolic uptake in the right midlung region. Surgical pathology demonstrated a benign granulomatous inflammation with foreign body reaction.

scan or nodule-enhancement CT. Biopsy may not be necessary in high risk patients with growing nodules. However, these patients may benefit from PET evaluation prior to surgery to identify distant metastases that would preclude surgical resection.

Biopsy is most helpful when a specific benign diagnosis is obtained as this obviates the need for further work-up. Bronchoscopy and transthoracic needle aspiration (TTNA) are the two options for performing a nodule biopsy. Due to the relatively low yield of bronchoscopy compared with TTNA, the latter is usually the preferred method. Bronchoscopy has yields in the range of 10–50% for nodules of 3 cm or smaller. Standard technique involves fluoroscopy and is often limited by the inability to see or localize the nodule at the time of the procedure. An exception to this is a nodule that has a bronchus leading directly to it; in this case yields may be high enough to warrant bronchoscopy as the procedure of choice. Recent studies have shown improved yields using bronchoscopic ultrasound or electromagnetic navigation for nodule localization. Despite promising results with these techniques, yields are still generally lower when compared with TTNA.

TTNA is typically performed while the patient is in the CT scanner and is limited by nodule size, respiratory motion, nodule depth, and patient cooperation. Yields for TTNA are in the range of 80–90% for nodules as small as 1 cm and can be higher for larger nodules. Pneumothorax occurs in approximately one in three procedures, and placement of a chest tube is required in about 33% of patients with

a pneumothorax. The use of small bore tubes with a Heimlich valve can minimize the impact of this complication.

What is the role of resection in the management of solitary pulmonary nodules?

Proceeding to resection for an indeterminate nodule may be appropriate in a subset of SPNs. These include nodules that are too small or too difficult for TTNA because of location, those that have a very high pretest probability of malignancy, demonstrate interval growth compatible with malignancy, or those that have a positive result on PET scan, nodule-enhancement CT, or tissue biopsy. After the discussion of management options, even some patients at low risk for malignancy will opt for surgical resection due to the anxiety associated with observation.

What is an appropriate management algorithm for solitary pulmonary nodules?

When a nodule is encountered on a plain radiograph or CT every effort should be made to obtain old films for comparison (Figure 6.9). If retrospective observation demonstrates that the nodule is stable for more than 2 years, then

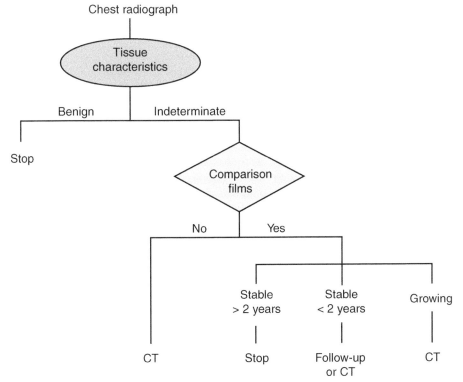

Figure 6.9
Decision algorithm for SPNs encountered on plain radiograph. Oval shaped branch point represents decision made based on radiographic findings, whereas diamond shaped branch points represent decisions made based on clinical information.

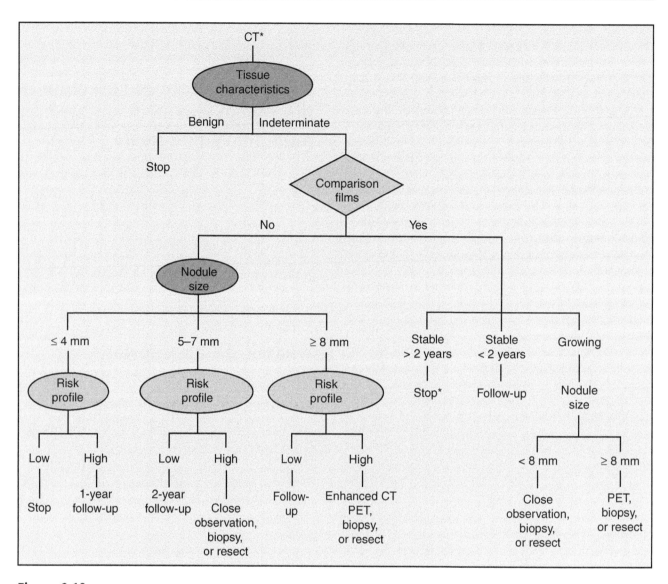

Figure 6.10
Decision algorithm for SPNs encountered on CT. *Ground glass partially solid nodules may require longer yearly follow-up to establish that they are benign. PET, positron emission tomography.

no further work-up is needed. If retrospective observation determines that a nodule is growing at a rate consistent with malignancy then one may proceed to biopsy or preoperative PET/CT evaluation.

CT evaluation of a nodule detected by plain radiograph is recommended when comparison films suggest that the nodule is new or growing, or there are no comparison films (Figure 6.10). The CT examination should be performed as a non-contrast examination with thin slices through the nodule. If at thin section the SPN has benign tissue characteristics, no further work-up is needed. If the nodule remains indeterminate, enhanced CT imaging is recommended provided appropriate criteria are met. As stated above this includes solid nodules 8 mm or larger in diameter which do not contain a central air bronchogram, eccentric calcification, or are located in an area affected

by imaging artifacts. Nodule-enhancement CT scan can occur during the initial CT examination.

The size of a SPN as well as a patient's clinical history profile (low or high risk as defined above in the Clinical consideration section) are the next features used in the management of SPNs. The smaller the size and the lower the risk profile, the lower the likelihood of a malignancy. Two average diameter sizes that are helpful to remember are 4 mm and 8 mm. The size of nodules can be categorized as 1–4 mm, 5–7 mm, and 8 mm or greater.

According to the Fleischner criteria, in patients who are low risk, nodules that are 4 mm or smaller need no additional work-up. This criterion is based on lung cancer screening studies, which have shown that small nodules have a very low likelihood of malignancy.[19,20] In high risk patients, these tiny nodules require a 1 year of follow-up.

If there is no change in size, no additional follow-up is needed. As stated above, the follow-up recommendations do not apply to patients with known malignancy at another organ site recognized to metastasize to the lung or to patients who are being evaluated for unexplained fever.

The management of nodules from 5 to 7 mm is limited to either serial follow-up imaging or surgical resection. Management of nodules that are 8 mm or larger has the option of undergoing biopsy or additional radiological imaging (nodule-enhancement CT or PET). All negative PET studies and negative nodule enhancement CT studies in high risk patients need follow-up imaging at 2 years to avoid false negative results. Negative nodule-enhancement CT studies in low risk patients have a high negative predictive value, but 2-year follow-up is still recommended. A positive nodule-enhancement CT examination should be followed by PET imaging or biopsy because of its relatively low specificity.

Conclusion

Imaging and image-guided intervention play an important role in the detection, evaluation, and management of SPNs. In some instances, imaging can be used to make a benign diagnosis, while in other cases it can be used to help determine pretest probability and how aggressively to work up a nodule that is indeterminate. Consideration of the patients' attitude towards a management plan is an important feature that must also be included in management decisions. The decision whether to follow, perform additional radiological studies, or proceed to biopsy should be based on the accumulated information from clinical history, imaging features helpful in determining likelihood of malignancy as well as the patient's desires in management and treatment options.

References

1. Ost D, Fein AM, Feinsilver SH. Clinical practice: the solitary pulmonary nodule. N Engl J Med 2003; 348: 2535–42.
2. Tan BB, Flaherty KR, Kazerooni EA et al. The solitary pulmonary nodule. Chest 2003; 123: 89S–96S.
3. Swensen SJ, Jett JR, Hartman TE et al. CT screening for lung cancer: five-year prospective experience. Radiology 2005; 235: 259–65.
4. Garland LH, Coulson W, Wollin E. The rate of growth and apparent duration of untreated primary bronchial carcinoma. Cancer 1963; 16: 694–707.
5. Revel MP, Merlin A, Peyrard S et al. Software volumetric evaluation of doubling times for differentiating benign versus malignant pulmonary nodules. AJR Am J Roentgenol 2006; 187: 135–42.
6. Jennings SG, Winer-Muram HT, Tann M et al. Distribution of stage I lung cancer growth rates determined with serial volumetric CT measurements. Radiology 2006; 241: 554–63.
7. Midthun DE, Swensen SJ, Jett JR. Diagnostic Workup of Screen Detected Nodules. In: Hirch F, Kato H, Mulshine J and Bunn P (Eds.) IASLC Textbook of Early Detection and Prevention of Lung Cancer. Taylor and Francis Group, 2005.
8. MacMahon H, Austin JH, Gamsu G et al. Guidelines for management of small pulmonary nodules detected on CT scans: a statement from the Fleischner Society. Radiology 2005; 237: 395–400.
9. Gadgeel SM, Ramalingam S, Cummings G et al. Lung cancer in patients < 50 years of age: the experience of an academic multidisciplinary program. Chest 1999; 115: 1232–6.
10. Gurney JW. Determining the likelihood of malignancy in solitary pulmonary nodules with bayesian analysis. Radiology 1993; 186: 405–13.
11. Siegelman SS, Zerhouni EA, Leo FP. CT of the solitary pulmonary nodule. AJR Am J Roentgenol 1980; 135: 1–13.
12. Henschke CI, Yankelevitz DF, Mirtcheva R et al. CT screening for lung cancer: frequence and significance of part solid and non-solid nodules. AJR Am J Roentgenol 2002; 178: 1053–7.
13. Li F, Sone S, Abe H et al. Malignant versus benign nodules at CT screening for lung cancer: comparison of thin section CT findings. Radiology 2004; 233: 793–8.
14. Kui M, Templeton PA, White CS et al. Evaluation of the air bronchogram sign on CT in solitary pulmonary lesions. J Comput Assist Tomogr 1996; 20: 983–6.
15. Woodring JH, Fried AM, Chuang VP. Solitary cavities of the lung: diagnostic implications of cavity wall thickness. AJR Am J Roentgenol 1980; 135: 1269–71.
16. Swensen SJ, Viggiano RW, Midthun DE et al. Lung nodule enhancement at CT: multicenter study. Radiology 2000; 214: 73–80.
17. Christensen JA, Nathan MA, Mullan BP et al. Characterization of the solitary pulmonary nodule: 18F-FDG PET versus nodule-enhancement CT. AJR Am J Roentgenol 2006; 187: 1361–7.
18 De Wever W, Ceyssens S, Mortelmans L et al. Additional value of PET-CT in the staging of lung cancer: comparison with CT alone, PET alone and visual correlation of PET and CT. Eur Radiol 2007; 17: 23–32.
19 Swensen SJ, Jett JR, Hartman TE. Lung cancer screening with CT: Mayo Clinic experience. Radiology 2003; 226: 756–61.
20. Henschke CI, Yankelevitz JF, Naidich JP. CT screening for lung cancer: suspiciousness of nodules according to size on baseline scans. Radiology 2004; 231: 164–8.

7

Interstitial lung diseases

Maureen Quigley, Athol U Wells, and David M Hansell

Introduction

Interstitial lung disease (ILD) encompasses a spectrum of conditions, with confusing nomenclature and varying prevalence. The commonest ILDs are the idiopathic interstitial pneumonias (IIP), sarcoidosis, and extrinsic allergic alveolitis (EAA). Clinical evaluation may be complicated by the variable presence of airway disease, pulmonary hypertension, opportunistic infection, and cardiac involvement.

High-resolution computed tomography (HRCT) is the single most useful imaging technique for the investigation and surveillance of ILD. HRCT can confirm, refine, and sometimes radically alter a presumptive diagnosis. Although the chest radiography still has a role in both diagnosis and monitoring (the optimal method for monitoring patients with ILD has yet to be definitely established), HRCT has greater accuracy in identifying ILD.

In this chapter, imaging techniques are summarized briefly. The value of HRCT in addressing key clinical questions is then considered in greater detail.

What imaging techniques are used in interstitial lung disease?

Chest radiography

The chest radiograph is an integral part in the investigation of patients with suspected or established lung disease. It is readily accessible, has a low radiation burden, and is inexpensive. The pattern of ILD on chest radiography may allow a specific histological diagnosis to be made, largely on the basis of the zonal distribution. Chest radiography also assists in detecting complications such as pneumonia, pneumothorax, and neoplastic disease. However, it has shortcomings in respect to sensitivity and specificity because almost half the lung volume is obscured behind the mediastinum

and diaphragm. Furthermore, millions of microscopic disease foci are required to generate an appreciable change in radiographic density.

All comparative studies between chest radiography and HRCT, describe HRCT as having greater accuracy in the diagnosis of ILD[1–3] and a range of accuracies have been quoted (Table 7.1).

The confidence with which a diagnosis of ILD is made is of relevance. When experienced radiologists examined the chest radiographs of a group of patients with histologically proven ILD, they made a confident diagnosis in less than one quarter of patients.[2] In some instances, a confident diagnosis can be made on chest radiography alone, an example of this is sarcoidosis. The chest radiograph is relatively insensitive to early disease and in a study of 458 patients with histologically proven lung disease, 44 (9.6%) had a normal chest radiograph.[4] Gaensler et al.[5] reported that 16% of patients with histopathological proof of diffuse ILD had a normal chest radiograph and in systemic lupus erythematosus, the superiority of HRCT to chest radiography has been conclusively demonstrated in the detection of ILD.[6]

Unlike HRCT, a chest radiograph seldom provides guidance as to the reversibility of disease. However, it is routinely employed as a monitoring tool in the evaluation of progressive fibrotic lung disease, although the value it adds to serial pulmonary function tests has not been formally evaluated.

High-resolution computed tomography

The technique of HRCT was first described in 1987.[7] It was devised to maximize the visualization of small parenchymal structures, as fine detail is lost in relatively thick sections (Figure 7.1). A typical HRCT examination provides images of 1 mm section thickness obtained 1 cm apart. With modern multidetector CT machines, volumetric

HRCT can be obtained in which there are no gaps between the sections but the radiation dose is at least three times that of standard interspaced HRCT. The decision to perform an interspaced or a volumetric HRCT is weighed between the information required from the scan and the individual's personal risk (notably their age) from the increased radiation. HRCT is a non-invasive, relatively accurate, diagnostic tool which has some prognostic value and can provide a baseline for monitoring disease. HRCT has significant advantages over chest radiography, in that there is no anatomical superimposition and contrast resolution is much higher. However, HRCT provides a greater radiation dose than a chest radiograph and an interspaced HRCT is equivalent to the radiation dose received from approximately 40 chest radiographs, with a volumetric HRCT delivering a dose equivalent to 200 chest radiographs.

Table 7.1 Summary of accuracy values quoted for chest radiography versus HRCT in the detection of biopsy-proven interstitial lung disease

Author and study group size (n)	Diagnostic accuracy of the chest radiograph (%)	Diagnostic accuracy of HRCT (%)
Mathieson et al. 1989[2] (n = 118)	57	76
Grenier et al. 1991[3] (n = 140)	63	75
Padley et al. 1991[1] (n = 86)	69	82

Both chest radiographs and HRCT are subject to observer variation and when different pathological processes produce the same gross morphological pattern, both may fail to achieve a specific diagnosis.

Diethylenetriamine penta-acetic acid clearance scan

Clearance of inhaled technetium 99m-labeled diethylenetriamine penta-acetic acid (DTPA) is an index of lung epithelial permeability.[8] Faster or 'increased' clearance may be a sensitive marker of inflammation,[9] and increased clearance has been linked with poor survival in idiopathic pulmonary fibrosis (IPF).[10] DTPA clearance results need to be interpreted in tandem with the cigarette smoking history, as tobacco smoking is independently associated with rapid DTPA clearance[11] and in patients with chronic obstructive airways disease, the isotope can be deposited in the central airways, which can give an artifactually normal clearance time.[12]

Increased DTPA clearance provides information about microscopic lung permeability, however, in IPF, abnormal clearance does not have a strong association with other more readily available parameters such as HRCT abnormalities, pulmonary function tests (PFTs), and bronchoalveolar lavage abnormalities.[13]

Magnetic resonance imaging

Magnetic resonance imaging (MRI) is not used for the routine imaging of ILD as the signal from the lung is limited by the inherent structural properties of the lung. Static imaging of the upper and lower respiratory tract is possible with hyperpolarized gas MRI. Both ³He and ¹²⁹Xe allow the

(a)

(b)

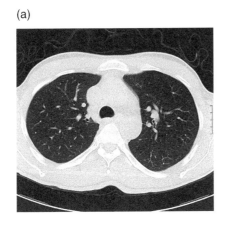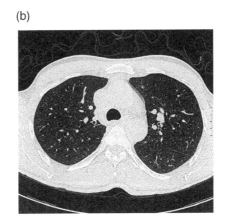

Figure 7.1
The difference between standard (thick) (a) and high-resolution computed tomography (HRCT) (b) is HRCT has superior parenchymal detail. No parencyhmal abnormality was identified in this middle-aged male patient. SOMATON Sensation 64 (Siemens Erlangen. Germany).

acquisition of diagnostic quality images that reflect airways and consequent ventilation abnormalities but this technique is not routinely used in clinical practice.

What radiation risks are associated with imaging procedures?

Chest radiography, HRCT, and DTPA scanning expose a patient to ionizing radiation and this has associated, albeit minor, risks. The International Commission on Radiological Protection has recommended the use of a conservative risk of 50 additional fatal cancers induced per million people of the general population exposed to 1 mSv of medical radiation[14] (the approximate effective dose of a typical interspaced HRCT). It should be stressed that this low risk, usually outweighed by the added clinical value of HRCT information, is significantly less than the risk of surgical lung biopsy. The overall mortality from surgical biopsy is around 1% (similar figures are quoted for thoracoscopic biopsy).[15] The mortality figure of 1% applies to a variety of respiratory conditions and this figure rises in the ventilated patient. The morbidity from surgical lung biopsy is reported as being between 10 and 20%.

Is interstitial lung disease present?

HRCT can understate or overstate the presence of ILD. Overstatement occurs when 'normal' changes within the parenchyma are over interpreted or when there is evidence of subclinical and unimportant 'disease'. There is little published work on the borderlands of normal and subclinical disease is almost ubiquitous in those with a cigarette smoking or connective tissue disease history.

When interpreting a HRCT scan, one of the hardest judgments can be the assessment of 'subtle' abnormalities and, in particular, the determination of their clinical relevance. Categorizing a HRCT as unequivocally abnormal can be difficult.[16] A good example of a HRCT sign that may be encountered in both health and disease is ground-glass opacity (GGO). GGO is based on a subjective assessment of lung parenchyma which appears lighter gray than expected; this perception can be created by altering image window settings, in patients scanned in the expiratory phase of respiration, and in those who are obese[17] or very young.[18]

At the other end of the density spectrum are small areas of low attenuation (black lung) which may represent air trapping at a lobular level and as can be seen in apparently healthy adults.[17] The extent of air trapping increases in

healthy non-smokers with increasing age.[19] The cause of subclinical air trapping is not known and it is seen in up to one-quarter of healthy individuals.[17]

Most thoracic radiologists have a working system for what they feel is acceptable for 'age-related' change but this is at best arbitrary. There are some changes that are clearly important in a young individual (such as a reticular pattern in the costophrenic angles) which may be of little importance in an 85-year old, representing the consequences of aging. The paucity of descriptions of normal age-related lung abnormalities stems from the ethical difficulty in acquiring a large enough data set of the aging population.

There are several contexts in which the detection of limited pulmonary parenchymal abnormalities are sufficiently common to pose real difficulties in the definition of clinically significant disease. HRCT abnormalities in 'healthy smokers' are an obvious example of this problem. Respiratory bronchiolitis is present in most current smokers and the rapidity with which it clears following smoking cessation is highly variable.[20] In a HRCT study of 175 healthy adult volunteers, the morphological effects of cigarette smoking was evaluated.[21] The group was divided into smokers, ex-smokers, and non-smokers, and all participants had normal pulmonary function tests and normal chest radiographs. Within the smoking group, 82% had HRCT abnormalities, most frequently consisting of subpleural micronodules, dependent areas of increased attenuation, and bronchial wall thickening, with parenchymal nodules and ground-glass attenuation exclusively observed in the smoking group and representing respiratory bronchiolitis (Figure 7.2). The clinical significance of these

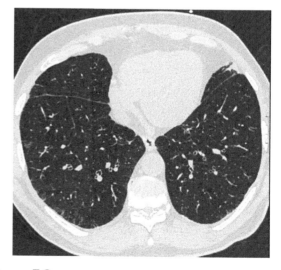

Figure 7.2
Probable smoking-related changes in a middle-aged man. A 1 mm HRCT section through the lower lobes showing mildly thickened airways with a subtle subpleural reticular pattern, these limited parenchymal abnormalities may represent limited interstitial fibrosis.

abnormalities is not always clear from CT findings in isolation, with the condition of respiratory bronchiolitis with associated interstitial lung disease (RBILD) requiring the presence of symptoms and pulmonary function impairment. Interestingly, only 57% of those who had never-smoked had a pristine HRCT.

In rheumatoid arthritis (RA), ILD may predate arthritic symptoms[22] and therefore patients with 'undeclared' RA can be erroneously included in groups of patients labeled with IPF. In those with RA, but no symptoms of respiratory disease, 29–49% have definite lung parenchymal abnormalities on HRCT[23–25] and as the lifelong prevalence of clinically significant diffuse lung disease has not approached 20% in any published RA cohort, it must be presumed that truly subclinical disease is being detected.[26] Pulmonary function tests (PFTs), bronchoalveolar lavage (BAL), clinical history, and DPTA scans may help in determining the clinical relevance of the subtly 'abnormal' HRCT.

Should diagnostic high-resolution computed tomography always be performed?

The initial investigation of a patient with ILD, involves eliciting a history, physical examination, chest radiography, PFTs, and serological evaluation. The decision to proceed to HRCT depends on whether a diagnosis is secure. In some instances, such as a patient with classical clinical and radiographic features of sarcoidosis, HRCT will not be required; the American Thoracic Society (ATS)/European Respiratory Society (ERS) statement on sarcoidosis, only indicates CT for those with atypical findings, for complications of the disease (e.g. fibrosis, bronchiectasis, aspergilloma), or for those with a normal chest radiograph who have suspected pulmonary disease.[27] More recently, respiratory physicians have increasingly tended to perform routine baseline scans in sarcoidosis, when disease is considered likely to persist, in order to establish baseline appearances with a view to future monitoring, but this use of HRCT has not yet been validated.

Some studies have endeavored to define the exact combination of symptoms and signs which would mean that HRCT was indicated; however, it is impossible to be so prescriptive, as patients may be asymptomatic with cryptic lung disease, e.g. in connective tissue disease where the incidence of subclinical disease is high. Nevertheless, the majority of patients with suspected ILD have a HRCT as part of their initial assessment. The real utility of the HRCT is its influence on diagnostic perception, notably in those that do not come to biopsy. In one study assessing the impact of HRCT on clinical decision-making in ILD,[28] chest physicians changed their diagnosis in over half the cases, once the HRCT result had been integrated with the clinical details. A HRCT diagnosis of IPF markedly improved diagnostic agreement between chest physicians. However, when the pre-HRCT diagnosis was sarcoid or extrinsic allergic alveolitis (EAA), the influence of HRCT was modest, reflecting the fact that the history and pre-test investigations are often very suggestive of the diagnosis in these conditions, especially when they have a typical presentation (e.g. known antigen exposure in the case of EAA). In this study, the HRCT results lowered the perceived need to biopsy, especially in IPF.[28]

When can high-resolution computed tomography appearances be viewed as pathognomonic?

HRCT diagnoses are never invariably pathognomonic in any single ILD as atypical appearances are always to be found in every disorder, in some patients. Moreover, it is always prudent for the clinician to ensure that the clinical context is appropriate, even when the CT diagnosis appears obvious. With these caveats, it is now clear that HRCT abnormalities are sufficiently diagnostic to make surgical biopsy unnecessary in a number of disorders. In 60–75% of IPF patients with 'typical' appearances, as discussed below, the diagnosis virtually never changes with a surgical biopsy, which can now be discarded in this context. Typical HRCT findings that obviate a surgical diagnostic procedure are also especially common in cystic lung disease (lymphangioleiomyomatosis, Langerhans cell histiocytosis), and lymphangitis carcinomatosis. In sarcoidosis and EAA, a highly confident HRCT diagnosis is possible in well over half of cases; however, particularly in these disorders, unusual variants are frequent and a compatible clinical presentation is essential. In other disorders, notably non-specific interstitial pneumonia (NSIP), a compatible HRCT picture is seldom sufficient in isolation and a confident diagnosis can only be made histologically in idiopathic disease. The common theme throughout the interstitial lung disorders is that if HRCT diagnoses are made in isolation, without consideration of the clinical presentation or observed course, misdiagnosis is an inevitable consequence.

When should a surgical biopsy be performed?

The complex decision on when to biopsy is influenced by many factors including the expertise of the local surgical service, the morbidity associated with the choice of treatment (when this varies according to the final diagnosis), the general health of the patient, the observed longitudinal behavior of the disease, and especially whether the clinical presentation is atypical. Taking account of the clinical picture is crucial to deciding when a surgical biopsy should be performed (Figure 7.3). There are certain disorders in which the HRCT features may be highly non-specific (e.g. randomly distributed ground-glass opacification as in desquamative interstitial pneumonia) and other conditions, such as NSIP, in which the spectrum of findings has yet to be fully characterized. This is particularly the case in pediatric ILD, in which the imaging repertoire is less defined than in adult disease.[29]

Although biopsies are sometimes performed for prognostic reasons, the single most frequent rationale is to guide the clinician in treatment and monitoring. ILD can usefully be subdivided into four primary scenarios: self-limited inflammatory disorders, stable or indolently progressive fibrotic disorders, aggressive inflammation in which outcome may be poor without intervention, and inexorably progressive fibrotic disease. In the first two categories, treatment is often unnecessary or can be minimized, especially when an underlying cause can be identified (as in EAA, drug-induced lung disease, or smoking). By contrast, aggressive intervention is often required in the remaining scenarios. A surgical biopsy is especially useful when the clinician is unable to make these crucial distinctions non-invasively. A crucial (and often under-utilized) advantage

of HRCT is the clear depiction of the range and distribution of morphological abnormalities, and this allows the surgeon to select biopsy sites across the spectrum of abnormalities, thus minimizing surgical 'sampling error'.

Are reports of high-resolution computed tomography diagnostic accuracy clinically robust?

The sensitivity of a test reflects the proportion of individuals with a disease, who have a positive test result. The true sensitivity is difficult to calculate as those who have the disease are never definitively identified. In the context of ILD, the population with the disease are usually defined by a retrospective review of a subgroup of referred patients, who have a histopathological diagnosis. Most series then quantify the proportion of patients who would have had their pathological condition accurately detected by HRCT. This is one of several biases that have to be factored in when interpreting studies of the 'accuracy' of HRCT.

Sensitivity

The landmark accuracy studies were performed in the late 1980s and early 1990s,[1-3] and they followed a standard format; the sensitivity of HRCT for the detection of a variety of ILDs was compared with that of plain chest radiography. The sensitivity of each was calculated by comparison with the histopathological gold standard, obtained by lung biopsy. The accuracy of HRCT in these early studies, was calculated with minimal clinical data[1,2,30] and many of these studies were designed in such a way that the HRCTs were viewed in isolation of clinical findings. A study by Grenier et al.[30] broke the mold of previous 'accuracy' studies and assessed the diagnostic value of clinical data, chest radiography, and HRCT, in the diagnosis of chronic diffuse ILD. When all three were assimilated, the correct diagnosis was reached against histological findings in 80% of cases.

Specificity

The specificity of a test is a measure of its ability to correctly assign the absence of disease (normality). The true 'specificity' of HRCT in the detection of ILD cannot be accurately defined as sizable numbers of normal individuals are rarely included in study cohorts. Furthermore, conditions which mimic ILD are rarely included (e.g. cardiac failure) and most studies are limited to the biased cohort of patients who come to surgical biopsy. Some of the patients in the surgical biopsy cohort may be in this group because of their atypical HRCT appearance and so the true specificity

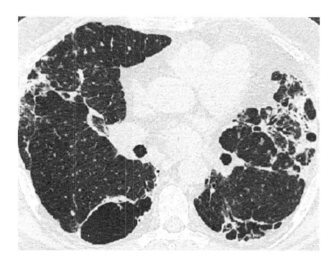

Figure 7.3
An example of the importance of assessing the longitudinal behavior of a presumptive diagnosis of a middle-aged male who was diagnosed (non-invasively) as having organizing pneumonia with fibrotic lung disease, when the patient failed to respond to therapy, a biopsy was taken from the lingula and this demonstrated adenocarcinoma (on the initial HRCT, the patchy consolidation in the lingula was interpreted as an area of organizing pneumonia).

of HRCT is not quantified in these studies. There is also bias within the surgical biopsy group, as the final diagnosis is affected by both sampling error and observer variability.

Most HRCT diagnostic studies effectively address the issue of specificity (and, by extension, positive predictive value). In some studies, typical HRCT appearances have a specificity of over 90% for a confident diagnosis of IPF, when made by experienced radiologists.[31–34] More recently, it has been reiterated that the diagnosis of ILD is most accurately made by consensus between the disciplines of respiratory medicine, radiology, and pathology;[35] the final step of this particular study was the synchronous review of the clinical, histopathological, and radiological information, and this led to all teams refining their diagnoses and improving their level of confidence.[35]

The 'histospecificity' of HRCT is a term used to express the overall accuracy of HRCT against a histological diagnosis and is influenced by both sensitivity and specificity. The 'histospecificity' of HRCT for all sub-groups of both ILD and especially IIP has not been comprehensively studied.

The majority of the data quoted are taken from large studies which have included all categories of IIP but, with the exception of IPF/NSIP, there are few studies focusing on individual pathologies. However, even in end-stage lung disease, a correct diagnosis can be made in up to 90% of cases[36] (Figure 7.4).

Earlier studies of IPF in the last century included histological patterns of both usual interstitial pneumonia (UIP) and NSIP. NSIP was first defined in the 1990s[37] but it was some years before it was viewed as a distinct entity, and it took even longer for typical HRCT variants of NSIP to be described. An early study of the diagnostic accuracy of HRCT in IIP found that the correct diagnosis was made in 71% of patients with IPF, 79% of those with organizing pneumonia (OP), 63% of those with desquamative interstitial pneumonia (DIP), 65% of those with acute interstitial pneumonia (AIP), and 9% of those with NSIP.[38] The strikingly low detection rate in NSIP has undoubtedly improved with accumulating radiological experience. However, when the differential diagnosis lies between IPF and

(a)

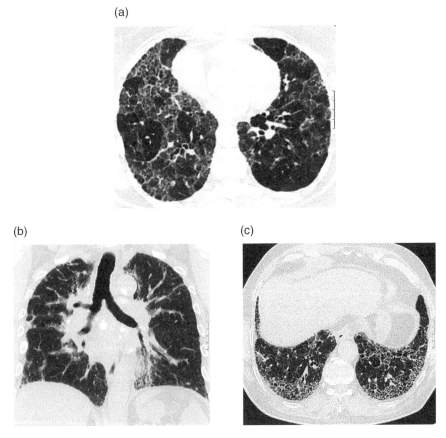

(b)

(c)

Figure 7.4
When there is marked fibrotic lung disease or even honeycombing present, a presumptive diagnosis of the etiological cause can be refined by ancillary features. (a) HRCT through the lower lobes showing spared secondary pulmonary lobules (decreased attenuation) interposed between areas of reticulation. The combination of fibrosis (reticular pattern) and evidence of small airways involvement (pulmonary lobules) is typical of chronic hypersensitivity pneumonitis. (b) Coronal section 5 mm HRCT through the carina of a middle-aged male patient. There is a fibrotic lung disease with calcified lymph nodes in a distribution which is typical of sarcoidosis. (c) HRCT section which shows the characteristic subpleural and basal honeycombing of usual interstitial pneumonia.

NSIP, clinicians and radiologists are more accurate in diagnosing IPF than NSIP, which tends to be over diagnosed.[35] A more recent study of HRCT histospecificity for IPF/NSIP reported 76% sensitivity and 85% specificity for NSIP versus 84% sensitivity and 77% specificity for IPF, but this is difficult to translate into normal practice as this study group only contained these two entities.[39]

Sarcoidosis represents a substantial subgroup in many CT accuracy studies[1–3,40] and it was correctly identified as the first choice diagnosis in 70% of patients by chest radiography and in 78% of patients by HRCT alone. Grenier et al.[30] found that when the diagnosis of sarcoidosis was made combining clinical and radiological information, it was made with a 90% sensitivity. The context of this result is important, as most patients with sarcoidosis do not have a HRCT and this result, therefore, has less immediate clinical relevance than the HRCT histospecificity for IPF.

Cigarette smoking is the commonest cause of inhalational disease and the accuracy of HRCT has not been fully explored with regard to respiratory bronchiolitis and respiratory bronchiolitis-interstitial lung disease (RBILD). Nevertheless, HRCT is precise in the diagnosis of another smoking-related lung disease, Langerhans cell histiocytosis, and when this diagnosis is made with a high level of confidence, it is between 90 and 100% accurate[3,41] (Figure 7.5).

There are few sources for the accuracy of HRCT in the diagnosis of EAA. Lynch et al.[42] reviewed the ability of HRCT to distinguish between hypersensitivity pneumonitis and IPF, this study found that when the diagnosis of EAA was made with a high level of confidence, it was correct in 12 out of 13 cases (92%).

The inhalation of mineral dusts has been the subject of quantitative and qualitative research because of the perceived need to evaluate occupational lung disease objectively. The HRCT diagnosis of silicosis has been reported as being 92% sensitive[30] and in another study, when the diagnosis was made with a high level of confidence, it was correct 100% of the time.[2] HRCT has a high sensitivity for asbestosis (96%) and it exceeds that of plain radiography,[43] nevertheless chest radiography is traditionally the modality chosen to screen for asbestos-related lung disease and there are no large studies with histopathological–radiological correlation for HRCT accuracy in asbestosis. Gamsu et al.[44] demonstrated the CT findings of early disease are not sensitive or specific for asbestosis and that histological disease can be present with a normal HRCT scan. The diagnosis of asbestosis should not be based on imaging alone and there are guidelines for the use of clinical and radiological information, together with exposure history, and an appropriate lag time between exposure and symptoms.

When the clinical and radiological findings are considered together, HRCT has been reported as being accurate in the diagnosis of lymphangitis carcinomatosis (100% sensitivity),[30] however, this estimate was from a small sample size (18 biopsy proven cases) and it is difficult to extrapolate these numbers to the entire cohort of patients with lymphangitis carcinomatosis.

Are high-resolution computed tomography diagnoses consistent between radiologists?

Interobserver variability is an important and often neglected concept. Until relatively recently, there has been little published work on the interobserver variation between radiologists. The majority of the current observational radiological studies now quote kappa values for variation between two, and rarely three, observers. Aziz et al.[45] studied diagnostic interobserver variation between eleven thoracic radiologists in ILD. Observer agreement for the first choice diagnosis was moderate for the entire cohort ($\kappa = 0.48$) and was good for cases from regional centers ($\kappa = 0.60$).

(a)

(b)

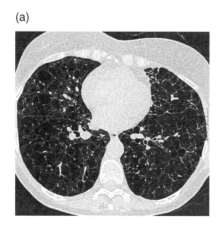
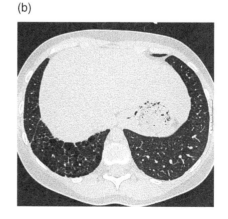

Figure 7.5
(a) Typical distribution of end-stage Langerhans cell histiocytosis: the advanced cystic lung destruction shows marked sparing of the extreme lung bases (b).

Interobserver variation was only fair for the cases from a tertiary referral hospital and this reflects the complexity of the case-mix seen in these centers ($\kappa = 0.34$).

A companion study investigated the variation between pathologists in ILD;[46] these experienced pulmonary pathologists ($n = 10$) were members of the UK interstitial lung disease panel. The overall kappa coefficient of agreement for the first choice diagnosis was fair at $\kappa = 0.38$, increasing to moderate ($\kappa = 0.43$) for patients with multiple biopsies.

These studies come from a specialist center and although the problems of less experienced clinical and radiological observers have been highlighted,[47] it is difficult to get a sense of the true interobserver variability 'at large' in nationwide clinical practice. In recognizing the ILD pattern, a further factor to consider is intraobserver variability and this affects both pathologists (personal communication with TV Colby) and radiologists.[48]

What is the gold standard for diagnosis in interstitial lung disease?

The gold standard for diagnosis has historically been based on histopathological examination of a lung biopsy specimen. However, this is no longer the case,[49] partly because observer variation between pulmonary pathologists has at last been acknowledged as an important limitation and partly because of biopsy sampling error. In one series the histological diagnosis would have differed between NSIP and UIP in one-quarter of patients, if single rather than multiple biopsies had been taken.[50] However, even when biopsies are representative and there is agreement between pathologists, the final diagnosis often changes when histological, HRCT, and clinical information are considered concurrently.[36] This happens most frequently in EAA (in which a variety of histological patterns is seen) and when the histological diagnosis is NSIP, but the final diagnosis is often IPF, EAA, or organizing pneumonia.

How should disease severity on high-resolution computed tomography be reconciled with functional impairment?

Historically, the severity of ILD has been staged using PFTs. The total diffusing capacity of the lung for carbon monoxide (Dlco) is a measure of both the surface area available for gas transfer and the integrity of that surface. A decrease in Dlco is a sensitive indicator of ILD but lacks specificity because Dlco can decrease in ILD, pulmonary vascular disease, cardiac conditions, and emphysema. In the IIPs, the extent of disease on HRCT has been most strongly linked to Dlco levels in many studies. However, a decreased Dlco is sometimes found in conjunction with a 'normal' HRCT. In those individuals with no explanation for decreased gas exchange, lung biopsy is inconsistently performed and thus there are no studies to explain the spectrum of pathological processes that might be found in this cohort. It is frequently assumed that these patients have emphysema, microscopic fibrosis, pulmonary hypertension, or capillaritis.

HRCT is less useful than PFTs in the clinical assessment of severity because HRCT scoring has not been routinely adapted to the provision of readily accessible absolute values. In research projects, estimations of the percentage of abnormal lung are often pivotal but numerical quantification is subjective and not routinely performed by non-academic radiologists. By contrast, PFTs are widely available. However, PFTs are sometimes misleading due to the wide range in normal values (80–120% of predicted). Thus, a disease process may decrease PFTs significantly within the normal range. A forced vital capacity (FVC) of 75% of the predicted value represents a reduction from baseline values of between 5% and 45%.

Furthermore, coexisting emphysema is found in up to 40% of IPF patients, leading to a spurious preservation of lung volumes and a disproportionate reduction in gas transfer. A composite physiological index (CPI) has been derived from disease extent observed by HRCT and it reconciles the functional severity with the global morphological extent of disease in IPF.[51] The CPI, which quantifies the functional defect due to IPF, while excluding that ascribable to emphysema, is more accurate in predicting mortality than individual lung function indices.

In routine practice, rapid evaluation HRCT provides useful approximate information of disease severity that can help to unravel the confounding factors discussed above. The clinical importance of minor reductions in PFTs can be more readily assessed and the observation of coexisting emphysema and pulmonary fibrosis allows patterns of functional impairment to be better understood.

Several investigators have found positive correlations between the extent of disease on HRCT and PFTs in sarcoidosis,[40,52–55] although the strength of correlations is little better than between chest radiographic scores and PFTs in two studies.[53,55] A role for HRCT in staging severity in sarcoidosis has yet to be established.

What is the prognostic role of high-resolution computed tomography?

The identification of reversible disease is a crucial clinical aim, especially when the diagnosis is uncertain. Generally,

HRCT findings of reticular abnormalities and distortion are irreversible, and this often allows clincans to avoid inappropriately aggressive treatment in an unrealistic attempt to produce regression of disease. By contrast, reversibility is more likely when ground-glass opacification and, especially, consolidation are prominent. However, it should be stressed strongly that these patterns do not always represent reversible disease, as ground-glass opacification often represents fine fibrosis and consolidation may represent malignancy or 'petrified' fibrosis. When ground-glass opacification is admixed with a reticular pattern or contains obvious traction bronchiectasis, a response to treatment should not be expected. In this regard, the term 'alveolitis on CT' (with connotations of inflammatory cell infiltration), as synonymous with prominent ground-glass opacification is seriously misplaced.

HRCT prognostic evaluation in ILD has focused on the IIPs and especially on IPF. Ground-glass opacification as a predictive sign was analyzed extensively in the 1990s and was found to increase the likelihood of survival and responsiveness to treatment.[56–61] In retrospect, this observation probably reflected the fact that GGO is the cardinal CT finding in NSIP[62] and is usually less extensive in IPF. Remy-Jardin et al.[63] correlated cases in which GGO was the dominant abnormality with the histological specimens of patients with ILD, and found GGO corresponded to inflammation in 65%, a combination of inflammation and fibrosis in 22%, and exclusively fibrosis in 13% (Figure 7.6). In this study, 85% of those with fibrosis had traction of airways (bronchiectasis or bronchiolectasis). Similarly, in patients with 'IPF' (in the pre-NSIP era), reticular patterns never regressed but GGO could increase or diminish with treatment.[58]

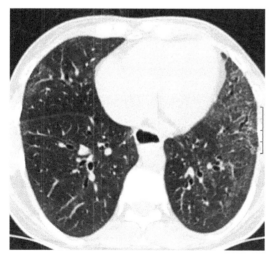

Figure 7.6
HRCT section at the level of the right atrium of a patient with systemic sclerosis showing widespread ground-glass opacity within which the airways are dilated and distorted, implying a fibrotic component, probably non-specific interstitial pneumonia.

These studies remain useful because in many patients with IIP, especially those with severe disease, biopsies are not performed and the differential diagnosis remains uncertain. However, the pattern of disease on HRCT is also useful in definite IPF. Although, as discussed above, the majority have 'typical' appearances, consisting of subpleural basal reticular abnormalities with little GGO, an important minority have prominent GGO and closely ressemble appearances often seen in NSIP. Patients with biopsy-proven UIP and a definite or probable diagnosis of IPF on HRCT, have increased mortality, compared with those who have biopsy-proven UIP and an HRCT pattern suggestive of NSIP.[34] Thus, although prominent GGO is not always indicative of reversible disease, it tends to be associated with a better outcome across the IIPs.

In IPF, a response to treatment is the exception and there is more clinical focus on identifying patients who are more likely to deteriorate relatively quickly. Prominent honeycombing is a malignant prognostic determinant and, when quantified as a 'CT fibrosis score' was shown to be accurate in predicting early and intermediate mortality.[57] Zisman et al.[64] extended these observations to IPF patients with IPF treated with cyclophosphamide and found that a better outcome was confined to those with lower CT fibrosis scores. In IPF, patients evaluated for lung transplantation, the CT fibrosis scores and reduction in Dlco before 40% of predicted were equally adverse prognostic factors.[65]

Abnormally rapid clearance of inhaled DTPA has also indicated a worse prognosis in IPF,[10] but had less prognostic significance in this study, requiring a larger cohort to achieve statistical significance than the HRCT observations discussed above. However, in patients with less rapidly progressive pulmonary fibrosis, as in scleroderma, normal DTPA clearance may be more useful in identifying stable disease.[66]

In other diffuse lung diseases, HRCT has no established role in defining prognosis. There have been conflicting reports about the reversibility of HRCT signs in sarcoidosis.[54,67] Nodules and alveolar/pseudoalveolar consolidation have been shown to regress in disease remission (inflammatory etiology), whereas septal/non-septal lines and lung distortion tend to have remained static (fibrotic etiology).[67] However, Remy-Jardin found that the profusion of lung changes in pulmonary sarcoidosis correlated poorly with functional impairment but did not reflect disease activity. This study failed to demonstrate any value for CT as a predictor for changes in functional impairment over time.[54,55]

What is the role of imaging in monitoring interstitial lung disease?

Historically, PFTs have had primacy in monitoring disease and this has changed little in the CT era. Serial change in

PFTs has important prognostic significance in NSIP/IPF[68] with a downward trend in Dlco, forced vital capacity (FVC), and forced expiratory volume in 1 second (FEV1) at 6 and 12 months strongly predicting mortality. Flaherty et al.[34] also found that a decline in FVC of 10% or more was associated with increased mortality in those with NSIP and UIP. Serial chest radiography has not been formally evaluated against PFTs in predicting outcome but is widely viewed as insensitive in progressive pulmonary fibrosis. By contrast, HRCT is sometimes too sensitive to change: HRCT monitoring has not yet been shown to add greatly to the monitoring and management of these patients. There is reported value in the longitudinal monitoring of FEV1, FVC, and Dlco, and fluctuations in these parameters informs the clinician about disease progression or response to treatment. Subtle HRCT changes can be too sensitive and have not been found useful in unselected patients, adding nothing to serial PFTs in predicting mortality in IPF and NSIP.[34] Serial HRCT is sometimes useful in confirming obvious change in selected patients when functional trends are marginal but should not be applied indiscriminately.

In conclusion, HRCT is generally accurate at identifying ILD and the morphological pattern of disease has prognostic value. Baseline clinical information must be integrated with HRCT appearances, to produce the most effective use of HRCT, and histopathological evaluation is reserved for those discordant cases in which biopsy is deemed appropriate.

References

1. Padley SP, Hansell DM, Flower CD, Jennings P. Comparative accuracy of high resolution computed tomography and chest radiography in the diagnosis of chronic diffuse infiltrative lung disease. Clin Radiol 1991; 44: 222–6.
2. Mathieson JR, Mayo JR, Staples CA, Muller NL. Chronic diffuse infiltrative lung disease: comparison of diagnostic accuracy of CT and chest radiography. Radiology 1989; 171: 111–6.
3. Grenier P, Valeyre D, Cluzel P et al. Chronic diffuse interstitial lung disease: diagnostic value of chest radiography and high-resolution CT. Radiology 1991; 179: 123–32.
4. Epler GR, McLoud TC, Gaensler EA, Mikus JP, Carrington CB. Normal chest roentgenograms in chronic diffuse infiltrative lung disease. N Engl J Med 1978; 298: 934–9.
5. Gaensler EA, Carrington CB. Open biopsy for chronic diffuse infiltrative lung disease: clinical, roentgenographic, and physiological correlations in 502 patients. Ann Thorac Surg 1980; 30: 411–26.
6. Fenlon HM, Doran M, Sant SM, Breatnach E. High-resolution chest CT in systemic lupus erythematosus. AJR Am J Roentgenol 1996; 166: 301–7.
7. Mayo JR, Webb WR, Gould R et al. High-resolution CT of the lungs: an optimal approach. Radiology 1987; 163: 507–10.
8. O'Brodovich H, Coates G. Pulmonary clearance of 99mTc-DTPA: a noninvasive assessment of epithelial integrity. Lung 1987; 165: 1–16.
9. Pantin CF, Valind SO, Sweatman M et al. Measures of the inflammatory response in cryptogenic fibrosing alveolitis. Am Rev Respir Dis 1988; 138: 1234–41.
10. Mogulkoc N, Brutsche MH, Bishop PW et al. Pulmonary (99m)Tc-DTPA aerosol clearance and survival in usual interstitial pneumonia (UIP). Thorax 2001; 56: 916–23.
11. Jones JG, Minty BD, Royston D. The physiology of leaky lungs. Br J Anaesth 1982; 54: 705–21.
12. Kaushik VV, Lynch MP, Dawson JK. Tc-DTPA clearance and rheumatoid arthritis-associated fibrosing alveolitis. Rheumatology (Oxford) 2002; 41: 712–3.
13. Antoniou KM, Malagari K, Tzanakis N et al. Clearance of technetium-99m-DTPA and HRCT findings in the evaluation of patients with Idiopathic Pulmonary Fibrosis. BMC Pulm Med 2006; 6: 4.
14. Mayo JR, Aldrich J, Muller NL. Radiation exposure at chest CT: a statement of the Fleischner Society. Radiology 2003; 228: 15–21.
15. Riley DJ. Risk of surgical lung biopsy in idiopathic interstitial pneumonias. Chest 2005; 127: 1485–6.
16. Dalal PU, Hansell DM. High-resolution computed tomography of the lungs: the borderlands of normality. Eur Radiol 2005; 1–10.
17. Webb WR, Stern EJ, Kanth N, Gamsu G. Dynamic pulmonary CT: findings in healthy adult men. Radiology 1993; 186: 117–24.
18. Koh DM, Hansell DM. Computed tomography of diffuse interstitial lung disease in children. Clin Radiol 2000; 55: 659–67.
19. Lee KW, Chung SY, Yang I et al. Correlation of aging and smoking with air trapping at thin-section CT of the lung in asymptomatic subjects. Radiology 2000; 214: 831–6.
20. Wells AU, Nicholson AG, Hansell DM, du Bois RM. Respiratory bronchiolitis-associated interstitial lung disease. Semin Respir Crit Care Med 2003; 24: 585–94.
21. Remy-Jardin M, Remy J, Boulenguez C et al. Morphologic effects of cigarette smoking on airways and pulmonary parenchyma in healthy adult volunteers: CT evaluation and correlation with pulmonary function tests. Radiology 1993; 186: 107–15.
22. Tansey D, Wells AU, Colby TV et al. Variations in histological patterns of interstitial pneumonia between connective tissue disorders and their relationship to prognosis. Histopathology 2004; 44: 585–96.
23. Remy-Jardin M, Remy J, Cortet B, Mauri F, Delcambre B. Lung changes in rheumatoid arthritis: CT findings. Radiology 1994; 193: 375–82.
24. Zrour SH, Touzi M, Bejia I et al. Correlations between high-resolution computed tomography of the chest and clinical function in patients with rheumatoid arthritis. Prospective study in 75 patients. Joint Bone Spine 2005; 72: 41–7.
25. Carotti M, Salaffi F, Manganelli P et al. The subclinical involvement of the lung in rheumatoid arthritis: evaluation by high-resolution computed tomography. Reumatismo 2001; 53: 280–8.
26. Wells AU. High-resolution computed tomography in the diagnosis of diffuse lung disease: a clinical perspective. Semin Respir Crit Care Med 2003; 24: 347–56.
27. Costabel U, Hunninghake GW. ATS/ERS/WASOG statement on sarcoidosis. Sarcoidosis Statement Committee.

American Thoracic Society. European Respiratory Society. World Association for Sarcoidosis and Other Granulomatous Disorders. Eur Respir J 1999; 14: 735–7.

28. Aziz ZA, Wells AU, Bateman ED et al. Interstitial lung disease: effects of thin-section CT on clinical decision making. Radiology 2005.

29. Bush A. Paediatric interstitial lung disease: not just kid's stuff. Eur Respir J 2004; 24: 521–3.

30. Grenier P, Chevret S, Beigelman C et al. Chronic diffuse infiltrative lung disease: determination of the diagnostic value of clinical data, chest radiography, and CT and Bayesian analysis. Radiology 1994; 191: 383–90.

31. Raghu G, Mageto YN, Lockhart D et al. The accuracy of the clinical diagnosis of new-onset idiopathic pulmonary fibrosis and other interstitial lung disease: A prospective study. Chest 1999; 116: 1168–74.

32. Hunninghake GW, Lynch DA, Galvin JR et al. Radiologic findings are strongly associated with a pathologic diagnosis of usual interstitial pneumonia. Chest 2003; 124: 1215–23.

33. Hunninghake GW, Zimmerman MB, Schwartz DA et al. Utility of a lung biopsy for the diagnosis of idiopathic pulmonary fibrosis. Am J Respir Crit Care Med 2001; 164: 193–6.

34. Flaherty KR, Thwaite EL, Kazerooni EA et al. Radiological versus histological diagnosis in UIP and NSIP: survival implications. Thorax 2003; 58: 143–8.

35. Flaherty KR, King TE Jr, Raghu G et al. Idiopathic interstitial pneumonia: what is the effect of a multidisciplinary approach to diagnosis? Am J Respir Crit Care Med 2004; 170: 904–10.

36. Primack SL, Hartman TE, Hansell DM, Muller NL. End-stage lung disease: CT findings in 61 patients. Radiology 1993; 189: 681–6.

37. Katzenstein AL, Fiorelli RF. Nonspecific interstitial pneumonia/fibrosis. Histologic features and clinical significance. Am J Surg Pathol 1994; 18: 136–47.

38. Johkoh T, Muller NL, Cartier Y et al. Idiopathic interstitial pneumonias: diagnostic accuracy of thin-section CT in 129 patients. Radiology 1999; 211: 555–60.

39. Bna C, Zompatori M, Poletti V et al. Differential diagnosis between usual interstitial pneumonia (UIP) and nonspecific interstitial pneumonia (NSIP) assessed by high-resolution computed tomography (HRCT). Radiol Med (Torino) 2005; 109: 472–87.

40. Bergin CJ, Bell DY, Coblentz CL et al. Sarcoidosis: correlation of pulmonary parenchymal pattern at CT with results of pulmonary function tests. Radiology 1989; 171: 619–24.

41. Bonelli FS, Hartman TE, Swensen SJ, Sherrick A. Accuracy of high-resolution CT in diagnosing lung diseases. AJR Am J Roentgenol 1998; 170: 1507–12.

42. Lynch DA, Newell JD, Logan PM, King TE Jr, Muller NL. Can CT distinguish hypersensitivity pneumonitis from idiopathic pulmonary fibrosis? AJR Am J Roentgenol 1995; 165: 807–11.

43. Aberle DR, Gamsu G, Ray CS, Feuerstein IM. Asbestos-related pleural and parenchymal fibrosis: detection with high-resolution CT. Radiology 1988; 166: 729–34.

44. Gamsu G, Salmon CJ, Warnock ML, Blanc PD. CT quantification of interstitial fibrosis in patients with asbestosis: a comparison of two methods. AJR Am J Roentgenol 1995; 164: 63–8.

45. Aziz ZA, Wells AU, Hansell DM et al. HRCT diagnosis of diffuse parenchymal lung disease: inter-observer variation. Thorax 2004; 59: 506–11.

46. Nicholson AG, Addis BJ, Bharucha H et al. Inter-observer variation between pathologists in diffuse parenchymal lung disease. Thorax 2004; 59: 500–5.

47. Nishimura K, Izumi T, Kitaichi M, Nagai S, Itoh H. The diagnostic accuracy of high-resolution computed tomography in diffuse infiltrative lung diseases. Chest 1993; 104: 1149–55.

48. Collins CD, Wells AU, Hansell DM et al. Observer variation in pattern type and extent of disease in fibrosing alveolitis on thin section computed tomography and chest radiography. Clin Radiol 1994; 49: 236–40.

49. Wells AU. Histopathologic diagnosis in diffuse lung disease: an ailing gold standard. Am J Respir Crit Care Med 2004; 170: 828–9.

50. Flaherty KR, Travis WD, Colby TV et al. Histopathologic variability in usual and nonspecific interstitial pneumonias. Am J Respir Crit Care Med 2001; 164: 1722–7.

51. Wells AU, Desai SR, Rubens MB et al. Idiopathic pulmonary fibrosis: a composite physiologic index derived from disease extent observed by computed tomography. Am J Respir Crit Care Med 2003; 167: 962–9.

52. Hansell DM, Milne DG, Wilsher ML, Wells AU. Pulmonary sarcoidosis: morphologic associations of airflow obstruction at thin-section CT. Radiology 1998; 209: 697–704.

53. Muller NL, Mawson JB, Mathieson JR et al. Sarcoidosis: correlation of extent of disease at CT with clinical, functional, and radiographic findings. Radiology 1989; 171: 613–8.

54. Remy-Jardin M, Giraud F, Remy J et al. Pulmonary sarcoidosis: role of CT in the evaluation of disease activity and functional impairment and in prognosis assessment. Radiology 1994; 191: 675–80.

55. Brauner MW, Grenier P, Mompoint D, Lenoir S, de CH. Pulmonary sarcoidosis: evaluation with high-resolution CT. Radiology 1989; 172: 467–71.

56. Lee JS, Im JG, Ahn JM, Kim YM, Han MC. Fibrosing alveolitis: prognostic implication of ground-glass attenuation at high-resolution CT. Radiology 1992; 184: 451–4.

57. Gay SE, Kazerooni EA, Toews GB et al. Idiopathic pulmonary fibrosis: predicting response to therapy and survival. Am J Respir Crit Care Med 1998; 157: 1063–72.

58. Wells AU, Rubens MB, du Bois RM, Hansell DM. Serial CT in fibrosing alveolitis: prognostic significance of the initial pattern. AJR Am J Roentgenol 1993; 161: 1159–65.

59. Wells AU, Hansell DM, Rubens MB et al. The predictive value of appearances on thin-section computed tomography in fibrosing alveolitis. Am Rev Respir Dis 1993; 148: 1076–82.

60. Muller NL, Staples CA, Miller RR et al. Disease activity in idiopathic pulmonary fibrosis: CT and pathologic correlation. Radiology 1987; 165: 731–4.

61. Wells AU, Hansell DM, Corrin B et al. High resolution computed tomography as a predictor of lung histology in systemic sclerosis. Thorax 1992; 47: 738–42.

62. MacDonald SL, Rubens MB, Hansell DM et al. Nonspecific interstitial pneumonia and usual interstitial pneumonia: comparative appearances at and diagnostic accuracy of thin-section CT. Radiology 2001; 221: 600–5.

63. Remy-Jardin M, Giraud F, Remy J et al. Importance of ground-glass attenuation in chronic diffuse infiltrative lung disease: pathologic-CT correlation. Radiology 1993; 189: 693–8.

64. Zisman DA, Lynch JP, III, Toews GB et al. Cyclophosphamide in the treatment of idiopathic pulmonary fibrosis: a prospective study in patients who failed to respond to corticosteroids. Chest 2000; 117: 1619–26.

65. Mogulkoc N, Brutsche MH, Bishop PW et al. Pulmonary function in idiopathic pulmonary fibrosis and referral for lung transplantation. Am J Respir Crit Care Med 2001; 164: 103–8.

66. Wells AU, Hansell DM, Harrison NK et al. Clearance of inhaled 99mTc-DTPA predicts the clinical course of fibrosing alveolitis. Eur Respir J 1993; 6: 797–802.

67. Brauner MW, Lenoir S, Grenier P et al. Pulmonary sarcoidosis: CT assessment of lesion reversibility. Radiology 1992; 182: 349–54.

68. Latsi PI, du Bois RM, Nicholson AG et al. Fibrotic idiopathic interstitial pneumonia: the prognostic value of longitudinal functional trends. Am J Respir Crit Care Med 2003; 168: 531–7.

8

Connective tissue disorders

Sujal R Desai and Athol U Wells

Introduction

Pulmonary involvement is remarkably common[1,2] in patients with connective tissue disorders and patients who present with respiratory symptoms pose a considerable challenge to the physician. Lung disease is now the most frequent cause of death in such patients. Hence, accurate evaluation of the lungs has become an increasingly important component of clinical practice. The growth in information technology has meant that patient awareness about lung disease and the expectations that disease will be treated have also increased. The result is that sensitive screening procedures, such as high-resolution computed tomography (HRCT), are often brought to bear and, perhaps not surprisingly, 'early' disease is frequently detected. The decision of whether to treat then becomes a problem with which the physician must grapple. Another difficulty is the plethora of different yet non-specific interstitial processes which overlap but may have different outcomes to those seen in the idiopathic interstitial pneumonias.[3,4] The clinical evaluation is further complicated by the variable presence of pulmonary vascular disease, airways disease, extra-thoracic pulmonary restriction, lung disease due to treatment of the underlying rheumatological disorder, and even possible cardiac involvement. In some connective tissue disorders, most notably rheumatoid arthritis, it is also known that different disease processes often coexist in an individual patient, confounding the quantification of the functional severity of disease.

In this chapter, we consider lung involvement in connective tissue disorders as a series of clinical problems. Important questions which commonly arise for the physician who cares for such patients include the issue of disease detection, evaluation of its clinical significance, the crucial dilemma of when to treat, and, finally, how best to monitor progress. This chapter attempts to consider the value, if any, of imaging tests in answering these potentially vexing clinical problems. However, before the specific issues are addressed, the next section revises the epidemiology and sometimes complex pathological nature of lung disease in patients with connective tissue disorders.

Epidemiological and histopathological aspects
Epidemiological considerations

It has always been difficult to be precise about the true prevalence of lung disease in patients with connective tissues disorders. There are a number of reasons why this has been so. First, the likelihood of lung involvement is truly disease dependent being relatively common in systemic sclerosis and rheumatoid arthritis but less prevalent in systemic lupus erythematosus. Second, there are issues about definition: in this regard systemic sclerosis is a good example since pulmonary involvement has been a criteria for diagnosis.[5] Third, the sophistication of methods used for detection of lung involvement (i.e. chest radiography versus HRCT) have influenced the reported prevalence in published series. Fourth, there are inevitably biases in published series depending on whether an unselected or referral population has been evaluated. A final problem is that 'early' lung disease may be truly subclinical and will escape detection.[6,7] Exertional dyspnea is an inconsistent marker of pulmonary disease. Furthermore, coexistent morbidity due to arthritis or myositis will limit exercise tolerance thereby masking lung disease in some patients, whereas in others, inefficient locomotion due to systemic disease may lead to exertional breathlessness even without pulmonary involvement.

Notwithstanding the above, it is clear that lung disease is probably most common in systemic sclerosis. Evidence of lung disease is apparent on chest radiographs in up to two-thirds of patients with systemic sclerosis,[8] a figure which would undoubtedly be higher if HRCT had been used for the detection of lung disease. In rheumatoid arthritis, although over 60% of patients are believed to have an element of interstitial fibrosis on histopathological examination,[9] only 5% have pulmonary fibrosis on chest radiography.[10,11] In polymyositis/dermatomyositis one-third of patients have clinically overt lung disease.[12] In one study, the majority of patients with polymyositis/dermatomyositis had respiratory symptoms which were attributed to community-acquired pneumonia.[13] However, there was evidence of established interstitial lung disease in a subset of 22 out of 70 patients who underwent surgical biopsy. In systemic lupus erythematosus, a small minority (typically less than 5%) of patients have clinical or chest radiographic evidence of interstitial lung disease at the outset and a similar proportion subsequently develops a disease which resembles fibrosing alveolitis.[14] As in other collagen vascular disorders, 'subclinical' lung involvement is more prevalent although signs of lung disease on CT are reported in up to one-third of patients.[15]

Histopathological issues

Historically, usual interstitial pneumonia (UIP) has been considered the most common histological pattern of lung disease. This pattern is recognized by the varying proportions of intermingled interstitial fibrosis, fibroblast foci, inflammation, and honeycombing merging with zones of normal lung.[3,4] One of the key diagnostic features is the temporal and spatial heterogeneity. Following the recent re-thinking of the diffuse interstitial lung diseases and specifically the idiopathic interstitial pneumonias,[3,4] it has been realized that histopathological patterns other than UIP are equally, if not more, prevalent in patients with connective tissue disorders. Thus, it is now known that non-specific interstitial pneumonia (NSIP), organizing pneumonia (OP), lymphocytic interstitial pneumonia (LIP), and acute interstitial pneumonia/diffuse alveolar damage all occur.[1,16] Indeed, in systemic sclerosis[17] and polymyositis/dermatomyositis,[13] NSIP is known to be the most common pattern. However, the histopathological evaluation of the lung in connective tissue disorders is rarely straightforward. It is well known, for example, that different histopathological processes may coexist in the same patient and this is particularly true in rheumatoid arthritis.[18] Another issue is that, in addition to fibrotic disease, airway involvement[19–24] is not uncommon and may give rise to a confusing pattern of physiological impairment. Finally, there is the further confounding factor that lung disease may be due to the drugs used in the treatment of the disease rather than the primary disorder.[25,26]

Key clinical questions in the management of patients with connective tissue disease

As indicated above, the physician involved in the care of patients with connective tissue disorders will generally seek answers to a number of key questions. In following sections these crucial questions are addressed and the value of imaging tests in these specific areas is considered critically.

Is lung disease present?

Confirming whether a patient with a connective tissue disorder has lung disease may be problematic for the physician. In general, clinical features are unlikely to be helpful and there are a number of specific issues.[10,16,21,27–29] One difficulty is that pulmonary symptoms are only liable to identify patients with relatively advanced lung disease. Furthermore, there is the problem that symptoms are generally variable and non-specific. Another issue is that underlying joint or muscle disease may limit activity and, in this way, might conceivably mask pulmonary involvement. Finally, because patients are increasingly aware of the possibility of lung involvement (in part explicable by the explosive growth of the Internet), respiratory symptoms may be reported even with limited (or indeed, absent) lung disease.

In contrast to clinical features, physiological tests have the advantage of greater objectivity. However, it must be appreciated that the process of interpretation of lung function tests in diffuse lung disease is complex. Lung volumes are a relatively blunt measure of functional impairment with a surprisingly broad normal predicted range (generally ranging from 80 to 120%). Indeed, a patient with spirometric volumes which border on the low-to-normal might have lost anything from zero to 35% of the baseline lung volume. Indices of gas transfer tend to be more sensitive but unfortunately only at the cost of a lower specificity. This is pertinent in connective tissue disorders, where interstitial fibrosis and pulmonary vascular disease may coexist;[18,30–34] a significant depression of diffusing capacity of the lung for carbon monoxide (Dlco) is required before pulmonary vascular disease is detectable by echocardiography.[35] Furthermore, minor reductions in gas transfer are very common, by their very nature non-specific, and thus difficult to interpret.

A number of other tests including bronchoalveolar fluid analysis,[36–41] measurement of autoantibody levels,[42–47] and measurement of the lung clearance of ^{99m}Tc-labeled diethylenetriaminepentaacetic acid (^{99m}Tc-DTPA)[48–51] have been used to detect lung disease in patients with connective tissue disorders. However, the specificity and, more importantly, significance of the 'signal' from these more sophisticated tests is difficult to gauge. Not surprisingly perhaps, these tests have not been readily incorporated into routine clinical practice.

Imaging tests have become central to the investigation of patients with suspected lung disease and, in this regard, the plain chest radiograph is usually the first radiological test to be requested by a physician. However, it has long been known by radiologists and physicians that plain chest radiography is an imperfect tool, plagued by issues of limited sensitivity,[52] accuracy,[53] and, in most instances, clinically unacceptable interobserver disagreement.[54–56] By comparison, because there is no anatomical superimposition (a major limitation of chest radiography) and contrast resolution is superior, CT is significantly superior in the detection of pulmonary pathology (Figure 8.1). Furthermore, it is clear that CT has a superior sensitivity for the detection of lung disease in a range of connective tissue disorders including systemic sclerosis,[57,58] rheumatoid arthritis,[48,59] systemic lupus erythematosus,[15,60] ankylosing spondylitis,[61,62] and Sjögren's syndrome.[63] In symptomatic subjects with 'early' systemic sclerosis abnormalities, for instance, pulmonary abnormalities were seen on CT in all but two of the 17 patients studied by Warrick et al.[58] This was contrasted against only 10/17 chest radiographs which were considered abnormal. There are parallel data for other connective tissue diseases. In the patients with rheumatoid arthritis studied by Gabbay et al.[48] there were features indicative of interstitial lung disease in a mere 6% of radiographs as compared with the signs of pulmonary involvement in one-third of patients as judged by CT. There were comparable results in another study which compared the findings on chest radiography and CT in a cohort of asymptomatic patients with either rheumatoid arthritis or ankylosing spondylitis.[62]

Clearly, it is difficult to be prescriptive about protocols for the detection of lung disease in connective tissue disorders. However, it is clear (despite the above discussion relating to sensitivity and accuracy) that the plain chest radiograph continues to have a role; indeed, it is only right that a physician should request a baseline chest radiograph and pulmonary function tests when patients with connective tissue disorders first present with respiratory signs and symptoms. In those patients who are symptomatic or for those in whom there is a suggestion of lung disease (based on the initial plain radiographic or functional assessment), CT evaluation is probably justified and particularly so for diseases such as systemic sclerosis and polymyositis/dermatomyositis where the prevalence of lung disease is known to be relatively high. However, whether HRCT should be used to 'screen' for lung disease in asymptomatic patients with systemic sclerosis and polymyositis/dermatomyositis is more contentious. In connective tissue disorders where the prevalence of lung disease is known to be lower (e.g. systemic lupus erythematosus and Sjögren's syndrome), screening HRCT examinations are probably not justified and should be reserved for patients with radiographic evidence of disease or symptoms.

What is the clinical significance of lung disease?

In contrast to the issue of disease detection, the question of determining the clinical significance of pulmonary involvement is more problematic for the physician. In principle, disease may be significant, because it is either extensive or intrinsically progressive. This question therefore amounts to a combination of staging disease severity and prognostic evaluation. These issues are considered separately below.

The issue of gauging disease severity

Staging the severity or extent of pulmonary damage is key to understanding the clinical significance of HRCT abnormalities. In this regard it is worth first considering the whole issue of subclinical lung disease. This is a particular concern in the connective tissue disorders since lung involvement of limited extent is not an infrequent finding and compounded by the fact that the physician may screen for lung disease. In rheumatoid arthritis, for example, lung disease is evident in up to 80% of patients on the basis of biopsy data.[64] However, against this, it must be stressed that clinically relevant lung disease is uncommon and that the majority of patients with limited disease do not have progressive involvement. Similar conclusions emerge from HRCT series. Of the 150 consecutive patients with rheumatoid arthritis in one series, only 19% had evidence of pulmonary fibrosis on HRCT.[65] More importantly, when groups were compared, there were no significant differences in the presence of respiratory symptoms between those patients

(a)

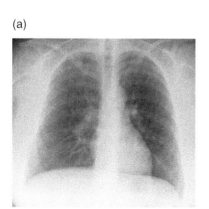

(b)

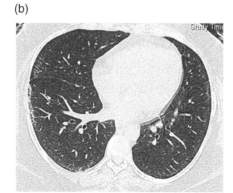

Figure 8.1
Chest radiograph and HRCT in a patient with rheumatoid arthritis. (a) There is no evidence of lung disease on the plain chest radiograph (even when reviewed in retrospect after HRCT). (b) Image at the level of the pulmonary venous confluence demonstrating a subpleural reticular pattern of relatively limited extent. The fibrosis is more conspicuous in the right lung.

with and those without lung disease. In another study of 75 consecutive patients with rheumatoid arthritis, there were HRCT abnormalities in approximately half the patients with no respiratory symptoms.[59] Limited lung involvement is almost the rule in the majority of patients with systemic sclerosis. In the largest study to date, in which the morphological abnormalities in well over 200 patients were quantified, the average extent of interstitial lung disease on CT was barely above 10%.[66] Clinically silent CT changes also occur in systemic lupus erythematosus. In the study by Bankier et al., all 48 consecutively evaluated systemic lupus erythematosus patients who had evidence of lung disease at CT were asymptomatic.[60] Clearly, the challenge for the physician is in deciding what represents 'significant' disease and the important message is that the physician cannot rely on imaging modalities alone to define a threshold disease extent above which disease can be considered clinically significant.

It is not surprising that pulmonary physicians continue to rely on functional tests to determine what is and what is not clinically important. However, the use of physiological tests for this purpose is not wholly precise. There are two separate potential limitations. First, because a wide range of individual functional parameters are routinely measured it is not always clear which, if any, should be regarded as the best measure of severity. Interestingly, CT has had a valuable indirect role in addressing this very question in patients with pulmonary fibrosis secondary to systemic sclerosis. By relating the severity of disease on CT to indices of functional impairment, Wells et al. showed that the percentage predicted Dlco was the best individual physiological correlate of the CT extent of interstitial lung disease.[67] This finding has some practical value for the physician since a single functional parameter (the percentage predicted Dlco) can now potentially be used as the key lung function variable in clinical staging. However, the reader will have realized that this approach is also problematic since no single discrete cut-off level of Dlco can be given above which lung disease becomes clinically significant. Furthermore, 'outlying' cases in which severely restricted lung volumes identify severe involvement (even though Dlco levels are only moderately reduced) are invariably present.

The second limitation to the use of functional tests when gauging clinical significance is that a multiplicity of pathological processes (with potentially opposing physiological effects) often coexist in connective tissue disease; although Dlco levels are clearly influenced by the presence and extent of interstitial fibrosis, a depression of Dlco may also reflect concurrent vascular disease. Similarly, lung volumes may be affected by lung fibrosis and extrapulmonary disease alike. For all the reasons given above, disease severity cannot be staged using pulmonary function tests in isolation and optimal assessment of disease severity must reconcile both functional and morphological findings.

The issue of judging prognostic significance

The re-classification of the idiopathic interstitial pneumonias by the consensus group of the American Thoracic and European Respiratory Societies has a potential bearing on a discussion about prognosis since the majority of histological entities recognized in the idiopathic pneumonias are also seen in patients with connective tissue disorders.[4,68] An important feature of the new classification is that the discrete histopathological patterns are associated with striking differences in survival, with patients having idiopathic pulmonary fibrosis (associated with a pattern of UIP) having the poorest outlook.[69–71] However, whether such distinctions are as prognostically useful in or may be readily extrapolated to the connective tissue disorders is more contentious. There are two possible reasons for this. First, it must be remembered that there are key differences between the connective tissue disorders and idiopathic interstitial pneumonias in the prevalence of these histopathological entities. With the possible exception of rheumatoid arthritis,[72,73] a pattern of NSIP is the dominant finding in many of the connective tissue disorders.[68] In the only large histological series of patients with lung disease due to systemic sclerosis, there was a high prevalence of NSIP (62/80, 78%) and low prevalence of a UIP pattern (6/80, 8%).[17] These data are supported by the results of a morphological study in which the CT appearances of lung disease in systemic sclerosis were more akin to NSIP than UIP[74] (Figure 8.2). The pattern of NSIP is also thought to predominate in polymyositis/dermatomyositis.[13] Notwithstanding this, it is important to remember that, as with the idiopathic pneumonias,[75] fibrotic disease also seems to predominate in the connective tissue disorders.[13,17]

The second important point is that, unlike idiopathic disease, the prognostic information provided by biopsy in connective tissue disorders may be only marginally additive. In systemic sclerosis, for example, survival appears not to be influenced significantly by histological findings (and thus, presumably, HRCT appearances), once baseline disease severity and serial physiological trends are accounted for.[17] This was elegantly demonstrated in the study by Bouros et al. in which 5-year survival did not differ significantly between patients with biopsy-proven NSIP and with UIP or 'end-stage' lung (91% versus 82%, respectively).[17] Indeed, in this study, a poor outcome was associated with a lower Dlco level and forced vital capacity at presentation. Furthermore, mortality in patients with a pattern of NSIP was linked to a lower initial Dlco, together with a serial decline in Dlco over 3 years and a higher eosinophil count in bronchoalveolar lavage fluid.[17] An earlier study, from a different institution, also showed the potentially important prognostic influence of Dlco levels, with a value at or below 40% predicted to be associated with a cumulative 5-year survival of under 10% in contrast to a survival above 75% at 5 years for levels above 40% predicted.[76] Interestingly,

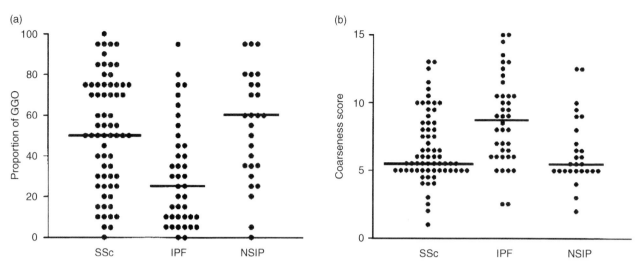

Figure 8.2
Scattergram plot comparing (a) the proportion of ground-glass opacification (GGO) and (b) the coarseness of fibrosis between patients with systemic sclerosis (SSc), idiopathic pulmonary fibrosis (IPF), and non-specific interstitial pneumonia (NSIP). There is no statistically seginificant difference between the proportions of ground-glass opacification and the coarseness of fibrosis between SSc and idiopathic NSIP. Reproduced with permission from Desai SR et al.[66] and the Radiological Society of North America.

this study also showed that some patients had an obstructive physiological defect and that this too was linked with increased mortality.

A small but important caveat to the discussion above is worth mentioning, since it would appear that the histological pattern of UIP has a better outcome when found in the context of a connective tissue disease than it has in patients with idiopathic disease. The suggestion is that this may be related to the lower profusion of fibroblastic foci in the UIP pattern associated with connective tissue disorders.[77] In their study of 108 patients, Flaherty et al. showed that during a median follow-up of 3.5 years, no deaths were recorded in the patients with connective tissue disease-associated UIP. This contrasted sharply with the 52 deaths in subjects with idiopathic disease.[77] Histological evaluation showed that the profusion of fibroblastic foci (a readily identifiable lesion denoting ongoing epithelial injury that leads to fibrosis) was higher in idiopathic UIP, even though the extent of fibrosis, as judged by HRCT, was not significantly different. Indeed, the profusion of fibroblastic foci was the key discriminative feature between idiopathic and connective tissue disease-related UIP.[77] An intriguing question (which was not formally tested) that arises from this study is whether, despite the similar extents of fibrosis, there are morphological differences (for example, the severity of honeycombing, the presence and/or severity of traction bronchiectasis) between idiopathic and connective tissue disease-associated UIP. Whilst it is not possible to draw firm conclusions because of the limited number of patients (99 patients with idiopathic UIP versus only nine with

connective tissue disease), these data do provide an insight into the possible different pathogenetic mechanisms and prognosis associated with the lung fibrosis in patients with idiopathic disease and connective tissue disorders.

It is also worth stating that in patients with idiopathic disease, CT features may modulate the information provided by biopsy.[78] Indeed, the prognostic evaluation may even be modified since a biopsy diagnosis of UIP with a discordant NSIP diagnosis on HRCT is associated with a better outcome than when both pathology and HRCT indicate a pattern of UIP.[78] However, as with the above discussion, there are no good data yet to suggest that this can be readily extrapolated to connective tissue disorders. In systemic sclerosis, the HRCT appearances of lung disease which, on average, are more like those of idiopathic NSIP (but may range from predominant and potentially treatable ground-glass attenuation to a predominant reticular pattern), do not necessarily translate into differences in survival which is in contrast to the situation with the idiopathic interstitial pneumonias.[79] Survival data, in relation to HRCT pattern, may subsequently emerge in larger series of other connective tissue disorders. However, given the predominance of NSIP in most connective tissue disorders, it appears unlikely that the HRCT subclassification of fibrotic disease will prove to be of any major prognostic significance. Even in rheumatoid arthritis, where the prevalence of the UIP pattern may be higher than in other connective tissue disorders, there is the confusion engendered by the finding that a UIP-like appearance on HRCT may be associated with NSIP histology.[72]

When and in whom should treatment be started?

Decisions regarding treatment are complex and unlikely to be made by the physician on the basis of clinical features, physiological indices, or radiological findings in isolation. However, on occasion, the HRCT findings may have some practical value. Based on HRCT signs, it is possible to recognize (albeit in relatively broad terms), the morphological caricatures of lung disease in individual connective tissue disorders. This exercise may have therapeutic implications in small subgroups of patients. In systemic sclerosis, for example, where the NSIP pattern predominates, there is bilateral ground-glass opacification with variable proportions of a reticular pattern and traction bronchiectasis[66] (Figure 8.3). In polymyositis/dermatomyositis features of organizing pneumonia (subpleural or bronchocentric foci of consolidation and ground-glass opacification, sometimes associated with signs of fibrosis) are the classical finding[80] (Figure 8.4). In patients with rheumatoid arthritis, HRCT findings more often reflect a pattern of UIP (a subpleural and basal reticular pattern with honeycombing) and less often the features of NSIP and organizing pneumonia.[72]

It will have been noted by the reader that the above argument is only applicable to patients with 'typical' HRCT findings. Clearly, a significant minority will not have the characteristic CT appearances and may also include patients with potentially reversible disease. For instance,

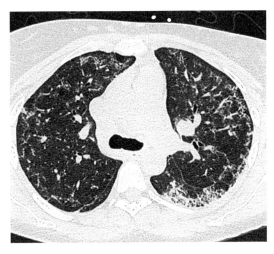

Figure 8.4
Organizing pneumonia in polymyositis. There are sub-pleural foci of consolidation but there is associated CT evidence of a reticular pattern suggesting admixed fibrosis.

ground-glass opacification on CT that is not associated with ancillary signs of fibrosis (i.e. parenchymal distortion, traction bronchiectasis, and an admixed reticular pattern) may indeed indicate treatable pathology.[81–83] In contrast, ground-glass opacification that has the above ancillary features is likely to indicate fine fibrosis below the limits of HRCT resolution. Pure ground-glass is a feature of lymphocytic interstitial pneumonia (which occurs most commonly in the context of Sjögren's syndrome and rheumatoid arthritis) or organizing pneumonia (typically present in rheumatoid arthritis and polymyositis and dermatomyositis), both of which may be responsive to treatment.

Another point that is worth mentioning (perhaps more relevant to the radiologist) is that when appearances are not typical of the known HRCT profile of an individual connective tissue disease, other differential diagnoses should be considered. Drug-induced lung disease, opportunistic infection because of immunocompromise, malignancy, and the plethora of vasculocentric and bronchocentric abnormalities generally seen with connective tissue disorders and specifically in rheumatoid arthritis should, where appropriate, always be considered in the differential diagnosis. Thus, the key message for the physician is that when HRCT findings are atypical, biopsy confirmation may become mandatory.

Whilst HRCT may guide treatment, it must again be stressed that the numbers of patients to whom this applies will be relatively small. The physician must therefore base treatment decisions on what is essentially traditional clinical evaluation. Such an assessment will take account of a number of factors. However, the physician will generally consider treatment if systemic disease has been present for under 5 years, when disease is considered severe on the basis of functional tests or HRCT estimates of the extent of disease

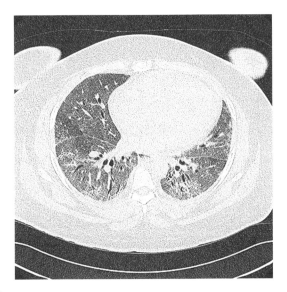

Figure 8.3
CT in a patient with systemic sclerosis and a pattern of fibrosis suggestive of non-specific interstitial pneumonia. There is predominant ground-glass opacification but there is a superimposed, more limited reticular pattern (without honeycombing). Dilatation of segmental and subsegmental airways (traction bronchiectasis) is also present.

or where there is symptomatic, radiographic, or functional evidence of recent deterioration. On this last point it is worth noting that in systemic sclerosis the onset of deterioration whilst on treatment may be a better indicator of prognosis than any other clinical feature at presentation.[17]

Can lung disease be monitored accurately?

Pulmonary function tests have traditionally been used to identify changes in disease severity. It has long been regarded as axiomatic that changes in pulmonary function tests are more reliable than changes in symptoms or chest radiography in reflecting the histological evolution of interstitial lung disease. Recently, serial pulmonary function tests have been more predictive of subsequent mortality in patients with fibrotic idiopathic interstitial pneumonia (i.e. IPF or fibrotic NSIP) than any baseline feature, including the histological diagnosis.[84] Serial chest radiography is notoriously insensitive to change, when compared with serial pulmonary function tests, based upon widespread anecdotal experience, although this question has not been formally addressed.

It might be expected that serial HRCT would add usefully to monitoring as it has the potential to detect relatively minor evolution of disease. However, herein lies the problem in that HRCT is sometimes too sensitive. In IPF, and in idiopathic fibrotic NSIP to a lesser extent, deterioration is expected and demonstration of subtle change on HRCT is not necessarily clinically useful. Strikingly, in a combined population of IPF and NSIP, serial change in pulmonary function indices were predictive of mortality whereas serial HRCT change was not.[85] Thus, it is clear that serial HRCT should not be performed by protocol, in the uncritical belief that it must necessarily inform prognostic evaluation.

However, in the absence of hard data, there is a growing consensus that monitoring the evolution of disease on HRCT is useful in carefully selected scenarios. First, pulmonary function changes are often marginal and difficult to interpret in individual cases. In connective tissue disorders, it is usually possible to limit disease progression with vigorous treatment unless disease is advanced. Therefore, it is often more important than in idiopathic disease to ascertain whether a marginal decline in Dlco, for example, represents progression of underlying pulmonary fibrosis. Crucial treatment decisions may depend upon this information. It should be understood that serial HRCT evaluation might be inconclusive. However, in other cases, it is obvious that there is real progression of disease on HRCT which is understated by a marginal decline in pulmonary function tests.

Second, serial imaging may also be helpful when there is an unexpectedly severe decline, based upon pulmonary function tests, symptoms, and chest radiography, particularly in the setting of connective tissue disease. In IPF, 'accelerated decline' is not uncommon and aggressive therapy at this point is seldom successful. By contrast, in connective tissue disorders a rapid functional deterioration due to diffuse alveolar damage is recognized but relatively infrequent (except in early polymyositis/dermatomyositis) and an alternative explanation should always be sought. Concurrent pulmonary vascular disease (due to pulmonary thromboembolism or an ablative vasculopathy), cardiac failure, opportunistic infection, drug-induced lung disease, and autoimmune alveolar hemorrhage are all variably treatable alternative causes of major reductions in pulmonary function tests. However, the differential diagnosis is especially difficult when there is a background of pulmonary fibrosis. Serial HRCT evaluation has two distinct roles in this context. The absence of major radiological change is useful, in the setting of a marked reduction in gas transfer, because this serves to identify occult pulmonary vascular disease as the likely culprit. By contrast, when HRCT change is marked, the pattern of change may serve to refine the above differential diagnoses, or, at least, to modify diagnostic likelihoods, guiding the clinician as to the next appropriate test or intervention.

In summary, serial HRCT evaluation is highly useful in selected scenarios, but should be applied case by case, and reserved for patients in whom important clinical dilemmas persist after routine serial evaluation.

Conclusions

The evaluation of patients with lung disease related to connective tissue disorders is a difficult undertaking, since the physician must contend with the vexing issues of disease detection, evaluating its significance, when best to treat, and, finally, how best to monitor progress. In this regard, it is clear that there is no single 'best' approach or test. HRCT is probably the most sensitive non-invasive test for the detection of lung disease and a histospecific diagnosis can sometimes be made. Evaluation of the significance of lung involvement (particularly when this is limited in extent) is more difficult on the basis of findings at HRCT. It is not yet clear whether the prognostic data relating to the idiopathic interstitial pneumonias can be readily extrapolated to the same patterns of lung disease when seen in the context of connective tissue disorders. Similarly, treatment decisions in individual patients are likely to be made on the basis of all available clinical information (functional, pathological, and imaging). However, because certain patterns on CT are considered to indicate potentially 'reversible' pathology, treatment may be instituted on occasion when further clinical data are either unhelpful or unlikely to be forthcoming. Finally, it seems likely that HRCT will have a role in the follow-up of patients (treated or otherwise) with established lung disease particularly when there is evidence of unexpectedly marked decline.

References

1. Colby TV, Carrington CB. Interstitial lung disease. In: Thurlbeck WM, Churg AM, eds. Pathology of the Lung, 2nd edn. New York: Thieme Medical Publishers, 1995: 589–737.

2. Travis WD, Colby TV, Koss MN et al. Connective tissue and inflammatory bowel disorders. In: Travis WD, Colby TV, Koss MN et al. eds. Non-neoplastic Disorders of the Lower Respiratory Tract, 1st edn. Washington DC: American Registry of Pathology and the Armed Forces Institute of Pathology, 2002: 291–320.

3. King TE Jr, Costabel U, Cordier JF et al. Idiopathic pulmonary fibrosis: diagnosis and treatment. International consensus statement. Am J Respir Crit Care Med 2000; 161: 646–64.

4. Travis WD, King TE Jr, and the Multidisciplinary Core Panel. American Thoracic Society/European Respiratory Society international multidiscplinary consensus classification of idiopathic interstitial pneumonias. Am J Respir Crit Care Med 2002; 165: 277–304.

5. Subcommittee for scleroderma criteria of the American Rheumatism Association Diagnostic and Therapeutic Criteria Committee. Preliminary criteria for the classification of systemic sclerosis (scleroderma). Arthritis Rheum 1980; 23: 581–90.

6. Wallaert B, Hatron P-Y, Grosbois J-M et al. Subclinical pulmonary involvement in collagen-vascular disease assessed by bronchovascular lavage: relationship between alveolitis and subsequent changes in lung function. Am Rev Respir Dis 1986; 133: 574–80.

7. Gilligan DM, O'Connor CM, Ward K et al. Bronchoalveolar lavage in patients with mild and severe rheumatoid lung disease. Thorax 1990; 45: 591–6.

8. Minai OA, Dweik RA, Arroglia A. Manifestations of scleroderma pulmonary disease. Clin Chest Med 1998; 19: 713–31.

9. Cervantes-Perez C, Toro-Perez AH, Rodriguez-Jurado P. Pulmonary involvement in rheumatoid arthritis. JAMA 1980; 243: 1715–9.

10. Walker WC, Wright V. Pulmonary lesions and rheumatoid arthritis. Medicine 1968; 47: 501–20.

11. Hyland RH, Gordon DA, Broder I et al. A systematic controlled study of pulmonary abnormalities in rheumatoid arthritis. J Rheumatol 1983; 10: 395–405.

12. Schwarz MI. The lung in polymyositis. Clin Chest Med 1998; 19: 701–12.

13. Douglas WW, Tazelaar HD, Hartman TE et al. Polymyositis-dermatomyositis-associated interstitial lung disease. Am J Respir Crit Care Med 2001; 164: 1182–5.

14. Eisenberg H, Dubois EL, Sherwin RP, Balchum OJ. Diffuse interstitial lung disease in systemic lupus erythematosus. Ann Intern Med 1973; 79: 37–45.

15. Fenlon HM, Doran M, Sant SM, Breatnach E. High-resolution chest CT in systemic lupus erythematosus. AJR Am J Roentgenol 1996; 166: 301–7.

16. Hunninghake GW, Fauci AS. Pulmonary involvement in the collagen vascular diseases. Am Rev Respir Dis 1979; 119: 471–503.

17. Bouros D, Wells AU, Nicholson AG et al. Histopathologic subsets of fibrosing alveolitis in patients with systemic sclerosis and their relationship to outcome. Am J Respir Crit Care Med 2002; 165: 1581–6.

18. Yousem SA, Colby TV, Carrington CB. Lung biopsy in rheumatoid arthritis. Am Rev Respir Dis 1985; 131: 770–7.

19. Geddes DM, Webley M, Emerson PA. Airway obstruction in rheumatoid arthritis. Ann Rheum Dis 1979; 38: 222–5.

20. Bégin R, Massé S, Cantin A, Ménard H-A, Bureau M-A. Airway disease in a subset of non-smoking rheumatoid patients: characterization of the disease and evidence for an autoimmune pathogenesis. Am J Med 1982; 72: 743–50.

21. Collins RL, Turner RA, Johnson AM, Whitley NO, McLean RL. Obstructive pulmonary disease in rheumatoid arthritis. Arthritis Rheum 1976; 19: 623–8.

22. Homma S, Kawabata M, Kishi K et al. Diffuse panbronchiolitis in rheumatoid arthritis. Eur Respir J 1998; 12: 444–52.

23. Newball HH, Brahim SA. Chronic obstructive airway disease in patients with Sjögren's syndrome. Am Rev Respir Dis 1977; 115: 295–304.

24. Franquet T, Díaz C, Domingo P, Giménez A, Geli C. Air trapping in primary Sjögren syndrome: correlation of expiratory CT with pulmonary function tests. J Comput Assist Tomogr 1999; 23: 169–73.

25. Winterbauer RH, Wilske KR, Wheelis RF. Diffuse pulmonary injury associated with gold treatment. N Engl J Med 1976; 294: 919–21.

26. Dayton CS, Schwartz DA, Sprince NL et al. Low-dose methotrexate may cause air trapping in patients with rheumatoid arthritis. Am J Respir Crit Care Med 1995; 151: 1189–93.

27. Piper WN, Helwig EB. Progressive systemic sclerosis: visceral manifestations in generalised scleroderma. Am Med Assoc Arch Dermatol 1955; 72: 535–46.

28. Silver RM, Miller KS. Lung involvement in systemic sclerosis. Rheum Dis Clin North Am 1990; 16: 199–216.

29. Hayakawa H, Sato A, Imokawa S et al. Bronchiolar disease in rheumatoid arthritis. Am J Respir Crit Care Med 1996; 154: 1531–6.

30. Kasukawa R. Pulmonary hypertension in connective tissue disease. Intern Med 1996 Jan; 35: 1–2.

31. Palevsky HI, Gurughagavatula I. Pulmonary hypertension in collagen vascular disease. Compr Ther 1999 Mar; 25: 133–43.

32. Fagan KA, Badesch DB. Pulmonary hypertension associated with connective tissue disease. Prog Cardiovasc Dis 2002 Nov; 45: 225–34.

33. Hoeper MM. Pulmonary hypertension in collagen vascular disease. Eur Respir J 2002 Mar; 19: 571–6.

34. Tanoue LT. Pulmonary hypertension in the collagen vascular diseases. Semin Respir Crit Care Med 2003 Jun; 24: 287–96.

35. Mukerjee D, George D, Knight C et al. Echocardiography and pulmonary function as screening tests for pulmonary arterial hypertension in systemic sclerosis. Rheumatology 2004; 43: 461–6.

36. Owens GR, Paradis IL, Gryzan S et al. Role of inflammation in the lung disease of systemic sclerosis: comparison with idiopathic pulmonary fibrosis. J Lab Clin Med 1986; 107: 253–60.

37. Witt C, Dorner T, Hiepe F et al. Diagnosis of alveolitis in interstitial lung manifestation in connective tissue diseases: importance of late inspiratory crackles, 67 gallium scan and bronchoalveolar lavage. Lupus 1996 Dec; 5: 606–12.

38. Spertini F, Aubert JD, Leimgruber A. The potential of bronchoalveolar lavage in the prognosis and treatment of connective-vascular diseases. Clin Exp Rheumatol 1996 Nov; 14: 681–8.

39. Behr J, Vogelmeier C, Beinert T et al. Bronchoalveolar lavage for evaluation and management of scleroderma disease of the lung. Am J Respir Crit Care Med 1996; 154: 400–6.

40. Manganelli P, Salaffi F, Pesci A. Clinical and subclinical alveolitis in connective tissue diseases assessed by bronchoalveolar lavage. Semin Arthritis Rheum 1997 Apr; 26: 740–54.

41. Witt C, Borges AC, John M et al. Pulmonary involvement in diffuse cutaneous systemic sclerosis: broncheoalveolar fluid granulocytosis predicts progression of fibrosing alveolitis. Ann Rheum Dis 1999 Oct 1; 58: 635–40.

42. De Clerck LS, Meijers KA, Cats A. Is MCTD a distinct entity? Comparison of clinical and laboratory findings in MCTD, SLE, PSS, and RA patients. Clin Rheumatol 1989 Mar; 8: 29–36.

43. Miyata M, Kida S, Kanno T et al. Pulmonary hypertension in MCTD: report of two cases with anticardiolipin antibody. Clin Rheumatol 1992 Jun; 11: 195–201.

44. Lee SL, Tsay GJ, Tsai RT. Anticentromere antibodies in subjects with no apparent connective tissue disease. Ann Rheum Dis 1993 Aug; 52: 586–9.

45. Friedman AW, Targoff IN, Arnett FC. Interstitial lung disease with autoantibodies against aminoacyl-tRNA synthetases in the absence of clinically apparent myositis. Semin Arthritis Rheum 1996 Aug; 26: 459–67.

46. Ihn H, Yamane K, Yazawa N et al. Distribution and antigen specificity of anti-U1RNP antibodies in patients with systemic sclerosis. Clin Exp Immunol 1999 Aug; 117: 383–7.

47. Ho KT, Reveille JD. The clinical relevance of autoantibodies in scleroderma. Arthritis Res Ther 2003; 5: 80–93.

48. Gabbay E, Tarala R, Will R et al. Interstitial lung disease in recent onset rheumatoid arthritis. Am J Respir Crit Care Med 1997; 156: 528–35.

49. Kon OM, Daniil Z, Black CM, du Bois RM. Clearance of inhaled technetium-99m-DTPA as a clinical index of pulmonary vascular disease in systemic sclerosis. Eur Respir J 1999 Jan 1; 13: 133–6.

50. Kaushik VV, Lynch MP, Dawson JK et al. Tc-DTPA clearance and rheumatoid arthritis-associated fibrosing alveolitis. Rheumatology 2002 Jun 1; 41: 712–3.

51. Okudan B, Sahin M, Ozbek FM, Keskin AU, Cure E. Detection of alveolar epithelial injury by Tc-99m DTPA radioaerosol inhalation lung scan in rheumatoid arthritis patients. Ann Nucl Med 2005; 19: 455–60.

52. Epler GR, McLoud TC, Gaensler EA, Mikus JP, Carrington CB. Normal chest roentgenograms in chronic diffuse infiltrative lung disease. N Engl J Med 1978; 298: 934–9.

53. Mathieson JR, Mayo JR, Staples CA, Müller NL. Chronic diffuse infiltrative lung disease: comparison of diagnostic accuracy of CT and chest radiography. Radiology 1989; 171: 111–6.

54. Garland LH, Cochrane AL. Results of an international test in chest roentgenogram interpretation. JAMA 1952; 149: 631–4.

55. Garland LH. Studies on the accuracy of diagnostic procedures. Am J Roentgenol Radium Ther Nucl Med 1959; 82: 25–38.

56. Tuddenham WJ. Problems in perception in chest roentgenology: facts and fallacies. Radiol Clin North Am 1963; 1: 277–89.

57. Harrison NK, Myers AR, Corrin B et al. Structural features of interstitial lung disease in systemic sclerosis. Am Rev Respir Dis 1991; 144: 706–13.

58. Warrick JH, Bhalla M, Schabel SI, Silver RM. High resolution computed tomography in early scleroderma lung disease. J Rheumatol 1991; 18: 1520–8.

59. Hassen Zrour S, Touzi M, Bejia I et al. Correlations between high-resolution computed tomography of the chest and clinical function in patients with rheumatoid arthritis: Prospective study in 75 patients. Joint Bone Spine 2005 Jan; 72: 41–7.

60. Bankier AA, Kiener HP, Wiesmayr MN et al. Discrete lung involvement in systemic lupus erythematosus: CT assessment. Radiology 1995 Sep 1; 196: 835–40.

61. Souza AS Jr, Müller NL, Marchiori E, Soares-Souza LV, de Souza Rocha M. Pulmonary abnormalities in ankylosing spondylitis: inspiratory and expiratory high-resolution CT findings in 17 patients. J Thorac Imaging 2004; 19: 259–63.

62. Ayhan-Ardic FF, Oken O, Yorgancioglu ZR, Ustan N, Gokharman FD. Pulmonary involvement in lifelong non-smoking patients with rheumatoid arthritis and ankylosing spondylitis without respiratory symptoms. Clin Rheumatol 2006; 25: 213–8.

63. Uffmann M, Keiner HP, Bankier AA et al. Lung manifestations in asymptomatic patients with primary Sjögren syndrome: assessment with high resolution CT and pulmonary function tests. J Thorac Imaging 2001; 16: 282–9.

64. Cervantes-Perez P, Toro-Perez AH, Rodriguez-Jurado P. Pulmonary involvement in rheumatoid arthritis. JAMA 1980; 243: 1715–9.

65. Dawson JK, Fewins HE, Desmond J et al. Fibrosing alveolitis in patients with rheumatoid arthritis as assessed by high resolution computed tomography, chest radiography, and pulmonary function tests. Thorax 2001; 56: 622–7.

66. Desai SR, Veeraraghavan S, Hansell DM et al. CT features of lung disease in systemic sclerosis: comparison with idiopathic pulmonary fibrosis and non-specific interstitial pneumonia. Radiology 2004; 232: 560–7.

67. Wells AU, Hansell DM, Rubens MB et al. Fibrosing alveolitis in systemic sclerosis: indices of lung function in relation to extent of disease on computed tomography. Arthritis Rheum 1997; 40: 1229–36.

68. Desai SR, Wells AU. Pulmonary manifestations of collagen vascular disorders. Eur Respir Monogr 2004; 30: 176–94.

69. Daniil ZD, Gilchrist FC, Nicholson AG et al. A histologic pattern of nonspecific interstitial pneumonia is associated with a better prognosis than usual interstital pneumonia in patients with cryptogenic fibrosing alveolitis. Am J Respir Crit Care Med 1999; 160: 899–905.

70. Bjoraker JA, Ryu JH, Edwin MK et al. Prognostic significance of histopathologic subsets in idiopathic pulmonary fibrosis. Am J Respir Crit Care Med 1998; 157: 199–203.

71. Nicholson AG, Colby TV, du Bois RM, Hansell DM, Wells AU. The prognostic significance of the histologic pattern of interstitial pneumonia in patients with the clinical entity of cryptogenic fibrosing alveolitis. Am J Respir Crit Care Med 2000; 162: 2213–7.

72. Tanaka N, Kim JS, Newell JD et al. Rheumatoid arthritis-related lung diseases: CT findings. Radiology 2004; 232: 81–91.

73. Lee HK, Kim DS, Yoo B et al. Histopathologic pattern and clinical features of rheumatoid arthritis-associated interstitial lung disease. Chest 2005 Jun 1; 127: 2019–27.

74. Flaherty KR, Travis WD, Colby TV et al. Histopathologic variability in usual and nonspecific interstitial pneumonias. Am J Respir Crit Care Med 2001 Nov 1; 164: 1722–7.

75. Flaherty KR, Toews GB, Travis WD et al. Clinical significance of histological classification of idiopathic interstitial pneumonia. Eur Respir J 2002 Feb; 19: 275–83.

76. Peters-Golden M, Wise RA, Hochberg MC, Stevens MB, Wigley FM. Carbon monoxide diffusing capacity as a predictor of outcome in systemic sclerosis. Am J Med 1984; 77: 1027–34.

77. Flaherty KR, Colby TV, Travis WD et al. Fibroblastic foci in usual interstitial pneumonia: idiopathic versus collagen vascular disease. Am J Respir Crit Care Med 2003; 167: 1410–5.

78. Flaherty KR, Thwaite EL, Kazerooni EA et al. Radiological versus histological diagnosis in UIP and NSIP: survival implications. Thorax 2003 Feb; 58: 143–8.

79. Wells AU, Hansell DM, Rubens MB et al. The predictive value of appearances on thin-section computed tomography in fibrosing alveolitis. Am Rev Respir Dis 1993; 148: 1076–82.

80. Ikezoe J, Johkoh T, Kohno N et al. High-resolution CT findings of lung disease in patients with polymyositis and dermatomyositis. J Thorac Imaging 1996; 11: 250–9.

81. Wells AU, Hansell DM, Corrin B et al. High resolution computed tomography as a predictor of lung histology in systemic sclerosis. Thorax 1992; 47: 738–42.

82. Remy-Jardin M, Giraud F, Remy J et al. Importance of ground-glass attenuation in chronic diffuse infiltrative lung disease: pathologic-CT correlation. Radiology 1993; 189: 693–8.

83. Collins J, Stern EJ. Ground-glass opacity at CT: the ABCs. AJR Am J Roentgenol 1997; 355–67.

84. Latsi PI, du Bois RM, Nicholson AG et al. Fibrotic idiopathic interstitial pneumonia: the prognostic value of longitudinal functional trends. Am J Respir Crit Care Med 2003 Sep 1; 168: 531–7.

85. Flaherty KR, Mumford JA, Murray S et al. Prognostic implications of physiologic and radiographic changes in idiopathic interstitial pneumonia. Am J Respir Crit Care Med 2003 Sep 1; 168: 543–8.

9

Immunologic diseases (other than asthma)

Alexander Bankier and Leopold Stiebellehner

Introduction

Immunological lung disorders other than asthma constitute a heterogeneous group of disorders. Most of which are of unknown origin. Their clinical and radiological manifestations, however, are surprisingly variable. Moreover, these manifestations can overlap, and the resulting diagnostic ambiguities often pose problems in a routine clinical context.

The aim of this chapter is to discuss the most common pathological entities belonging to this group, with an emphasis on either congruence or disparity of clinical and radiological findings, and to improve clinical decision-making.

Diagnostic clinical approach to immunological lung diseases

The patient with suspected immunological lung disease presents a formidable diagnostic challenge to physicians and an organized approach is critical. In general all patients should have an extensive history taken and undergo physical examination and laboratory and pulmonary function testing. However, confirming whether a patient with an immunological disease has lung involvement may be problematic for the physician.

What is the role of imaging in the diagnosis of immunological lung diseases?

Imaging tests are central to the investigation of patients with suspected immunological lung disease. The standard chest radiograph still remains the

Conventional chest radiographs

Radiographic studies primarily consist of chest radiography and/or computed tomography (CT). The conventional chest radiograph is usually the first radiological test to be requested by a physician. Radiographic imaging can provide initial diagnostic clues in evaluating immunological lung diseases. Various radiographic patterns may be diagnostic when supported by the clinical presentation, for example, multiple cavitary pulmonary nodules or masses in a middle-aged patient with upper airway disease (severe sinusitis), fever, and hemoptysis represent a combination of findings highly suggestive of Wegener's disease.

The chest radiograph is also helpful in following the course of a long-term illness and evaluating the patient's response to therapy.

Computerized tomography scan

Chest CT is useful in patients who have respiratory symptoms but normal or questionable radiographic findings. It is more sensitive than conventional chest radiography in those patients who present with hemoptysis and, particularly, for pulmonary vasculitis where the prevalence of lung disease is known to be relatively high. It may be helpful in the assessment of subtle parenchymal abnormalities not visible on conventional radiographic studies such as localized or diffuse alveolar infiltrates, bronchial and peribronchial involvement, and small pleural effusions.

Wegener's granulomatosis
Epidemiological and clinical features

The etiology of Wegener's granulomatosis (WG) is unknown. Its prevalence is 3 : 100 000 in the US. WG can occur at any age; however, the mean age at diagnosis is currently between 40 and 55 years. Men and women are equally affected, but airway involvement is more frequent in women.

The most common clinical symptoms of WG are sinusitis, rhinitis, and otitis media. Other common clinical symptoms include perforation of the nasal septum, and voice changes that are often combined with stridor, hearing loss, vertigo, and chondritis. Respiratory manifestations of WG may include dyspnea, wheezing, hemoptysis, and chest pain. Renal symptoms can include proteinuria, microscopic hematuria, and an elevated serum creatinine level. Musculoskeletal manifestations include myalgias, joint pain, and joint swelling. Furthermore, conjunctivitis, scleritis, episcleritis, and the occurrence of orbital pseudotumors have been reported. The classical Wegener triad includes sinus, lung, and renal disease.[1] However, WG can affect any part of the body, and systemic involvement in the disease process is the rule rather than the exception.

In patients with WG circulating anti-neutrophil cytoplasmic antibody (cANCA) is usually directed against proteinase-3, an antigen found in neutrophils. Of patients with active WG 70–90% have positive cANCA. This finding strongly supports the diagnosis of WG. However, because of the high toxicity of medical therapy for WG, any definitive diagnosis should be based on biopsy specimen from paranasal sinuses, lung, or kidneys.[2]

Treatment and prognosis

The mean survival time without therapy is 5 months. With therapy, the mean survival at 24 months is 80%. The disease can relapse in up to 50%, and side-effects of medical therapy can occur in up to 42% of patients. The most common cause of death is renal failure.[2]

Medical therapy consists in the systemic administration of glucocorticoids and cyclophosphamide. Although these treatments are successful in most patients, they increase the risk of the occurrence of transitional cell carcinoma and myeloproliferative disorders.[1,2]

Imaging features

The most common plain radiographic manifestations of WG are single or multiple pulmonary nodules. The nodules can be either sharp or ill-defined, the latter suggesting surrounding hemorrhage. Up to 50% of the nodules and resulting masses can cavitate. These cavities are often thick walled. Rapid enlargement of the cavities on follow-up examinations suggests hemorrhage or superinfection. The nodules can be of variable sizes and show a tendency to coalesce. Solitary nodules are slightly more frequent than multiple nodules. Spontaneous regression of nodules has been reported. WG can also manifest as focal consolidation and as air space disease, which commonly results from either hemorrhage or infection. Peripheral airway stenosis can result in segmental or lobar atelectasis. Subglottic stenosis can be present, but remains difficult to detect on plain radiographs. Pleural effusion occurs in 20% of patients. Pneumothorax and both hilar and mediastinal adenopathy are rare. Under therapy, a complete normalization of the radiographic alterations can occur within 2–6 weeks.[3]

On CT, the nodules can be solid or cavitated (Figure 9.1). Like metastases the nodules can have a feeding vessel. A wedge-shaped consolidation that arises from the nodules can result from peripheral infarction. Some nodules may display a halo sign caused by surrounding bleeding. Upper airway stenosis is far better detected by CT than by chest radiography. Furthermore, the trachea and bronchi can be concentrically thickened, with thickening being either focal or occupying longer airway segments.[4,5]

Differential diagnosis

The main radiological determination is the differential diagnosis of WG from metastatic disease. Metastases from squamous cell carcinoma or sarcoma often cavitate and may resemble nodules seen in WG. In such cases, the presence of a potential malignancy must be excluded. Septic emboli and tuberculous lesions may also resemble the nodules seen in WG. In septic emboli, however, blood cultures will be positive for a given infectious agent, and the radiographic evolution of the nodules will be more rapid than in WG. Rheumatoid nodules may also cavitate and can therefore mimic WG. Such nodules will, however, be associated with a clinical history of joint disease. The largest group from

(a)

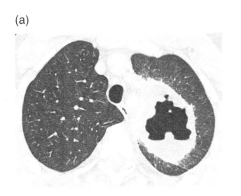

(b)

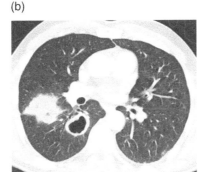

Figure 9.1
CT in a patient with Wegener's granulomatosis. CT shows both large and thick-walled cavitated nodules (a), and small cavitated nodules as well as consolidations (b). Despite their considerable size, the lesions regressed under therapy.

which a differential diagnosis should be made includes the pulmonary-renal syndromes. In microscopic polyangiitis no necrotizing granulomatous inflammation will be seen. In Churg–Strauss syndrome there will be peripheral blood eosinophilia and evidence of an antineutrophil cytoplasmic antibody vasculitis. In Goodpasture's syndrome there will be pulmonary hemorrhage, glomerulonephritis, and evidence of antiglomerular basement membrane antibodies. In polyarteritis nodosa lung involvement is less common than in WG, and there will be evidence of renal infarcts or other renal disorders. In systemic lupus erythematosus there will be evidence of antinuclear antibodies, and both pulmonary hemorrhage and serositis will prevail over pulmonary nodules. Finally, in lymphomatoid granulomatosis (B cell lymphoma) there often will be evidence of central or peripheral nerve involvement, and of skin disease.[1,2]

Imaging recommendations for the clinician

Most patients with suspected WG will inevitably undergo conventional radiography. The clinician should nevertheless be aware that this method is relatively insensitive in the detection of WG-associated disease in subtle or early cases. The conventional radiograph can, however, be helpful for ruling out other potential differential diagnoses. The much more sensitive CT is the imaging modality of choice. Not only can CT depict small parenchymal lesions, but also it allows direct visualization of the airways. A conventional CT protocol is usually sufficient to suggest the diagnosis. The administration of contrast material is not mandatory. If WG is suspected on the basis of the clinical presentation, it might be helpful to include the glottis into the anatomic area covered by CT to allow assessment of a potential subglottical involvement. Up-to-date multidetector CT scanners with acquisition of isotropic voxels also allow multiplanar reconstruction of the airways which might prove helpful in cases that remain ambiguous on transverse sections.

What the clinician wants to know from the radiologist

- Are the radiological findings suggestive of WG?
- Is there pure parenchymal involvement?
- Is there concomitant airway involvement?
- If yes, does this potentially require intervention (e.g. stent placement)?
- Is there evidence of complications, such as hemorrhage or infection?
- Is there evidence of alterations that may be prone to complications (e.g. large cavities that might be colonized by *Aspergillus* spp)?

- On follow-up examinations, what is the radiological rate of progression/regression of the disease?

What the radiologist wants to know from the clinician

- Are the clinical findings suggestive of WG?
- Which clinical and laboratory findings do or do not support the diagnostic suspicion of WG?
- Are there potential alternative diagnoses supported by the clinical presentation of the patient?
- Is the classical WG triad present?
- Are there clinical or laboratory findings suggestive of complications, such as hemorrhage or infection?
- For follow-up examinations, what is the clinical rate of progression/regression of the disease?

Eosinophilic pneumonia
Epidemiological and clinical features

Eosinophilic pneumonia (EP) occurs in an acute (AEP) and a chronic (CEP) form. For both AEP and CEP the exact etiology is unknown, but it is speculated that both diseases represent a hypersensitivity reaction to an unknown antigen. The prevalence of the disease is 1 : 1 000 000 in the US, with AEP being increased in military deployments. While AEP shows no gender predilection, CEP affects women twice as often as men. AEP occurs at all ages, however, CEP has a peak incidence in the fourth decade of life.

AEP presents with an acute onset including fever, shortness of breath, myalgias, and pleuritic chest pain. Hypoxemic respiratory failure may occur and can evolve to life-threatening levels of severity. The disease may be more common in smokers than in non-smokers. Peripheral eosinophilia can be absent, but there usually is a marked increase in eosinophils within the bronchoalveolar lavage fluid, with a relative rate exceeding 40%.

CEP has an insidious onset with fever, malaise, weight loss, dyspnea, and cough. Around 50% of patients with CEP also have asthmatic symptoms. Of patients with CEP 90% are non-smokers. Peripheral eosinophilia is evident in over 90% of patients, while the increase of eosinophils on bronchoalveolar lavage is less striking than in AEP.[6]

Treatment and prognosis

Both AEP and CEP are often misdiagnosed as pneumonia, given an 'apparent' response to antibiotic therapy. This can delay the diagnosis for months or even years. Both AEP and CEP, however, show a rapid response to corticosteroids, and usually there is rapid clearing of clinical and radiographic abnormalities within several days. Complete resolution should occur in no more than 7–10 days. Relapse of the disease is unusual in AEP, but commonly occurs in CEP.[6]

Imaging features

On chest radiographs AEP shows a combined alveolar and interstitial pattern, often with a lower lobe predominance. There is rapid progression of the radiographic abnormalities. Small pleural effusions tend to be common. AEP can then mimic pulmonary edema. The rapid resolution of abnormalities after administration of corticosteroids is typical. On CT bilateral and predominantly lower lobe ground-glass opacities can be seen. On thin sections these ground-glass opacities can be admixed with septal thickening, thereby producing a so-called 'crazy paving' pattern. There is smooth interlobar septal thickening and thickening of the bronchovascular bundles. Occasionally, localized areas of consolidation can be detected. Small nodules are comparatively rare, but small pleural effusions are common. Band-like opacities paralleling the chest wall and crossing pleural fissures are nearly pathognomonic of the disease.[6,7]

On chest radiographs, CEP manifests with bilateral, nonsegmental, homogeneous consolidations that show peripheral distribution and upper lobe predominance. In more advanced cases CEP may involve the entirety of one lung. The typical case of CEP is described as the 'photographic negative' of pulmonary edema. In the absence of treatment the radiographic abnormalities are usually persistent over time, but cases of transient and fleeting infiltrates have also been reported. When recurrent, the infiltrates are often seen in the same location of the lung. Pleural effusions are rare. Under therapy, the most peripheral infiltrates are usually the first ones to clear. As the peripheral areas clear, residual band-like opacities may be seen. With CT the strikingly peripheral infiltrates are detected more frequently than on conventional images (Figure 9.2). Infiltrates are often accompanied by ground-glass opacities, thereby giving rise to a halo sign. As in AEP, a 'crazy paving' pattern can be seen.[7,8]

Differential diagnosis

The most important group from which a differential diagnosis should be made is other eosinophilic lung diseases. In simple pulmonary eosinophilia (Löffler's syndrome) opacities are more often fleeting than persistent. Commonly, there is resolution within 1 month. Eosinophilic lung diseases due to specific causes can mimic AEP. The key to the correct diagnosis is the exclusion of potential causes, such as drugs, parasitic infection, fungal infection, and the hypereosinophilic syndrome. The Churg–Strauss syndrome may be radiographically indistinguishable from CEP, but is accompanied by systemic disease in most cases. Systemic manifestations of the syndrome that do not occur in CEP include gastrointestinal (pain, diarrhea, bleeding), cardiac (heart failure, pericarditis), renal (renal insufficiency), and musculoskeletal (arthralgias) symptoms.

In cryptogenic organizing pneumonia (COP), the peripheral localization of infiltrates may mimic CEP, but in COP the lower lung zones are more commonly affected. The manifestations of COP can also be centered around the bronchovascular bundles. Pulmonary infarcts show a peripheral distribution similar to CEP, but infarcts tend to be more subtle and less confluent than CEP. Moreover, they show a lower lobe predominance and are often wedge-shaped. Aspiration pneumonia occurs in gravity-dependent lung regions and is commonly associated with small airways disease that can manifest as a tree-in-bud pattern. Finally, diffuse pulmonary hemorrhage presents with diffuse pulmonary consolidations, but, unlike AEP and CEP, these consolidations tend to evolve into reticular interstitial patterns. A history of renal disease, and anemia and hemoptysis is common in such cases.[6–8]

Imaging recommendations for the clinician

Virtually all patients with suspected AEP or CEP will undergo conventional chest radiography. In combination with a typical history and evident radiographic manifestations, the presence of the disease can be strongly suggested. In such cases, AEP mimics pulmonary edema, and CEP

(a) 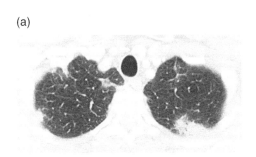   (b)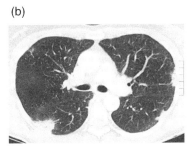

Figure 9.2
CT in a patient with chronic eosinophilic pneumonia. CT shows multiple consolidations with a strikingly peripheral distribution (a) and (b). Some of the consolidations show air bronchograms.

displays the 'photographic negative' of pulmonary edema. In milder or less typical cases, however, conventional radiography might not be sensitive enough for disease detection. In such cases, the clinician should promptly proceed to CT in order not to delay the diagnosis. CT will reveal subtle findings invisible on chest radiography and may serve as both a useful guide to further bronchoscopic evaluation and a sensitive documentation for follow-up. For CT the administration of contrast material is not required. The optimal approach is probably to acquire thin sections either sequentially or in a continuous manner, and in full suspended inspiration. Expiratory sections are of little diagnostic value. The review of multiple old films is often suggestive of the correct diagnosis.

What the clinician wants to know from the radiologist

- Are the radiographic and CT abnormalities suggestive of either AEP or CEP?
- Where are the abnormalities and how have they evolved?
- What is a good site for either bronchoalveolar lavage or biopsy?
- Are there signs of associated disease (e.g. asthma in CEP)?

What the radiologist wants to know from the clinician

- Are the clinical findings and the history compatible with either AEP or CEP?
- Are there other potential causes for eosinophilic lung disease, such as drugs, parasitic infections, or fungal infections?
- Is there a history of recent respiratory infection?

Diffuse alveolar hemorrhage

Epidemiological and clinical features

Diffuse alveolar hemorrhage encompasses a number of variable clinical syndromes that have diffuse alveolar hemorrhage (DAH) as a common manifestation. According to the differences between the syndromes, the epidemiological characteristics are also variable. Most commonly, the syndromes are classified according to the immune status of the individuals. In immunocompetence the syndromes included

are Goodpasture's syndrome (antibasement membrane antibody disease, ABMABD), WG, systemic lupus erythematosus (SLE) vasculitis, microscopic angiitis, and idiopathic pulmonary hemosiderosis (IPH). In immunosuppression the entities are bone marrow transplantation (BMT) and leukemia.[9]

The most common clinical signs and symptoms are cough, hemoptysis, and dyspnea. Many patients will suffer from iron-deficiency anemia. Of patients with microscopic polyangiitis 80% will be perinuclear (p)-ANCA positive, and 85–98% of patients with active WG will be c-ANCA positive. In patients with Goodpasture's syndrome or ABMABD symptoms may follow an influenza-like illness. In patients after BMT symptoms usually occur during the marrow engraftment period, i.e. 10–21 days after transplantation.

Treatment and prognosis

Immune complex diseases and inflammatory vasculitis are treated with immunosuppression and corticosteroids. Patients after BMT receive early instituted high dose corticosteroids. The 5-year survival in IPH averages 15 years. SLE with DAH has a mortality rate of 40–60%. In microscopic polyangiitis, the 5-year survival is about 70%. WG has a mortality rate of 80% if untreated, but up to 75% of patients will experience a complete remission during therapy.

Imaging features

The overall chest radiographic finding is the acute occurrence of bilateral, diffuse, or predominantly basilar consolidations in an anemic patient. With the persistence of bleeding, or the recurrence of episodes, reticular opacities and areas of fibrosis may develop. Patients with Goodpasture's syndrome, IPH, and microscopic polyangiitis show a substantial overlap of both clinical and imaging findings. The presence of antibasement membrane antibodies, the degree of renal involvement, and the patient's age can help to distinguish these entities. WG often manifests with multifocal peripheral consolidations or cavitating nodules. The capillaritis form of the disease predisposes to DAH, and pleural effusions and enlarged lymph nodes are uncommon in this manifestation. In SLE vasculitis, a triad of anemia, acute bilateral consolidations, and hemoptysis supports DAH, which occurs in 2% of all patients with SLE. The term 'lupus pneumonitis' is often used, but this term also comprises diffuse alveolar damage, infection, and the cellular variant of non-specific interstitial pneumonia. After BMT 20% of patients develop DAH, with the characteristic time course after engraftment. In leukemia extensive bilateral consolidations most often occur secondary to hemorrhage, with infection, edema, and leukemic involvement seen in decreasing order.

On CT, IPH, ABMABD, and microscopic angiitis manifest as extensive bilateral areas of ground-glass opacities and consolidations in an acute clinical setting (Figure 9.3). Sparing of the lung periphery and of the costophrenic angles is characteristic. Over the 48 hours following the acute event, intra- and interlobular thickening may appear, thereby producing a 'crazy-paving' pattern. The CT abnormalities should resolve over 7–14 days after the initial event, as hemorrhage is steadily removed by macrophages. Repeated episodes of hemorrhage, however, can lead to fibrosis, and small nodules, resulting in reticulations and ground-glass opacities. WG often shows cavitary nodules and multifocal areas of consolidation which extend to the periphery of the lung.[9]

Differential diagnosis

The differential diagnosis should be made from edema, infection, and other forms of hemorrhages. In cardiogenic edema there often is cardiomegaly. Opacities are bilateral and symmetric. There is evidence of pleural effusion and septal thickening. In non-cardiogenic edema, there is a diffuse distribution of ground-glass opacities and/or consolidations. Other than edema fluid, hemorrhage will not alter with changes in patient position. Infection is clinically accompanied by fever, chills, cough, and elevated white blood cell counts. Radiographic consolidations tend to be multifocal and asymmetric. Under therapy, most infections will resolve, and not evolve to reticular patterns.[9]

Imaging recommendations for the clinician

In a matching clinical context, chest radiography is commonly sufficient to document the evidence of pathology in the acute setting. However, CT is more sensitive than chest

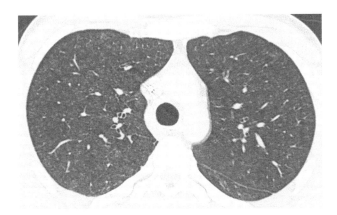

Figue 9.3
CT in a patient with diffuse alveolar hemorrhage. CT shows diffuse small, subtle, and ill-defined opacities, so-called 'air space' nodules.

radiography in detecting DAH and following its evolution from ground-glass opacities through consolidation and septal thickening up to potential lung fibrosis.

What the clinician wants to know from the radiologist

- Are the findings compatible with DAH?
- Is there evidence of other disease that might require further investigations?

What the radiologist wants to know from the clinician

- Are there clinical symptoms suggestive of DAH?
- Which entity is likely to have caused DAH?

Pulmonary amyloidosis
Epidemiological and clinical features

Pulmonary amyloidosis (PA) can be either primary or secondary. Primary PA is related to amyloid light chains and considered as AL-type. Secondary PA is related to amyloid A and alpha-globulin, and considered as AA-type. Primary PA is characterized by excessive deposition of protein secreted by B lymphocytes or plasma cells. Secondary PA is characterized by extracellular protein deposition caused by underlying chronic inflammatory diseases. According to its morphological and anatomical manifestations, PA is also classified into systemic and localized. Localized thoracic manifestations can be tracheobronchial, nodular, diffuse, lymphatic, and pleural.[10,11]

The clinical manifestations largely depend on the underlying form of PA. With the tracheobronchial form many patients are asymptomatic. Symptomatic patients will present with wheezing, dyspnea, hemoptysis, and recurrent pneumonia. The nodular form usually is asymptomatic, but can occasionally be accompanied by cough and hemoptysis. The diffuse form commonly manifests with dyspnea and respiratory insufficiency. Primary PA is also termed myeloma associated. Indeed, most patients with amyloid have a monoclonal spike. Conversely, less than 25% of patients with monoclonal gammopathy develop amyloidosis. On the other hand, 10% of patients with multiple myeloma develop amyloidosis. Secondary PA can follow inflammation (rheumatoid arthritis, cystic fibrosis, osteomyelitis, Crohn's disease), and malignancies (renal cell carcinoma, thyroid carcinoma, Hodgkin's disease). The so-called 'senile'

PA is asymptomatic in virtually all patients, and 90% of cases occur in patients over 90 years of age.[10,11]

Treatment and prognosis

The prognosis of the disease depends upon the underlying manifestation. For diffuse disease, the prognosis is poor, and survival averages 2 years. To date, there is no treatment for diffuse forms. In individual cases, surgical resection might be considered to alleviate symptoms of tracheo-bronchial obstruction. However, disease often recurs.

Imaging features

Like the clinical features, the radiological features of PA will largely depend upon the form of disease present in the individual patient. On conventional chest radiographs, the tracheobronchial form can manifest as focal or diffuse tracheal thickening. Subglottical manifestation of the disease is common, and multiple concentric or excentric strictures might be evident. Foci of calcification are seen in 30% of patients. In the pulmonary nodular form, single or multiple pulmonary nodules can be seen. Their size can range from 5 mm to 5 cm. Of these nodules 20% will be calcified. Growth of the nodules is very slow and therefore may require long follow-up periods to become detectable. The nodules are sharply defined, peripheral, round or lobulated. Cavitary nodules are exceedingly rare. In the diffuse form, miliary nodules with predominantly basal distribution are seen. In advanced disease, nodularity might evolve to a diffuse linear or reticular pattern that can be combined with honeycombing. If lymph nodes are affected, several anatomical stations of lymph nodes may become pathological. Nodules may calcify. Rarely are the heart and the pleura affected.[12,13]

On CT, tracheobronchial abnormalities such as airway wall thickening, intraluminal nodules, and submucosal foci of calcification are well delineated. Parenchymal abnormalities seen on CT include diffuse micronodular, reticulonodular, or linear patterns. Calcifications are seen in 20–50% of nodules. Rarely, these nodules may cavitate. Thickening of the bronchovascular bundles is seen more frequently than ground-glass opacities and honeycombing (Figure 9.4). Affected lymph nodes can display stippled, diffuse, or eggshell calcifications.[12,13]

Differential diagnosis

The main differential diagnosis for tracheobronchial amyloidosis is from primary benign and malignant tumors. These tumors are usually focal, but not diffuse. In tracheopathia osteochondroplastica nodules are located only along the anterior and lateral walls of the trachea, whereas amyloidosis is circumferential. In relapsing polychondritis usually no nodules are seen. In rhinoscleroma a positive culture for *Klebsiella* spp. may rule out PA. For the nodular form, the differential diagnosis encompasses the entire spectrum of benign and malignant pulmonary nodules. For the diffuse form, the differential diagnosis includes the entire spectrum of interstitial lung disease, and notably pulmonary fibrosis, cryptogenic organizing pneumonia, and remnants after drug toxicity. In diffuse lung calcification the differential diagnosis includes granulomatous infection, alveolar microlithiasis, metastatic calcification, silicosis, and sarcoidosis. In adenopathy the differential diagnosis includes lymphomas, sarcoidosis, tuberculosis, and metastases.[12,13]

Imaging recommendations for the clinician

The conventional chest radiograph is often sufficient to document the extent of thoracic involvement. In ambiguous or suspected cases, however, CT may be used. CT, and notably thin-section CT, is more sensitive in detecting tracheobronchial involvement, lymphadenopathy, the presence of calcifications, and subtle parenchymal abnormalities. The administration of contrast material is not mandatory. Expiratory CT sections can be helpful to confirm airway

(a)

(b)

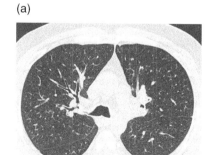
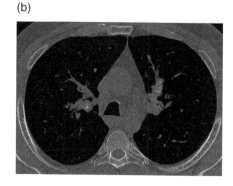

Figure 9.4
CT in a patient with pulmonary amyloidosis. On soft tissue window (a), bronchial narrowing and multiple bronchial stenoses with diffuse bronchial wall thickening is seen. On bone window (b) calcifications in proximity of the bronchial structures can be detected.

involvement in cases of distally located tracheobronchial amyloidosis.

What the clinician wants to know from the radiologist

- Is there any finding, alone or in combination, that might be suggestive of PA?
- Is the conventional chest radiograph sufficient to confirm the diagnosis, or should the patient proceed to CT?

What the radiologist wants to know from the clinician

- What is the clinical presentation of the patient?
- What are the clinical findings suggesting the presence of PA?
- In secondary cases, what is the underlying disease?

Hypersensitivity pneumonitis
Epidemiological and clinical features

The frequency of hypersensitivity pneumonitis (HP) is unknown, given that personal habits can substantially alter the appearance and course of the disease. In 95% of patients, HP occurs in non-smokers. The disease is an allergic reaction to airborne organic particles. More than 200 different organic antigens have been identified as potential causative agents for HP. There are acute, subacute, and chronic forms of the disease, with the three forms showing considerable overlap as to their clinical presentation.[14,15]

Acute HP often manifests as a flu-like syndrome with dyspnea, chest tightness, and dry or mildly productive cough. The peak intensity of symptoms is 3–6 hours after the exposure. If exposure is over, the symptoms may clear within 24–48 hours. In subacute and chronic forms, the clinical manifestations are indistinguishable from other forms of chronic inflammatory lung disease. Clinical symptoms often improve if exposure is avoided. Subtypes of HP are classified according to the origin of specific antigens. These subtypes include so-called farmer's lung, pigeon breeder's lung, humidifier lung, and mushroom lung.[16,17]

Treatment and prognosis

Treatment depends largely on avoiding the antigens responsible for the disease. Patients should be removed from any environment suspected to cause HP. Steroids may support healing after the removal of antigens. The prognosis of acute and subacute HP is good, provided that contacts with antigens are avoided. The prognosis of chronic HP is poor and similar to that of idiopathic pulmonary fibrosis.[14,15]

Imaging features

On conventional radiography, 90% of patients with acute HP have no abnormalities. In the remaining 10% of patients, a fine reticulonodular pattern can be seen. There may also be bilateral air space consolidation of the lower lobes that is commonly misdiagnosed as pneumonia. In subacute HP the radiograph will be abnormal in 90% of patients. Lung density is increased, and ill-defined nodules may be detected. Also, there may be an obscuration of vascular margins. In chronic HP, the key finding is fibrosis with volume loss and architectural distortion. The most common locations are the middle parts of the lungs. There is neither pleural disease nor adenopathy. The disease often spares the costophrenic angles.[14,15]

CT, and notably thin-section CT, is more sensitive than chest radiography for the detection of abnormalities. In acute HP small and ill-defined air space nodules are the most common finding. Bilateral air space consolidation may also occur and on chest radiographs, could be mistaken for pneumonia. In subacute HP ground-glass opacities in patchy distribution and ill-defined centrilobular nodules are the most common findings (Figure 9.5). Mosaic perfusion may create the so-called 'headcheese' sign. Lung cysts may occur. The disease has a middle and lower lung predominance. In chronic HP there is honeycombing, traction bronchiectasis, and architectural distortion. Reticular opacities may also be seen. The distribution is random, and both a peribronchiolar and a subpleural predominance has

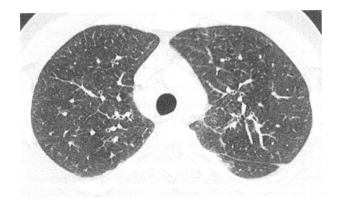

Figure 9.5
CT in a patient with hypersensitivity pneumonitis. CT shows subtle but diffuse ground-glass opacities in the upper parts of the lungs. These opacities are accompanied by subtle interstitial markings.

been described.[17] The disease dominates in the middle and upper lung. Often, the costophrenic angles are less severely affected.[15,16]

Differential diagnosis

The main differential diagnosis of HP is from idiopathic pulmonary fibrosis. Idiopathic pulmonary fibrosis, however, shows a typical anatomical distribution with the lung bases and the costophrenic angles being the zones the most severely affected. In non-specific interstitial pneumonia honeycombing is minimal or absent. Respiratory broncholitis occurs only in smokers, predominates in the upper lung zones, and is often associated with centrilobular emphysema. Sarcoidosis shows a peribronchiovascular distribution, and frequently there is adenopathy. In silicosis there is a history of professional exposure. Scleroderma often diplays a widened esophagus.[14–17]

Imaging recommendations for the clinician

In the acute phase conventional radiography is relatively insensitive in the detection of abnormalities. Thin-section CT is far more sensitive. Therefore, thin-section CT is not only the modality of choice for detecting patients with HP, but also for following the evolution of HP from ground-glass opacities to consolidation and, eventually, honeycombing suggestive of pulmonary fibrosis.

The correct diagnosis requires the constellation of clinical, radiographic, physiological, pathological, and immunological criteria. A high clinical index of suspicion must be maintained in clinically typical cases that occur after exposure to a known antigen. Patients with a histopathological diagnosis of non-specific interstitial pneumonia should always also be evaluated for HP.

What the clinician wants to know from the radiologist

- Is the chest radiograph normal?
- If not, are the findings suggestive of HP? When in the course of the disease should CT occur?
- What is an adequate site for lavage or biopsy?

What the radiologist wants to know from the clinician

- What is the clinical presentation?
- Is there a known antigen?
- Has there been previous allergic disease?

Allergic bronchopulmonary aspergillosis

Epidemiological and clinical features

Allergic bronchopulmonary aspergilosis (ABPA) is a hypersensitivity reaction to *Aspergillus fumigatus* that occurs after colonization of the bronchial tree. ABPA manifests with cough, sputum production, fever, and malaise. Sputum is commonly thickened and may contain aspergillus hyphae. A negative skin test with aspergillus antigen excludes the diagnosis of ABPA. The disease occurs in 1–2% of patients with asthma, and in up to 10% of patients with cystic fibrosis. ABPA is associated with peripheral blood eosinophilia, with cutaneous reactivity to *Aspergillus* spp. with an increased total serum IgE concentration, with serum precipitating antibodies to aspergillus antigens, and with increased serum antibodies of IgE and/or IgG. ABPA may be combined with cryptogenic organizing pneumonia and with chronic eosinophilic pneumonia.[18,19]

Treatment and prognosis

Of exacerbations 35% are asymptomatic, but may result in lung damage. Recurrent ABPA may result in widespread lung destruction, mainly manifested as fibrosis and bronchiectasis. Oral corticosteroids are the treatment of choice, but inhaled steroids show little to no effect. Addition of oral itraconazole to the steroid treatment may result in resolution of pulmonary consolidations and clinical symptoms. Patients with associated allergic fungal sinusitis may benefit from surgical resection of obstructing nasal polyps and inspissated mucus. Allergic fungal sinusitis may require endoscopic sinus surgery to improve drainage. Serial measurements of serum IgE levels have been shown to be useful in monitoring the response to therapy.[18,19]

Imaging features

Conventional radiography shows mucoid impaction. This manifests as tubular and sometimes finger-in-glove-like increased opacities with bronchial distribution. The opacities can also be Y-shaped. Central and predominantly cystic bronchiectases another common finding.[20,21]

On thin-section CT, bronchiectasis often affects multiple lobes. Bronchiectases can be either cystic or saccular, and represent ballooned bronchi that may contain air–fluid levels. Varicose bronchiectasis may have a bullous appearance, with dilated bronchi and interspersed constrictions. Lobulated masses, ground-glass opacities, and centrilobular lobules are less common findings.[20,21]

Differential diagnosis

Both bronchogenic carcinoma and bronchial carcinoids can manifest as bronchial lesions, both with and without air–fluid levels. In malignomas associated adenopathy is common, and there is no history of allergies or cystic fibrosis. Cystic fibrosis and other forms of bronchiectasis can be differentiated from ABPA by the different clinical presentation. Bronchial atresia may look very similar to ABPA, but the patients often show hyperinflation of the affected lung and have no history of allergies or cystic fibrosis. Onchocentric granulomatosis is a rare hypersensitivity lung disease that may be caused by *Aspergillus* spp. Radiographically the disease may be indistinguishable from ABPA. In suspected tuberculosis the presence of cavitary disease may be a clue to the correct diagnosis.[18,19,21]

Imaging recommendations for the clinician

Mucoid impaction and bronchiectasis, both with upper lobe predominance, in combination with an adequate clinical history, may be a clue to the diagnosis. In typical and advanced disease conventional chest radiograph might suffice to establish the diagnosis. Subtle findings will require CT. CT is also required in the follow-up of clinically ambiguous patients. Administration of contrast material and expiratory sections are not required.

What the clinician wants to know from the radiologist

- Are the findings suggestive of ABPA?
- What are other potential diagnoses?
- On follow-up, is there a progression of bronchiectasis or fibrosis?

What the radiologist wants to know from the clinician

- What is the clinical history of the patient?
- Is there evidence of cystic fibrosis or bronchiectasis?
- Was a sputum culture performed?
- Is eosinophilia present?
- Is there a positive skin test for aspergillus antigens?

References

1. DeRemee RA. Wegener's granulomatosis. Curr Opin Pulm Med 1995; 1: 363–7.
2. Hoffman GS, Kerr GS, Leavitt RY et al. Wegener granulomatosis: an analysis of 158 patients. Ann Intern Med 1992; 116: 488–98.
3. Aberle DR, Gamsu G, Lynch D. Thoracic manifestations of Wegener granulomatosis: diagnosis and course. Radiology 1990; 174: 703–9.
4. Screaton NJ, Sivasothy P, Flower CD, Lockwood CM. Tracheal involvement in Wegener's granulomatosis: evaluation using spiral CT. Clin Radiol 1998; 53: 809–15.
5. Daum TE, Specks U, Colby TV et al. Tracheobronchial involvement in Wegener's granulomatosis. Am J Respir Crit Care Med 1995; 151: 522–6.
6. Allen JN, Davis WB. Eosinophilic lung diseases. Am J Respir Crit Care Med 1994; 150:1423–38.
7. Johkoh T, Muller NL, Akira M et al. Eosinophilic lung diseases: diagnostic accuracy of thin-section CT in 111 patients. Radiology 2000; 216: 773–80.
8. Mayo JR, Muller NL, Road J, Sister J, Lillington G. Chronic eosinophilic pneumonia: CT findings in six cases. AJR Am J Roentgenol 1989; 153: 727–30.
9. Hansell DM. Small-vessel diseases of the lung: CT-pathologic correlates. Radiology 2002; 225: 639–53.
10. Gillmore JD, Hawkins PN. Amyloidosis and the respiratory tract. Thorax 1999; 54: 444–51.
11. Falk RH, Comenzo RL, Skinner M. The systemic amyloidoses. N Engl J Med 1997; 337: 898–909.
12. Pickford HA, Swensen SJ, Utz JP. Thoracic cross-sectional imaging of amyloidosis. AJR Am J Roentgenol 1997; 168: 351–5.
13. Prince JS, Duhamel DR, Levin DL, Harrell JH, Friedman PJ. Nonneoplastic lesions of the tracheobronchial wall: radiologic findings with bronchoscopic correlation. Radiographics 2002; 22 Spec No: S215–30.
14. McLoud TC. Occupational lung disease. Radiol Clin North Am 1991; 29: 931–41.
15. Matar LD, McAams HP, Sporn TA. Hypersensitivity pneumonitis. AJR Am J Roentgenol 2000; 174: 1061–6.
16. Gurney JW. Hypersensitivity pneumonitis. Radiol Clin North Am 1992; 30: 1219–30.
17. Hartman TE. The HRCT features of extrinsic allergic alveolitis. Semin Respir Crit Care Med 2003; 24: 419–26.
18. Moss RB. Allergic bronchopulmonary aspergillosis. Clin Rev Allergy Immunol 2002; 23: 87–104.
19. Franquet T, Muller NL, Gimenez A et al. Spectrum of pulmonary aspergillosis: histologic, clinical, and radiologic findings. Radiographics 2001; 21: 825–37.
20. Franquet T, Muller NL, Oikonomou A, Flint JD. Aspergillus infection of the airways: computed tomography and pathologic findings. J Comput Assist Tomogr 2004; 28: 10–16.
21. Khan AN, Jones C, Macdonald S. Bronchopulmonary aspergillosis: a review. Curr Probl Diagn Radiol 2003; 32: 156–68.

10

Thromboembolic disease

Douglas R Lake, Joseph J Kavanagh, and U Joseph Schoepf

Introduction

Acute pulmonary embolism (PE) is a common disorder with significant morbidity and mortality. The reliable diagnosis of acute PE has long been a vexation for clinicians and there has always been a need for a robust test or series of tests for its diagnosis. The clinical presentation of acute PE ranges from the 'silent' (asymptomatic) clot to catastrophic and life-threatening embolization. Perhaps because of this the estimation of the exact prevalence of acute PE has always been difficult to predict. However, acute PE is believed to affect close to 650 000 Americans every year and thought to account for around 50 000 deaths. While these numbers are alarming, the true incidence of PE is likely to be higher because an unknown number of patients with this condition remain either undiagnosed or misdiagnosed. Moreover even when symptomatic, patients generally present with non-specific complaints such as dyspnea, pleuritic chest pain, cough, and occasionally hemoptysis. Not surprisingly, unless the index of clinical suspicion is high, the diagnosis is commonly overlooked.

In this chapter, the value of imaging tests (and specifically computed tomography (CT)) in the diagnosis of acute PE is discussed. The topic is approached from the viewpoint of the clinician and the common clinical questions posed in regard to acute PE are covered. Whilst the focus of the chapter is on the role of multidetector row CT (MDR CT), the discussion begins with a brief review of the non-radiological evaluation and other imaging tests brought to bear in patients with suspected acute PE.

Is there a role for diagnostic algorithms and other tests in acute pulmonary embolism?

Given the known difficulties in making an accurate diagnosis and the absence of a single reliable test, physicians have necessarily developed and relied on a combination of clinical experience and investigations. In this regard, the attraction of a diagnostic algorithm, utilizing aspects of the clinical evaluation and various tests (both invasive and non-invasive) is obvious. There are a number of such algorithms which help the physician to determine the clinical pre-test probability of acute PE. To a greater or lesser degree, such algorithms provide a logical pathway prior to formal pulmonary artery imaging. An important component of most algorithms is the determination of clinical pre-test probability and one of the most widely accepted systems (a seven-feature bedside evaluation for quantifying pre-test probability) was proposed by Wells et al.[1] (Table 10.1). The value of the Wells scoring system is that, in combination with D-dimer testing, over 50% of patients with a low pre-test probability for PE might be identified and excluded from further unnecessary investigation. Naturally, the success of such a scoring system is critically dependent on the high sensitivity (reportedly around 97%) of the enzyme-linked immunosorbent assay for D-dimer levels and the high negative predictive value (99.6%)[2] which are strongly concordant with the results of CT angiography in a high percentage of cases.[3] Thus, a Wells score of 4.0 or less, combined with a negative D-dimer indicates that acute PE is unlikely (1.7% rate of acute PE in the validation group). Wells et al. have concluded reasonably that in this group further diagnostic work-up is probably unnecessary. Their study noted that this low rate of PE is far less than the rate of PE in patients with normal ventilation-perfusion (V/Q) scintigraphy and comparable with the rate of PE in patients with traditional catheter-based pulmonary angiography. However, it must be emphasized that a positive D-dimer assay is non-specific and hence of limited value particularly in the in-patient setting.

While awaiting results of D-dimer assay, most physicians will consider requesting chest radiography and electrocardiography before more sophisticated imaging. Supplementary investigations are of potential value in the detection or exclusion of important alternative diagnoses

Table 10.1 Clinical pre-test probability of pulmonary embolism (PE). If total score is ≤ 4.0 and the patient has a negative D-dimer, the PE rates within the study groups were < 2.5%

Clinical signs and symptoms of DVT (i.e. leg swelling and pain with palpation of deep veins)	3.0 points
An alternative diagnosis is less likely than PE	3.0 points
Heart rate > 100 bpm	1.5 points
Immobilization or surgery in the prior 4 weeks	1.5 points
Previous DVT/PE	1.5 points
Hemoptysis	1.0 point
Malignancy (on treatment, treated in last 6 months or palliative)	1.0 points

DVT, deep venous thrombosis. From Wells et al.[1]

such as myocardial infarction, congestive heart failure, and pneumonia. Chest radiographs in patients with proven PE are often normal or show only minor non-specific abnormalities including subsegmental atelectasis and small pleural effusions.[4] Wedge-shaped air-space opacities (pulmonary infarcts) and regional hypoperfusion are more specific findings but are much less frequently encountered. However, the real value of chest radiography (discussed in greater detail below) may be in the triage of patients with cardiopulmonary disease that should preclude radionuclide scanning; the high prevalence of 'indeterminate' results at V/Q scanning has always been a frustration for physicians. In patients with acute PE, the electrocardiogram may be normal but might sometimes suggest an alternative cause for chest pain or rarely show signs of right-heart strain with negative T-waves in the precordial leads, right bundle-branch block, the so-called (but seldom seen) 'S1Q3T3' pattern, or Qr in lead V1.[5–7] Other laboratory tests have shown variable utility in the diagnosis of acute PE. Arterial blood gas sampling is probably not a useful triage tool in patients with suspected PE[8] since hypoxemia is wholly non-specific. Similarly the alveolar–arterial gradient may be normal in as many as 20% of patients with proven PE.[9]

It will be gathered from the above discussion and personal experience that imaging tests remain a cornerstone in the diagnostic work-up of patients with suspected PE. Conventional pulmonary angiography, V/Q scanning, and compression Doppler ultrasonography of the lower limb veins have, at various times, been in vogue but more recently have had complementary roles in the diagnosis of acute PE.[10,11] In this regard, CT pulmonary angiography (particularly since the advent of MDR-CT machines) is emerging as the primary diagnostic modality at many institutions. Indeed, it might be argued that MDR-CT should

now be considered the 'gold standard' investigation for the diagnosis and exclusion of PE.

What are the advantages of computed tomography pulmonary angiography?

CT has a number of inherent strengths in comparison with alternative imaging strategies such as ultrasound, V/Q scanning, and conventional (invasive) catheter angiography. The primary advantages of CT pulmonary angiography, especially since the advent of MDR-CT, are speed and the now relatively widespread availability. It is a fact that a complete examination of the pulmonary arteries can be performed within a reasonably comfortable single breath hold. When coupled with CT of the lower limb veins, such examinations may be used to confirm or confidently exclude acute PE and/or lower-extremity deep venous thrombosis (DVT). The additional value of CT pulmonary angiography is that in patients who present with symptoms that are not due to PE, an alternative diagnosis (such as congestive heart failure, pneumonia, interstitial lung disease, or pulmonary malignancy) is not infrequently suggested by the radiologist.[12]

The diagnosis of PE is dependent on the detection of a variety of characteristic CT signs (summarized in Table 10.2) (Figure 10.1): filling defects in a well opacified arterial branch are the typical CT appearance of pulmonary emboli. Occasionally complete vessel cut-off is seen and the vessel proximal to the occlusion may be seen to be enlarged. The non-diagnostic secondary signs include peripheral wedge-shape areas of increased density (reflecting pulmonary infarction and eponymously termed Hampton's hump) (Figure 10.2), or relative oligemia involving an affected pulmonary segment (the Westermark sign).[13]

There are now good data which confirm the diagnostic utility of CT pulmonary angiography. Studies which have

Table 10.2 Diagnostic and ancillary CT findings in acute pulmonary embolism

Intraluminal filling defects (polo mint/lifesaver sign or tram-track sign)

Total cut-off of vascular enhancement

Enlargement of an occluded vessel

Pleurally based, wedge-shaped areas of increased attenuation

Linear atelectasis

Pleural effusion

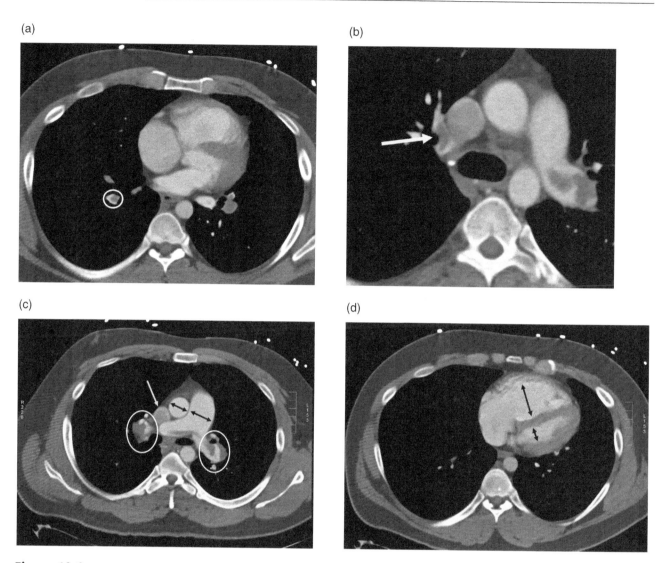

Figure 10.1

CT signs of acute pulmonary embolism in two patients. (a) There is a filling defect in a segmental right lower lobe arterial branch (circled): central low attenuation is highlighted by contrast-enhanced blood in the vessel (the so-called 'polo mint' or 'livesaver' signs). The left lower lobe segemental vessel is completely occluded. (b) Targeted image through the mediastinum with emboli in the right upper lobe (arrow) and left main pulmonary arteries. (a-f) Integrated findings and prognosis of PE findings and prognosis of PE with optimized bolus protocol. Figures 10.1(a-f) demonstrate nearly all the findings of PE and important prognostic implications. (a) Lifesaver sign. Segmental left lower lobe pulmonary embolus (white circle – 10.1(a) shows the classic "lifesaver" or "polo mint" sign of a dark thombus outlined by white contrast on axial images. The long axis of the embolus is perpendicular to the plane of scanning. Also note large segmental emboli in the left lower lobe pulmonary arteries. (b) "Railway-track" sign of PE. Axial CT image from a pulmonary angiogram 1(b) demonstrates segmental right upper lobe pulmonary embolus. Note that the embolus lies within the plane of imaging. Also note the left main PE. (c) Note the enlargement of the main pulmonary artery versus the aorta (double headed black arrows), a secondary sign of poor prognosis (Fleischner sign) as a result of the bilateral saddle pulmonary emboli (white circles). Also note the relative hypodense SVC (grey arrow) secondary to using only 40 mL of contrast media followed immediately by 100 mL of normal saline as a flush. (d) Note the enlargement of the right ventricle (10.1(d) long double-headed black arrow) versus the left ventricle (10.1(d) short double-headed black arrow) versus the left ventricle (10.1(d) short double-headed black arrow black arrow) where the RV/LV ratio exceeds 1.5 and independently indicates a significant embolic event. There is straightening of the interventricular septum and slight bowing into the left ventricle, indicating right ventricular strain. (e) An axial image demonstrate reflux of contrast into the hepatic veins also suggesting right ventricular strain. (f) A coronal image which is produced as a curved planar reformatted image to better depict the bilateral saddle embolus (10.1(f) – white arrows) that occurrred in this patient also demonstrates reflux of contrast down the inferior vena cava into the hepatic vein (10.1(f) – dotted white arrow).

(e)

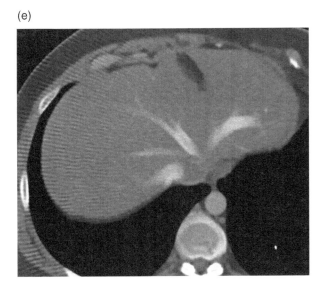

(f)

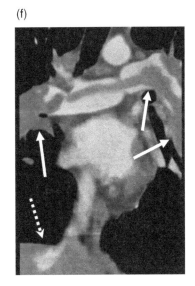

Figure 10.1 (Continued)

(a)

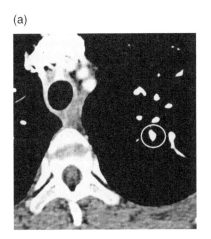

(b)

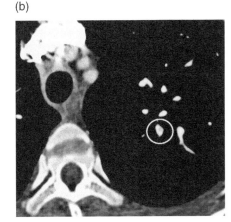

Figure 10.2

(a-b): window-level artifact. Axial images just above the takeoff of the arch vessels all in the same patient at different settings demonstrate the importance of appropriate window width and window level setttings. The first axial image is set at a mediastinal window width and level setting of 400/40, which is commonly used for analyzing the mediastinum. The embolus (10.2(a) – white circle) is impossible to see. However at PE-specific window/level setting (10.2(b) – white circle) of 700/100, the pulmonary embolus is well seen.

compared CT pulmonary angiography with the results of conventional angiography have shown that the negative predictive value of CT pulmonary angiography (exceeding 95%) for the exclusion of acute PE, are entirely acceptable.[14–16] These data are bolstered by a recent meta-analysis, of 3500 patients with negative CT pulmonary angiography, which confirmed a negative predictive value of 99%.[17] Clearly, this compares favorably with the results of conventional pulmonary angiography and the high negative predictive value of a normal V/Q scan.[18]

Another potential benefit of CT angiography, which is exploited at some institutions, is that the venous system (CT venography (CTV)) can be interrogated at the same session. The technique of CTV has reportedly varying sensitivities and specificities of 70–97% and 96–100%, respectively, mirroring Doppler sonography[19,20] but with the potential added benefit of imaging the iliac veins and inferior vena cava which are not included in the routine ultrasound examination.

What are the detrimental effects of computed tomography pulmonary angiography?

The potential disadvantages of CT pulmonary angiography with MDR-CT must be borne in mind by the referring physician. The most important of these has to be radiation exposure. However, the problem of indeterminate examinations, issues related to intravenous access, and contrast allergies are sometimes also problematic.

The carcinogenic effects of ionizing radiation to the female breast, thyroid, and eye are often not considered or occasionally deemed irrelevant in the acute setting. However, in a recent review of over 1300 MDR-CT studies for PE, it was shown that 60% of such studies are performed on women and that the calculated effective minimum radiation dose to the breast on a 60-kg woman was 2.0 rad (20 mGy) per breast. It is also worth stressing that the average from routine two-view screening mammography is a fraction of this dose at 0.3 rad (3 mGy). To put this into some kind of perspective, MDR-CT imparts a radiation dose equilavent to 10–25 two-view mammograms and between 100 and 400 chest radiographs.[21] While the potential latent carcinogenic effects of this dose are not known, a study of 1030 women with scoliosis who underwent multiple thoracic spine radiographic examinations as young girls revealed a nearly two-fold statistically increased risk for incident breast carcinoma.[22]

While the sensitivity of MDR-CT for the detection of acute PE is comfortingly high it must be remembered that indeterminate studies do occur in between 0.5 and 10.8% of patients with suspected acute PE. In one recent study the causes of an indeterminate study were motion artifact (74%), poor contrast bolus (40%), parenchymal disease (12%), and body habitus (7%).[23] In reviewing 237 indeterminate studies and comparing with 25 control studies, the average Hounsfield (HU) attenuation value of the indeterimate studies was 245 HU versus 340 HU for the control group. At follow-up of these indeterminate studies, 4.2% were positive for PE, therefore empiric treatment for PE or follow-up examination might be appropriate after an indeterminate MDR-CT PE study.

MDR-CT for PE requires a method of administering a high-pressure rapid bolus of intravenous contrast. However, obtaining appropriate intravenous access for this bolus, which is performed with a power-injector, can be problematic. No central venous catheters state manufacturer approval for the amount of pressure produced by the power-injector, which can approach 300 psi when injecting non-ionic contrast media at 4 ml/s. At our institution, 18–20-gauge intravenous Angiocath™ (Beckton, Dickinson and Co, Sandy, Utah, USA) catheters, and 5–6-French PowerPICC® and PowerHohn (Bard Access Systems, Salt Lake City, Utah, USA) devices are commonly power-injected while smaller-bore and multilumen devices are avoided. With the newer devices emerging and increasing imaging utilization there will be a continued drive for intravenous devices which can tolerate greater pressure loads.

While the incidence of contrast reactions has decreased with the near-universal use of non-ionic contrast media, ten severe reactions (0.02%) and one death were reported after reviewing 41 060 non-ionic contrast media administrations.[24] When comparing all reported patient reactions, 0.2% of patients reported reactions to non-ionic contrast media versus a relatively lower rate for gadolinium of 0.0003–0.07% for magnetic resonance imaging (MRI) examinations. Contrast extravasation remains a rare but important problem cause of morbidity occurring in 0.25–0.6% of cases.

What prognostic information might be gleaned from the results of computed tomography pulmonary angiography?

In addition to the diagnostic role of CT pulmonary angiography, there is potential prognostic information in the results of MDR-CT in patients with PE. Thus, it might become possible to stratify patients with acute PE according to risk based on MDR-CT datasets. Such data might, in turn, be of value in management and determining prognosis. Specific findings include the ratio of the diameter of the short axis of the right ventricle in relation to the diameter of the short axis of the left ventricle (RV/LV ratio), bowing of the interventricular septum, and reflux of contrast into the hepatic veins (Table 10.3) (Figure 10.3) can be assessed to help stratify the risk of right ventricular dysfunction, cardiogenic shock, and circulatory collapse. Specifically, it is believed that an RV/LV ratio exceeding 1.0 has a high specificity and positive predictive value for right ventricular dysfunction when compared with echocardiographic findings. Additionally, an RV/LV ratio exceeding 1.5 indicates a severe episode of PE. Bowing of the interventricular septum has also been shown to be an indicator of the severity of pulmonary arterial obstruction and the likelihood of subsequent admission to the ICU, but is not specific for acute PE as any of a number of causes of chronic pulmonary arterial obstruction will lead to bowing of the interventricular septum. Finally, reflux of contrast into the hepatic veins has been shown to be a predictor of mortality because it represents an indirect sign of tricuspid valve insufficiency, regurgitation, and later right heart failure in cases of severe PE.[25]

What are the alternatives to computed tomography pulmonary angiography in the evaluation of patients with thromboembolic disease?

With MDR-CT assuming a central role in the imaging of acute PE (supplemented, where appropriate, with CTV for imaging of the lower extremities), other imaging modalities have assumed a complementary role. In this regard, ultrasound is considered the gold standard test for detecting venous thrombosis in the lower limb veins. Traditional catheter angiography has been steadily relegated in importance for a diagnois of PE but remains the primary modality for the treatment of massive pulmonary embolism.

As hinted above, the chest radiograph and traditional V/Q scan have both assumed a secondary role to MDR-CT in the diagnosis of PE. In a recent article, the role of the chest radiograph as a triage tool to determine whether patients should receive V/Q scan or CT was explored.[26] In this study, 370 patients with suspected PE were either referred for V/Q scanning or CT pulmonary angiography based on the findings of the initial chest radiograph. Specifically, those with a normal chest radiograph underwent V/Q scanning whereas those with abnormal findings at chest radiography were referred for CT pulmonary angiography. In this study there was a relatively high rate of low-probability scans in patients with an initial normal chest radiograph. The authors also made the useful practical point that the V/Q scan remained a useful examination for those with chronic renal insufficiency or contrast allergy.

Novel MRI techniques have been developed for imaging of the pulmonary circulation. In a recent study, 48 consecutive symptomatic patients underwent chest radiography, contrast-enhanced MDCT pulmonary angiography, MR angiography (MRA) with sensitivity encoding (SENSE),

V/Q scintigraphy, and traditional catheter pulmonary angiography.[27] Indeed, conventional pulmonary angiography was used as the gold standard because only a four-channel MDR-CT unit was used in the trial. The sensitivity and specificity of MRA with SENSE on a per-vascular zone basis were 83% and 97%, and on a per-patient basis 92% and 94%, respectively. The authors also noted that the overall specificity and accuracy of MRA (94% and 94%, respectively) were greater than those of V/Q scanning (78% and 78%, respectively, $P < 0.05$).

Several technical limitations to this MR technique were highlighted and included equipment availability, rapidity of examination, and difficulty of monitoring the patient in the MR environment. Imaging-based limitations leading to a relatively high rate of false positive diagnoses were also noted including susceptibility artifacts from alveolar air, flow artifacts from contrast in pulmonary veins, superimposition of pulmonary veins and pulmonary arteries, and image degradation by respiratory motion artifact. However, MRA remains a developing alternative in patients with chronic renal insufficiency, contrast allergy, or in young patients to reduce the potential risk of radiation-induced neoplasm.

Table 10.3 CT pulmonary angiographic signs with potential prognostic implications

RV/LV ratio > 1
Leftward bowing of the interventricular septum
Reflux of contrast into hepatic veins

RV/LV ratio, right ventricular short axis to left ventricular short axis ratio.

What are the implications for treatment from the results of computed tomography pulmonary angiography?

A full discussion of the treatment of PE is well beyond the scope of this text. However, a focused review of

(a) (b)

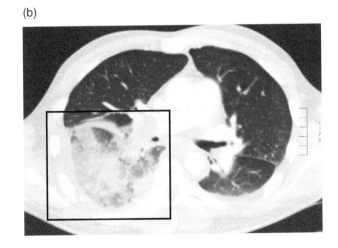

Figure 10.3

(a-b) CT Hampton Hump. Two axial images from CT pulmonary angiography demonstrate large right lower lobe hilar pulmonary embolus (10.3(a) white square) and accompanying ground glass opacification of the superior segment of the right lower lobe likely representing hemorrhage and infarct, the so-called CT Hampton-Hump (10.3(b) - black square).

medical management for non-massive PE, therapeutic options available as relevant to interventional radiology (Tables 10.4–10.6), and a discussion of the isolated subsegmental pulmonary embolus (ISSPE) follow below. Where applicable, evidence-based recommendations on the treatment of PE are provided.

For objectively confirmed acute non-massive PE, subcutaneous low-molecular weight heparin (LMWH) or intravenous unfractionated heparin (UFH) both receive a grade 1A evidence-based recommendation, with subcutaneous LMWH favored over intravenous UFH except in cases of acute renal failure.[30] A vitamin-K antagonist such as warfarin should be administered on treatment day 1 with either LMWH or UFH and continued until the international normalized ratio (INR) has stabilized at > 2.0.[30] Treatment of PE and DVT often overlap considerably and should be considered manifestations of the same disease process. Patients considered to be at high risk of PE should be anticoagulated while undergoing diagnostic testing (grade 1C+).[30] It is important to note that in most patients with PE, anticoagulation with thrombolytics is not recommended (grade 1). However, in selected cases and unstable patients, systemic thrombolytics may be prescribed (grade 2B). Furthermore, because patient survival depends upon rapid recanalization of the pulmonary arterial system and reduction in right ventricular afterload, mechanical thrombectomy is suggested in high-risk patients in whom thrombolytic therapy is contraindicated or in those whom the critical status does not allow sufficient time to infuse thrombolytic therapy (grade 2C).[30]

Catheter-based thrombolysis is known to accelerate clot breakdown and speeds reduction in afterload. Available techniques include catheter-based thrombolysis, percutaneous mechanical thrombus fragmentation, or indeed a combination of the two techniques. Indications for interventional radiological assessment and catheter-based therapy are given in Table 10.5.[28] Catheter-based direct medicinal thrombolysis involves obtaining femoral venous access, positioning a catheter in the obstructing embolus and infusing a thrombolytic medication such as urokinase, recombinant tissue plasminogen activator (rt-PA), or heparin. Percutaneous mechanical thrombus fragmentation can also be performed via low-profile access from femoral venous access. The two devices used most commonly include the Angiojet® thrombectomy catheter (Possis, Minneapolis, Minnesota, USA) and the Amplatz thrombectomy device (ATD; Microvena, White Bear Lake, Minnesota, USA). The Angiojet device is a double-lumen catheter through which a smaller lumen injects a high-velocity stream of saline into a larger lumen. The device is advanced over a wire and is therefore steerable into areas of PE. The high-pressure injection creates a local low-pressure environment around the catheter which promotes fragmentation of the clot. The ATD works via a different mechanism in that it has a recessed impeller housed within

Table 10.4 Indications for aggressive intervention in PE (one or more must be present)

Arterial hypotension (90 mmHg systolic or drop of 40 mmHg)

Cardiogenic shock with peripheral hypoperfusion and hypoxia

Circulatory collapse with need for cardiopulmonary resuscitation

Echocardiographic findings indicating right ventricular afterload stress and/or pulmonary hypertension

Diagnosis of precapillary pulmonary hypertension (mean partial arterial pressure 20 mmHg in presence of normal partial arterial pressure occlusion pressures)

Widened arterial–alveolar O_2 gradient (50 mmHg)

Clinically severe PE with a contraindication to anticoagulation or thrombolytic therapy

From Uflacker.[28]

Table 10.5 Subsets of patients in whom small PE might require treatment

Inadequate cardiopulmonary reserve

Coexisting acute deep venous thrombosis

Recurrent PE, possibly due to thrombophilia to prevent chronic PE and pulmonary artery hypertension

Table 10.6 Subsets of patients with small/questionable PE in whom treatment risk may outweigh benefit

Symptomatic patients with PE limited to subsegmental vessels, no DVT, and adequate cardiopulmonary reserve

Indeterminate MDCT or V/Q scanning result, no DVT, and adequate cardiopulmonary reserve

Asymptomatic patients with incidentally discovered small emboli, no DVT, and adequate cardiopulmonary reserve

Patients with contraindications to anticoagulation (intracranial hemorrhage, recent surgery, or trauma) with isolated subsegmental PE or indeterminate MDCT with no DVT

V/Q, ventilation-perfusion; MDCT, multidetector CT. Adapted from Goodman et al.[29]

a metal capsule. The impeller creates a vortex within the vessel which pulverizes the thrombus and recirculates smaller fresh clots which migrate peripherally and reduce afterload because the cross-sectional area of the peripheral pulmonary arterial vasculature is several times that of the central pulmonary vasculature. The greatest efficacy will probably be achieved in those critically ill patients where both direct medicinal thrombolysis and mechanical thrombus fragmentation techniques are utilized, but this has not yet been validated in clinical trials.

One of the vexing problems in the treatment of acute PE lies at the other end of the spectrum. The small, often incidental subsegmental PE in the absence of DVT remains a management challenge. This entity is becoming more common and recent research performed on four-detector MDCT units noted a 3.4% rate of PE in asymptomatic patients,[31] and in non-selected patients referred for MDR-CT for possible PE approximately 5% had isolated subsegmental PE. Some authors reduce the emphasis on this entity by suggesting that the pulmonary circulation normally functions as a filter for small emboli to prevent passage into the more systemic circulation and note that up to 20% of otherwise healthy accident victims have macroscopic emboli at autopsy. However, the opposite view is that there are historical data which confirm a mortality rate of between 18 and 38% for untreated PE.[32] However, this notwithstanding, it has been argued that small PE, in certain patient populations, do not always warrant treatment (Table 10.6). Recently an outcome study of 1435 consecutive patients imaged on eight- and 16-detector MDCT units examined clinician management and patient outcome following isolated subsegmental pulmonary emboli and indeterminate MDR-CT PE studies. Three-month follow-up data showed that 37% of the patients with isolated subsegmental pulmonary emboli and 85% of the indeterminate patients received no anticoagulation therapy. Importantly only two patients, in each subgroup, re-presented with signs and/or symptoms of PE but were negative at follow-up MDR-CT imaging.[32] These results suggest that treatment might safely be withheld in certain patient populations (Table 10.7), especially when considering that the mortality and morbidity of anticoagulant therapy are 1% and 7%, respectively, per treatment year. However, Goodman suggests follow-up ultrasound may be prudent after 1 week to exclude DVT in patients with isolated subsegmental pulmonary emboli.

Conclusions

CT pulmonary angiography is now well established as the imaging modality of choice for the rapid and accurate evaluation of patients with suspected acute PE. MDR-CT can also contribute important prognostic information regarding the cardiopulmonary status and overall outcome. If the results of CTV are included in the clinical evaluation, MDR-CT has the potential to become a 'one-stop-shop' for excluding venous thromboembolism.

References

1. Wells PS, Anderson DR, Rodger M et al. Derivation of a simple clinical model to categorize patients probability of pulmonary embolism: increasing the models utility with the SimpliRED D-dimer. Thromb Haemost 2000; 83: 416–20.
2. Dunn KL, Wolf JP, Dorfman DM et al. Normal D-dimer levels in emergency department patients suspected of acute pulmonary embolism. J Am Coll Cardiol 2002; 40: 1475–8.
3. Abcarian PW, Sweet JD, Watabe JT et al. Role of a quantitative d-dimer assay in determining the need for CT angiography of acute pulmonary embolism. AJR Am J Roentgenol 2004; 182: 1377–81.
4. Elliott CG, Goldhaber SZ, Visani L et al. Chest radiographs in acute pulmonary embolism. Results from the international cooperative pulmonary embolism registry. Chest 2000; 118: 33–8.
5. Ferrari E, Imbert A, Chevalier T et al. The ECG in pulmonary embolism: predictive value of negative T waves in precordial leads: 80 case reports. Chest 1997; 111: 537–43.
6. Daniel KR, Courtney DM, Kline JA. Assessment of cardiac stress from massive pulmonary embolism with 12-lead ECG. Chest 2001; 120: 474–81.
7. Kucher N, Walpoth N, Wustmann K et al. QR in V1: an ECG sign associated with right ventricular strain and adverse clinical outcome in pulmonary embolism. Eur Heart J 2003; 24: 1113–9.
8. Stein PD, Goldhaber SZ, Henry JW et al. Arterial blood gas analysis in the assessment of suspected acute pulmonary embolism. Chest 1996; 109: 78–81.
9. Stein PD, Goldhaber SZ, Henry JW. Alveolar-arterial oxygen gradient in the assessment of acute pulmonary embolism. Chest 1995; 107: 139–43.
10. Prologo JD, Glauser J. Variable diagnostic approach to suspected pulmonary embolism in the ED of a major academic tertiary care center. Am J Emerg Med 2002; 20: 5–9.
11. Stein PD, Kayali F, Olson RE. Trends in the use of diagnostic imaging in patients hospitalized with acute pulmonary embolism. Am J Cardiol 2004; 93: 1316–7.
12. Kim KI, Muller NL, Mayo JR. Clinically suspected pulmonary embolism: utility of spiral CT. Radiology 1999; 210: 693–7.
13. Han D, Lee KS, Franquet T et al. Thrombotic and non-thrombotic pulmonary arterial embolism: spectrum of imaging findings. Radiographics 2003; 23: 1521–39.
14. Krestan CR, Klein N, Fleischmann et al. Value of negative spiral CT angiography in patients with suspected acute PE: analysis of PE occurrence and outcome. Eur Radiol 2004; 14: 93–8.
15. Musset D, Parent F, Meyer G et al. Diagnostic strategy for patients with suspected pulmonary embolism: a prospective multicentre outcome study. Lancet 2002; 360: 1914–20.
16. Qanadli SC, Hajjam ME, Mesurolle B et al. Pulmonary embolism detection: prospective evaluation of dual-section helical CT versus selective pulmonary arteriography in 157 patients. Radiology 2000; 217: 447–55.
17. Quiroz R, Kucher N, Zou KH et al. Clinical validity of a negative computed tomography scan in patients with suspected pulmonary embolism – a systematic review. JAMA 2005; 293: 2012–17.

18. Blachere H, Latrabe V, Montaudon M et al. Pulmonary embolism revealed on helical CT angiography: comparison with ventilation-perfusion radionuclide lung scanning. Am J Roentgenol 2000; 174: 1041–7.

19. Taffoni MJ, Ravenel JG, Ackerman SJ. Prospective comparison of indirect CT venography versus venous sonography in ICU patients. Am J Roentgenol 2005; 185: 457–62.

20. Loud PA, Katz DS, Bruce DA et al. Deep venous thrombosis with suspected pulmonary thromboembolism: detection with combined CT venography and pulmonary angiography. Radiology 2001; 219: 498–502.

21. Parker MS, Hui FK, Camacho MA et al. Female breast radiation exposure during CT pulmonary angiography. Am J Roentgenol 2005; 185: 1228–33.

22. Morin DM, Lonstein JE, Stovall M et al. Breast cancer morality after diagnostic radiography: findings from the U.S. scoliosis cohort study. Spine 2000; 25: 2052–63.

23. Jones SE, Wittram C. The indeterminate CT pulmonary angiogram: imaging characteristics and patient clinical outcome. Radiology 2005; 237: 329–37.

24. Cochran ST, Bornyea K, Sayre JW. Trends in adverse events after IV administration of contrast media. Am J Roentgenol 2001; 176: 1385–8.

25. Ghaye B, Ghuysen A, Bruyere PJ. Can CT pulmonary angiography allow assessment of severity and prognosis in patients presenting with pulmonary embolism? What the radiologist needs to know. Radiographics 2006; 26: 23–40.

26. Daftary A, Gregory M, Daftary A et al. Chest radiograph as a triage tool in the imaging-based diagnosis of pulmonary embolism. Am J Roentgenol 2005; 185: 132–4.

27. Ohno Y, Higashino T, Takenaka D et al. MR angiography with sensitivity encoding (SENSE) for suspected pulmonary embolism: comparison with MDCT and ventilation–perfusion scintigraphy. Am J Roentgenol 2004; 183: 91–8.

28. Uflacker R. Interventional therapy for pulmonary embolism. J Vasc Interv Radiol 2001; 12: 147–64.

29. Goodman LR. Small pulmonary emboli: what do we know? Radiology 2005; 234: 654–8.

30. Buller HR, Agnelli G, Hull RD et al. Antithrombotic therapy for venous thromboembolic disease: The Seventh ACCP Conference on Antithrombotic and Thrombolytic Therapy. Chest 2004; 126; 401–28.

31. Storto ML, DiCredico A, Guidol F et al. Incidental detection of pulmonary emboli on routine MDCT of the chest. AJR AM J Roentgenol 2005; 184: 264–7.

32. Eyer BA, Goodman LR, Washington L. Clinicians' response to radiologists' reports of isolated subsegmental pulmonary embolism or inconclusive interpretation of pulmonary embolism using MDCT. Am J Roenhtgenol 2005; 184: 623–8.

11

Pleural sepsis

Fergus V Gleeson and YC Gary Lee

Introduction

Pleural infection is an age-old problem which, through the ages, has claimed many lives including those of the famous physicians Guillaume Dupuytrens and Sir William Osler.[1] It has been estimated that pleural sepsis affects over 65 000 patients each year in the UK and USA, with a mortality approximating 20%[2] and a hospital cost of $500 million. As might perhaps be expected, the incidence of pleural infection is believed to be higher in developing countries.[3,4] Furthermore, the incidence of empyema, at least in children, is rising.[5,6] In adults, the prevalence of HIV, wider use of immunosuppressants, and organ transplantation have meant that pleural infection continues to be a common and significant clinical problem.

Pleural infection refers to the presence of 'complicated' parapneumonic effusions and empyema. Sterile pleural effusions are common, especially after pneumonia, and are referred to as 'simple' parapneumonic effusions. However, when there is secondary infection, such effusions are termed 'complicated' parapneumonic effusions and are characterized by a low fluid pH and glucose, and often have septations visible on ultrasound. Empyema refers to an advanced stage of pleural infection where frank pus is present in the pleural space.

The diagnosis of pleural infection is a clinical challenge. The disease can affect any age, gender, and ethnic background, and the clinical presentation may be entirely nonspecific. Delays in establishing a diagnosis of pleural infection are common and intervals of up to 6 weeks following the onset of pleural sepsis are not uncommonly reported,[7] especially in the developing world.[8] Although systemic antimicrobial therapy has had an impact in reducing mortality from pleural infection, antibiotics alone are often insufficient. Nevertheless, the best management of pleural infection remains controversial. Advances in radiological technology in recent decades have made imaging an integral component of the clinical management of pleural infection. In this chapter, we discuss the management of pleural infection as a series of key clinical questions, and whether and how input from imaging tests can significantly improve the care of patients with pleural sepsis.

Which techniques are of use in establishing the presence of a parapneumonic effusion?

Pleural infection is almost inevitably characterized by the presence of a pleural effusion. Thus, the detection of a pleural fluid is the first step in the recognition of pleural infection. The majority of cases of pleural infection occur as a sequel to pneumonia and can affect any age group. Indeed, as many as 40% of patients with pneumonia will develop a pleural effusion.[9] However, it is worth mentioning that pleural infection can also complicate esophageal rupture, thoracic (open or closed) trauma, and iatrogenic procedures, such as surgery (especially lung resection).[10] 'Spontaneous' bacterial empyema is rare.

A high index of clinical suspicion is generally required to make an early and accurate diagnosis of a parapneumonic effusion. In most reported series, the symptoms of a parapneumonic collection include cough and fever, which are more a manifestation of the pneumonic process rather than the pleural involvement per se. As such, the pleural component is frequently overlooked. In the elderly, fever may not be a prominent feature.[11] It is also worth stressing that immunosuppressed patients may have disproportionately mild symptoms relative to the severity of the pleural infection. The bedside diagnosis of a pleural effusion, especially in the presence of pneumonia, is not straightforward. The sign of percussive dullness, incidentally described in the 18th century by Auenbrugger, remains the standard for the clinical detection of pleural effusion. However, these signs are often indistinguishable, even to experienced physicians, from those of the underlying consolidation and atelectasis.

Following on from the above discussion it is clear that physicians rely critically on radiological tests, such as chest radiography or pleural ultrasonography, for the identification of a pleural/parapneumonic effusion. It is noteworthy that the volume of the parapneumonic fluid is highly variable and cannot be used to predict infective etiology.[1] With simple parapneumonic effusions and in the absence of pleural adhesions the fluid collects, is 'free', and accumulates in the most dependent part of the pleural space. On the standard erect chest radiograph, this normally means the posterior or, less commonly, the lateral costophrenic recess. A small volume of fluid (often as little as 50 ml) will manifest as minor blunting of the posterior recess on the lateral radiograph, whereas a somewhat larger volume (approximately 200 ml) is usually needed before any abnormality is visible on the standard posteroanterior chest radiograph.[12] Traditionally, a lateral decubitus chest radiograph has been considered the optimal plain radiographic technique for the diagnosis of small volumes of pleural fluid. However, this has been superseded by the ready availability and improved quality of ultrasound. Larger pleural effusions will produce the characteristic 'meniscus' sign, and if very large (for example, when occupying over 50% of the hemithorax), may result in contralateral mediastinal shift. As with clinical examination, the presence of adjacent pneumonic consolidation renders the detection of small to moderate volumes of pleural fluid difficult. Thus, where there is clinical concern, an ultrasound of the thorax should be requested. Ultrasound is a valuable tool for the detection of pleural fluid. Although the clinical significance of very small collections is debatable, volumes as small as 5 ml can be detected using ultrasound.[13] Another advantage of ultrasound is that, unlike clinical evaluation or plain chest radiography, pleural fluid can be readily distinguished from adjacent consolidated/atelectatic lung or an elevated hemidiaphragm. A number of different methodologies have been devised for the quantification of pleural fluid but the more pragmatic visual estimation and classification of effusion as small, moderate, or large is nearly always sufficient.[14]

Computed tomography (CT) has no added value in the diagnosis of a pleural effusion. However, there is little doubt that because of its superior sensitivity, CT may detect smaller volumes of fluid than seen on chest radiographs. If loculated pleural fluid is present, CT has the advantage (over both chest radiography and ultrasound) of being able to differentiate between pulmonary abscess and empyema:[15] the presence of an acute angle to the chest wall/pleural surface, the absence of the so-called 'split pleura' sign, the lack of adjacent passive atelectasis, and a variable wall thickness all favor the diagnosis of abscess over empyema (Figure 11.1). Magnetic resonance imaging (MRI) is sensitive to small volumes of pleural fluid. However, because of a variety of issues, MRI has no routine or practical role in the diagnosis of pleural fluid in patients with suspected parapneumonic effusions or empyema.

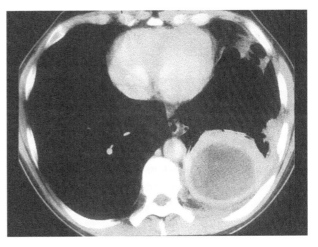

Figure 11.1
Contrast-enhanced CT through the lower zones demonstrates an intrapulmonary abscess rather than an empyema: there is a thicker wall than that which is normally seen with an empyema. In addition, the angle of contact between the collection and the pleural surface is acute.

Can the diagnosis of pleural infection be established by imaging tests?

Over 3000 patients per million population develop a pleural effusion each year[17] and parapneumonic effusions are the most common cause, accounting for about one-third of all exudative effusions. After confirming the presence of a pleural effusion, the physician is faced with two key clinical questions. The first is whether a pleural collection is infected or due to one of the other common causes such as congestive heart failure or malignancy. The second clinical concern, which follows from the first, is whether a parapneumonic effusion is sterile (simple parapneumonic effusion) or infected (complicated parapneumonic effusion or empyema), the latter almost always requires more urgent intervention. Attempts to answer the above questions have been made with partial success using non-invasive radiological tests. A clue to the diagnosis of a complicated parapneumonic effusion or empyema may come from the plain chest radiograph. The presence of septations and pleural adhesions in complicated parapneumonic effusion or empyema, results in loculation of pleural fluid on the chest radiograph and the effusion will not have the characteristic signs of 'free flowing' fluid in the pleural space with a typical meniscus.[18] On occasion a loculated effusion may appear as a pleural or, when loculated within a fissure, an apparently intrapulmonary mass.[18] The demonstration of loculation on chest radiograph should alert the radiologist to the diagnosis of a complicated parapneumonic effusion or empyema. Similarly, pockets of gas or air–fluid levels within a pleural collection are suspicious features; a caveat to this, for the plain film diagnosis, is in patients with pre-existing adhesions which might be a consequence of prior pleural pathology secondary to trauma, surgery, or an earlier episode of pleural infection. In such patients simple pleural collections might also appear loculated and thus mimic the appearances of a more complicated collection. In practice, due consideration to the history and supportive findings from blood tests (for example the white cell count, erythrocyte sedimention rate, and C-reactive protein levels) should point to the correct diagnosis.

In addition to its role in the detection of pleural fluid, ultrasound may suggest whether the effusion is transudative and simple or exudative and complicated. As a general rule transudative effusions are anechoic and non-septated, whereas exudative effusions may either be anechoic and non-septated or septated and echoic[14] (Figure 11.2). However, it must be emphasized that ultrasound features will not obviate diagnostic aspiration of the pleural fluid. Furthermore, there are conflicting data on whether ultrasound is of any value in detemining the likely duration of in-patient admission, the success of tube drainage, and the need for surgery.[19–21]

The diagnostic utility of contrast-enhanced CT has also been evaluated in patients with suspected complicated parapneumonic effusions and empyema.[19,22–24] When present, the 'split pleura' sign (thickened enhancing visceral and parietal pleural layers separated by pleural fluid) is easily identifiable on CT (Figure 11.3). Thickening and enhancement of the parietal pleura (with increased pleural thickening seen in those with more severe disease) is seen in 80–100% of patients with empyema, although this sign is not useful in determining the likely success of chest tube drainage.[19] The other CT features of empyema include

increased thickness and attenuation of the adjacent extrapleural fat. These signs also do not correlate with the duration or severity of the illness.[19] Septations are not usually evident on CT although their presence may be inferred if the effusion contains multiple pockets of gas[18] (Figure 11.4). Another potential benefit of CT is that a proximal endobronchial lesion (which might be causative or associated with the pneumonia) may be identified. Lymph node enlargement is common in patients with empyema undergoing CT but does not reflect the severity of the illness nor the presence of an underlying malignancy.[25,26] As previously mentioned, MRI is exquisitely sensitive to small volumes of pleural fluid and, in contrast to CT, may demonstrate septations as well as parietal pleural thickening[18] (Figure 11.5). However, the higher cost compared with CT, relative lack

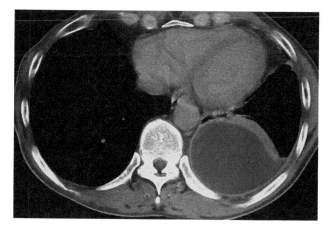

Figure 11.3
Contrast-enhanced CT through the lower zone showing pleural enhancement, an increase in extrapleural fat thickness and attenuation and the 'split pleura' sign.

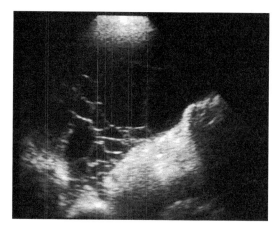

Figure 11.2
An ultrasound image demonstrating a markedly septated parapneumonic effusion. The appearance strongly suggests the presence of an exudative collection, a finding confirmed on subsequent biochemical analysis.

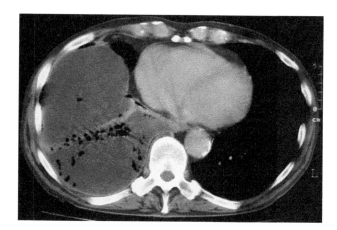

Figure 11.4
CT in patient with an empyema in the right hemithorax. Although no discrete septae are seen there are multiple pockets of gas from which it might be suspected that the collection is septated.

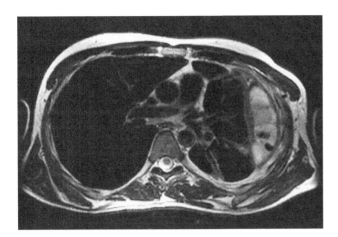

Figure 11.5
A T2-weighted MR image through the upper zone
demonstrating a small loculated parapneumonic effusion
on the left. There is high signal and the collection contains
septations and pockets of gas.

of availability (particularly in the UK and many countries
in Europe), and technical issues related to the imaging of
critically ill patients has meant that MRI is of limited
practical utility in these patients.

In practice, despite the advances in imaging technology,
the diagnosis of an infected parapneumonic effusion
requires biochemical analyses of aspirated pleural fluid.[27]
Parapneumonic effusions are usually exudative (i.e. there is
an elevated pleural fluid protein and lactate dehydrogenase
levels) and there is a prominent neutrophilia. Complicated
parapneumonic effusions are defined by a low pH (< 7.20)
and glucose, together with significant inflammatory cell
influx. Empyema is confirmed by the presence of frank
pus or by positive microbial culture of the pleural fluid.
Although aspiration and pleural fluid analysis are prerequi-
sites for a diagnosis of a complicated parapneumonic effusion
or empyema, it is important to remember that the aspirate
only reflects pleural fluid content at one point in time and in
septated effusions, in any one locule. As regards the latter,
Maskell et al.[28] have recently shown that fluid content may
vary between locules and that, if pleural fluid analysis does
not reflect the clinical and radiographic status, aspiration
may need to be repeated with samples taken from other
locules.

A causative organism is isolated in only about 60% of
pleural fluid samples using conventional laboratory culture methods. In this context, the use of broad range 16S
recombinant-DNA polymerase chain reactions may increase
the chance of identifying pathogens (especially Gram-positive
organisms) from pleural fluid.[29] In a recent UK series, the
commonest organisms of empyema were *Streptococcus
milleri* and *Strep. pneumoniae* in cases of community-
acquired pleural infection, and *Staphylococcus aureus* (including methicillin-resistant *Staph. aureus*) in patients with

hospital-acquired infection.[30] The bacteriology is likely to
vary among regions and countries; thus, physicians must
be aware of local epidemiological data guide treatment.

What is the role of image-guided thoracocentesis and drain insertion?

The two key aspects of the management pleural sepsis are
control of infection and drainage of infected material.
Thus, it is widely accepted that once a diagnosis of pleural
infection is made, broad spectrum systemic antibiotics
should be initiated. Furthermore, attempts must be made to
correct malnutrition.[31] Evaluation of underlying clinical
predisposing factors (for instance, poor dentition and
immunodeficiency) should be also made wherever clinically
appropriate.

The optimal method of aspiration of pleural fluid (whether
for diagnosis or treatment) has been debated. When aspiration is undertaken for diagnostic purposes, a number of
studies have shown ultrasound-guided aspiration is not
only safer but also more likely to be successful than aspiration without image guidance.[32,33] This is particularly true in
patients with effusions of small volume. In principle, repeated
(image-guided) thoracocentesis would serve the same purpose
and has been shown effective in animal experiments[34] as
well as in one small clinical study.[35] However, this approach
is currently not practiced and would require further evaluation before being adopted. For the purposes of therapeutic
drainage, the most common practice is for the insertion of
an intercostal catheter. Interestingly, the closed method of
chest tube drainage was first described by Hewitt as early as
in 1876.[36] Although 'blind' bedside insertion of an intercostal catheter remains a reasonably common practice, this
approach is increasingly being replaced by image-guided
chest tube placement.[18] With image-guided drain insertion,
optimal placement of the catheter in the largest infected
collection can be achieved. A Seldinger technique (in which
the drainage catheter is safely rail-roaded over a guide wire)
is preferred over blunt dissection.[18]

Ultrasound guidance is perhaps the most commonly
used technique for image guidance. With ultrasound the
tube may be directed into the dominant pocket of fluid.
This is of practical importance in patients with small or
awkwardly positioned collections. The complication rates
following image guidance are satisfyingly low.[18] Although
ultrasound is the most commonly used modality, CT guidance may be of value for pleural collections (e.g. collections
positioned behind the scapula or lying medially adjacent to
the heart, descending aorta, or paraspinally) that are poorly
visualized.

Traditionally, large bore chest tubes have been favored for
the drainage of pus. However, this practice was previously

untested in clinical studies. In the Multicenter Intrapleural Sepsis Trial (MIST)[2] of 430 patients, a retrospective post-hoc analysis demonstrated no significant difference in the clinical outcome (avoidance of surgery or death) in patients treated with small bore (i.e. thinner than 16 French gauge) catheters or larger chest drains. Several observational series have also suggested that pigtail catheters are effective for the drainage of pus.[37,38] Furthermore, there is the important observation that patients find small bore catheters more comfortable. It should also be remembered that in patients with multiple large loculations more than one catheter may be required to adequately evacuate pus.

Various adjunctive intrapleural therapies have also been proposed.[39] In particular, fibrinolytic agents have been used, the hypothesis is that loculations may be lyzed and drainage of infected pleural fluid enhanced. Initial studies showed that although intrapleural administration of streptokinase or urokinase significantly increased drainage volumes,[40–43] patient outcome was not necessarily improved.[44] Indeed, there are interesting data from animal studies which suggest that intrapleural streptokinase can itself provoke fluid accumulation (even in the normal pleural cavity) and that this may account for the apparent increase (up to nine-fold) in pleural fluid drainage following fibrinolytic therapy.[39] Accordingly, in the double-blind randomized MIST[2] study, streptokinase infusion did not reduce mortality or the need for salvage surgical drainage. Similar findings have been reported in the single-center study from South Africa in which there was no improvement in the same outcome measures following 3 days of treatment with intrapleural streptokinase.[45] Alternative fibrinolytic agents, such as tissue plasminogen activator and DNase (which has been shown to reduce pus viscosity in vitro[46,47] and has been effective in isolated case reports)[48] are currently under investigation.

Are imaging tests of value in assessing progress?

Failure of standard treatment (as judged by persistent symptoms, fever, leukocytosis, and raised inflammatory markers such as C-reactive protein) is an indication for surgical intervention. It has been shown in retrospective studies that those referred late for surgery have more complications and lower success rates from video-assisted thoracoscopic surgery (VATS), and longer hospital stays.[49–54] A review of 44 retrospective studies comprising a total 1369 patients found that early surgery reduced the duration of fever and hospitalization.[55]

Surgical drainage of infected pleural fluid, which has failed conventional treatment, is considered the 'definitive' treatment. However, VATS drainage has been shown to be equally effective but less invasive (and thus associated with a shorter in-patient stay and complication rate) as compared

with open thoracotomy in both adults and children.[56–59] VATS is the procedure of choice in patients with pleural sepsis, including those with HIV disease,[60] although the procedure is technically not feasible in up to 21% of patients where conversion to open thoracotomy drainage may be required.[49] Radiological features on CT do not predict which patients require conversion to thoracotomy decortication.[61]

More aggressive surgical approaches (permanent open drainage, muscle flap closure, or even extrapleural pneumonectomy)[62] have been described for refractory cases of chronic empyema, especially those associated with a bronchopleural fistula (including post-pneumonectomy). Fortunately, these cases are rare. The role of 'primary surgical treatment' as the first line for empyema is unclear. To date, only one published randomized trial of 20 patients has compared primary VATS with conservative chest tube drainage and declared benefit from early surgery.[63] A non-randomized study of 37 children has also come to similar conclusions.[64] No significant cost differentials exist between primary VATS and conservative chest tube drainage in published health economic analyses.[65,66]

Contrary to popular belief, radiological clearance of pleural collection is not a good indicator of disease progress. In the presence of satisfactory clinical improvement, the lack of radiological clearance should not be considered an indication for surgery. Numerous longitudinal studies have shown that radiological opacity of pleural infection improves in both adult[45] and pediatric patients[67,68] over the subsequent months without the need of surgery. Likewise, restrictive changes in pulmonary function tests usually improve in parallel over time; very few patients have functional impairment from residual pleural fibrosis.

Conclusions

Imaging tests have an established role in the management of patients with pleural sepsis. When the clinical question is whether or not there is pleural fluid, plain chest radiography and ultrasound are the prime investigations; as little as 5 ml of pleural fluid may be detected at ultrasound. The diagnosis of a parapneumonic effusion (simple or otherwise) is more problematic and generally depends on microbiological and, more importantly, biochemical analysis. However, there may be valuable diagnostic clues from ultrasound and CT studies. In most institutions, ultrasound is also probably the first-line test when image-guided drain insertion is required.

References

1. Maskell NA, Davies RJO. Effusions from parapneumonic infection and empyema. In: Light RW, Lee YCG, eds. Textbook of Pleural Diseases. London, UK: Arnold Press, 2003; 310–28.

2. Maskell NA, Davies CW, Nunn AJ et al. U.K. Controlled trial of intrapleural streptokinase for pleural infection. N Engl J Med 2005; 352: 865–74.

3. Cohen M. Challenges in pleural disease management in Central America. Intl Pleural Newsl 2005; 3: 8.

4. Hailu S. Paediatric thoracic empyema in an Ethiopian referral hospital. East Afr Med J 2000; 77: 618–21.

5. Byington CL, Spencer LY, Johnson TA et al. An epidemiological investigation of a sustained high rate of pediatric parapneumonic empyema: risk factors and microbiological associations. Clin Infect Dis 2002; 34: 434–40.

6. Thompson A, Reid A, Shields M, Steen H, Taylor R. Increased incidence in childhood empyema thoracis in Northern Ireland. Ir Med J 1999; 92: 438.

7. Chu MW, Dewar LR, Burgess JJ, Busse EG. Empyema thoracis: lack of awareness results in a prolonged clinical course. Can J Surg 2001; 44: 284–8.

8. Nadeem A, Bilal A, Shahkar S, Shah A. Presentation and management of empyema thoracis at Lady Reading Hospital, Peshawar. J Ayub Med Coll Abbottabad 2004; 16: 14–7.

9. Hamm H, Light RW. Parapneumonic effusion and empyema. Euro Respir J 1997; 10: 1150–6.

10. Davies CWH, Gleeson FV, Davies RJO. The British Thoracic Society guidelines on the management of pleural infection. Thorax 2003; 58: ii18–ii28.

11. Tsai TH, Jerng JS, Chen KY, Yu CJ, Yang PC. Community-acquired thoracic empyema in older people. J Am Geriatr Soc 2005; 53: 1203–9.

12. Blackmore CC, Black WC, Dallas RV et al. Pleural fluid volume estimation: a chest radiograph prediction rule. Acad Radiol 1996; 3: 103–9.

13. Gryminski J, Krakowa P, Lypacewicq G. The diagnosis of pleural effusion by ultrasonic and radiologic techniques. Chest 1976; 70: 33–7.

14. Mayo PH, Doelken P. Pleural ultrasonography. Clin Chest Med 2006; 27: 215–27.

15. Stark DD, Federle MP, Goodman PC et al. Differentiating lung abscess and empyema: radiography and computed tomography. AJR Am J Roentgenol 1983; 141: 163–7.

16. Sahn SA, Light RW. The sun should never set on a parapneumonic effusion. Chest 1989; 95: 945–7.

17. Marel M, Zrustova M, Stasny B, Light RW. The incidence of pleural effusion in a well-defined region. Epidemiologic study in central Bohemia. Chest 1993; 104: 1486–9.

18. Qureshi NR, Gleeson FV. Imaging of pleural disease. Clin Chest Med 2006; 27: 193–213.

19. Kearney SE, Davies CW, Davies RJ, Gleeson FV. Computed tomography and ultrasound in parapneumonic effusions and empyema. Clin Radiol 2000; 55: 542–7.

20. Huang HC, Chang HY, Chen CW, Lee CH, Hsiue TR. Predicting factors for outcome of tube thoracostomy in complicated parapneumonic effusion for empyema. Chest 1999; 115: 751–6.

21. Chen KY, Liaw YS, Wang HC, Luh KT, Yong PC. Sonographic septation: a useful prognostic indicator of acute thoracic empyema. J Ultrasound Med 2000; 19: 837–43.

22. Donnelly LF, Klosterman LA. CT appearance of parapneumonic effusions in children: findings are not specific for empyema. AJR Am J Roentgenol 1997; 169: 179–82.

23. Waite RJ, Carbonneau RJ, Balikkian JP et al. Parietal pleural changes in empyema: appearances at CT. Radiology 1990; 175: 145–50.

24. Aquino SL, Webb WR, Gushiken BJ. Pleural exudates and transudates: diagnosis with contrast enhanced CT. Radiology 1994; 192: 803–8

25. Haramati LB, Alterman DD, White CS, Kerr AS. Intrathoracic lymphadenopathy in patients with empyema. J Comput Assist Tomogr 1997; 21: 608–11.

26. Kearney SE, Davies CW, Tattersall DJ, Gleeson FV. The characteristics and significance of thoracic lymphadenopathy in parapneumonic effusion and empyema. Br J Radiol 2000; 73: 583–7.

27. Light RW. Pleural Diseases. 4th ed. Baltimore: Lippincott, Williams & Wilkins, 2001.

28. Maskell NA, Gleeson FV, Darby M et al. Diagnostically significant variations in pleural fluid pH in loculated parapneumonic effusions. Chest 2004; 126: 2022–4.

29. Saglani S, Harris KA, Wallis C, Hartley JC. Empyema: the use of broad range 16S rDNA PCR for pathogen detection. Arch Dis Child 2005; 90: 70–3.

30. Chapman SJ, Davies RJ. Recent advances in parapneumonic effusion and empyema. Curr Opin Pulm Med 2004; 10: 299–304.

31. Yilmaz E, Dogan Y, Aydinoglu AH, Gurgoze MK, Aygun D. Parapneumonic empyema in children: conservative approach. Turk J Pediatr 2002; 44: 134–8.

32. Diacon AH, Brutsche MH, Soler M. Accuracy of pleural puncture sites: a prospective comparison of clinical examination with ultrasound. Chest 2003; 123: 436–41.

33. Jones PW, Moyers P, Rogers JT et al. Ultrasound-guided thoracentesis: is it a safer method? Chest 2003; 123: 418–23.

34. Sasse S, Nguyen T, Teixeira LR, Light R. The utility of daily therapeutic thoracentesis for the treatment of early empyema. Chest 1999; 116: 1703–8.

35. Shoseyov D, Bibi H, Shatzberg G et al. Short-term course and outcome of treatments of pleural empyema in pediatric patients: repeated ultrasound-guided needle thoracocentesis vs chest tube drainage Chest 2002; 121: 836–40.

36. Hewitt C. Drainage for empyema. Br Med J 1876; 1: 317.

37. Pierrepoint MJ, Evans A, Morris SJ, Harrison SK, Doull IJ. Pigtail catheter drain in the treatment of empyema thoracis. Arch Dis Child 2002; 87: 331–2.

38. Shankar S, Gulati M, Kang M, Gupta S, Suri S. Image-guided percutaneous drainage of thoracic empyema: can sonography predict the outcome? Eur Radiol 2000; 10: 495–9.

39. Lee YCG. Ongoing search for effective intrapleural therapy for empyema: Is streptokinase the answer? Am J Respir Crit Care Med 2004; 170: 1–2.

40. Banga A, Khilnani GC, Sharma SK et al. A study of empyema thoracis and role of intrapleural streptokinase in its management. BMC Infect Dis 2004; 29: 19.

41. Cochran JB, Tecklenburg FW, Turner RB. Intrapleural instillation of fibrinolytic agents for treatment of pleural empyema. Pediatr Crit Care Med 2003; 4: 39–43.

42. Tuncozgur B, Ustunsoy H, Sivrikoz MC et al. Intrapleural urokinase in the management of parapneumonic empyema: a randomized controlled trial. Int J Clin Pract 2001; 55: 658–60.

43. Bouros D, Schiza S, Tzanakis N et al. Intrapleural urokinase versus normal saline in the treatment of complicated parapneumonic effusions and empyema. A randomized, double-blind study. Am J Respir Crit Care Med 1999; 159: 37–42.

44. Chin NK, Lim TK. Controlled trial of intrapleural streptokinase in the treatment of pleural empyema and complicated parapneumonic effusions. Chest 1997; 111: 275–9.

45. Diacon AH, Theron J, Schuurmans MM, Vande Wal BW, Bolliger CT. Intrapleural streptokinase for empyema and complicated parapneumonic effusions. Am J Respir Crit Care Med 2004; 170: 49–53.

46. Simpson G, Roomes D, Heron M. Effects of streptokinase and deoxyribonuclease on viscosity of human surgical and empyema pus. Chest 2000; 117: 1728–33.

47. Light RW, Nguyen T, Mulligan ME, Sasse SA. The in vitro efficacy of varidase versus streptokinase or urokinase for liquefying thick purulent exudative material from loculated empyema. Lung 2000; 178: 13–8.

48. Simpson G, Roomes D, Reeves B. Successful treatment of empyema thoracis with human recombinant deoxyribonuclease. Thorax 2003; 58: 365–6.

49. Hope WW, Bolton WD, Stephenson JE. The utility and timing of surgical intervention for parapneumonic empyema in the era of video-assisted thoracoscopy. Am Surg 2005; 71: 512–4.

50. Chen LE, Langer JC, Dillon PA et al. Management of late-stage parapneumonic empyema. J Pediatr Surg 2002; 37: 371–4.

51. Kalfa N, Allal H, Montes-Tapia F et al. Ideal timing of thoracoscopic decortication and drainage for empyema in children. Surg Endosc 2004; 18: 472–7.

52. Waller DA, Rengarajan A, Nicholson FH, Rajesh PB. Delayed referral reduces the success of video-assisted thoracoscopic debridement for post-pneumonic empyema. Respir Med 2001; 95: 836–40.

53. Huang FL, Chen PY, Ma JS et al. Clinical experience of managing empyema thoracic in children. J Microbiol Immunol Infect 2002; 35: 115–20.

54. Melloni G, Carretta A, Ciriaco P et al. Decortication for chronic parapneumonic empyema: results of a prospective study. World J Surg 2004; 28: 488–93.

55. Gates RL, Caniano DA, Hayes JR, Arca MJ. Does VATS provide optimal treatment of empyema in children? A systematic review. J Pediatr Surg 2004; 39: 381–6.

56. Waller DA, Rengarajan A. Thoracoscopic decortication: a role for video-assisted surgery in chronic postpneumonic pleural empyema. Ann Thorac Surg 2001; 71: 1813–6.

57. Podbielski FJ, Maniar HS, Rodriguez HE, Hernan MJ, Vigneswaran WT. Surgical strategy of complex empyema thoracis. JSLS 2000; 4: 287–90.

58. Cohen G, Hjortdal V, Ricci M et al. Primary thoracoscopic treatment of empyema in children. J Thorac Cardiovasc Surg 2003; 125: 79–83.

59. Klena JW, Cameron BH, Langer JC, Winthrop AL, Perez CR. Timing of video-assisted thoracoscopic debridement for pediatric empyema. J Am Coll Surg 1998; 187: 404–8.

60. Khwaja S, Rosenbaum DH, Paul MC et al. Surgical treatment of thoracic empyema in HIV-infected patients: severity and treatment modality is associated with CD4 count status. Chest 2005; 128: 246–9.

61. Roberts JR. Minimally invasive surgery in the treatment of empyema: intraoperative decision making. Ann Thorac Surg 2003; 76: 225–30.

62. Shiraishi Y, Nakajima Y, Koyama A et al. Morbidity and mortality after 94 extrapleural pneumonectomies for empyema. Ann Thorac Surg 2000; 70: 1202–6.

63. Wait MA, Sharma S, Hohn J, Dal Nogare A. A randomized trial of empyema therapy. Chest 1997; 111: 1548–51.

64. Chen CY, Chen JS, Huang LM et al. Favorable outcome of parapneumonic empyema in children managed by primary video-assisted thoracoscopic debridement. J Formos Med Assoc 2003; 102: 845–50.

65. Meier AH, Smith B, Raghavan A et al. Rational treatment of empyema in children. Arch Surg 2000; 135: 907–12.

66. Thourani VH, Brady KM, Mansour KA, Miller JIJ, Lee RB. Evaluation of treatment modalities for thoracic empyema: a cost-effectiveness analysis. Ann Thorac Surg 1998; 66: 1121–7.

67. Satish B, Bunker M, Seddon P. Management of thoracic empyema in childhood: does the pleural thickening matter? Arch Dis Child 2003; 88: 918–21.

68. Kohn GL, Walston C, Feldstein J et al. Persistent abnormal lung function after childhood empyema. Am J Respir Med 2002; 1: 441–5.

12

Pulmonary sepsis

Tomás Franquet, Jacob Sellarés, and Antoni Torres

Introduction

Despite advances in diagnosis and treatment, respiratory tract infection continues to be a major cause of morbidity and mortality. The major routes of pulmonary infection are hematogenous spread, direct inoculation, and contiguous spread. Appropriate and prompt diagnosis is made with imaging and relevant microbiological studies.

Characteristic imaging findings and isolation of the causative organism are the main tools for the correct diagnosis. Imaging evaluation in pulmonary infections is essentially confined to chest radiography and computed tomography (CT).[1-3] Although plain radiographic evaluation is generally the initial modality used, CT may help to demonstrate pulmonary abnormalities not seen on conventional films. Significant disease is required to generate visible changes in radiographic density or an obviously abnormal radiographic pattern. Several factors may render early pulmonary infection invisible on chest radiograph.

Pneumonia is the leading cause of death due to infectious disease.[4] More than 6 million cases of bacterial pneumonia occur each year in the US and the incidence of pneumonia is increasing. The spectrum of organisms known to cause respiratory infections is broad and constantly increasing as new pathogens are identified and an increasing number of patients have decreased immunity due to disease or medications. In the US, it has been estimated that there are 1.1 million cases of community-acquired pneumonia (CAP) requiring hospitalization each year.[4] Nosocomial pneumonia is the most important hospital-acquired infection as it is associated with the highest mortality rate of nosocomial infections.[5] In addition to direct patient care costs, pneumonia is responsible for over 50 million days of restricted activity from work and is the sixth leading cause of death in the US with a mortality rate of 13.4 per 100 000.[6]

In the past two decades there has been not only an increase in the prevalence of various infections but also the recognition of several important new viral pathogens. These include hantaviruses, human metapneumovirus, avian influenza A viruses, and coronavirus associated with severe acute respiratory syndrome (SARS).[7-14]

In this chapter, we discuss and illustrate the main problems in diagnosis and the common imaging findings of CAP, hospital-acquired pneumonia (HAP), pneumonia in immunocompromised patients, and mycobacterial infections.

Clinical approach in the management of patients with thoracic infection and sepsis: the problem of disease detection

Diagnosis of pneumonia requires clinical acumen, appropriate microbiological tests, and imaging. It should be suspected in a febrile patient with cough and crackles. The clinician evaluating a patient with a known or suspected diagnosis of pulmonary infection faces a diagnostic challenge because the infection may be caused by a variety of different organisms that may present with similar clinical symptoms and signs, and result in similar radiographic manifestations. Furthermore, the radiographic manifestations of a given organism may be variable depending on the immunological status of the patient and the presence of pre- or coexisting lung disease.

The number of immunocompromised patients has increased considerably in the past three decades because of three main phenomena: the AIDS epidemic, advances in cancer chemotherapy, and expanding solid organ and hematopoietic stem cell transplantation. At the onset of the AIDS epidemic, in the early and mid-1980s, there was 50–80% mortality for each episode of *Pneumocystis jiroveci* pneumonia (PCP). Since routine prophylaxis was instituted in 1989, there has been a declining incidence of PCP in the AIDS population[15-17] and a decrease in mortality in mild to moderate cases.[18] However, other infections including bacterial pneumonia, fungal infection, cytomegalovirus (CMV), *Mycobacterium avium* complex (MAC), and tuberculosis remain a significant cause of morbidity and mortality in these patients.[15–18] The role of imaging is to identify the presence, location, and extent of pulmonary abnormalities, the course and evolution of pneumonia, the presence of associated complications, and detection of additional or alternative diagnosis.

What is the role of chest radiography in the diagnosis and follow-up of thoracic infections?

The main applications of radiology in pneumonia are oriented to detection, characterization, and follow-up.[2] Confirming whether a patient has a pneumonia can be a challenge for the clinician. The most useful imaging modalities for the evaluation of patients with known or suspected pulmonary infection are chest radiography and CT. Chest radiography must be routinely undertaken in patients with 'presumptive' pneumonia to make the diagnosis. The American Thoracic Society guidelines recommend that posteroanterior (PA) (and lateral when possible) chest radiographs be obtained whenever pneumonia is suspected in adults.[19] The role of chest radiography is as a screening tool for the detection of abnormalities consistent with pneumonia and for monitoring response to therapy. Other roles for the chest radiograph include assessment of disease extent, detection of complications (i.e. cavitation, abscess formation, pneumothorax, pleural effusion), detection of additional or alternative diagnoses, and, in some cases, to guide invasive diagnostic procedures (Figure 12.1).

In most cases the radiographic findings are suggestive or consistent with the diagnosis of pneumonia and sufficiently specific in the proper clinical context to preclude the need for additional imaging.[1–3,20] However, a normal chest radiograph should not exclude the diagnosis of pneumonia because the radiograph can lag behind the clinical findings by several days. There is wide disagreement among physicians on the presence or absence of CAP on chest radiographs, and a chest radiograph that shows 'no pneumonia' may not be sufficient to rule out the diagnosis.[21] In one large series, approximately 10% of patients with proven pulmonary infection had an apparently normal chest radiograph. Early and definitive diagnosis of pulmonary infection is essential to guide therapy and may have an impact on the patient's prognosis.

Radiographic evidence of pneumonia generally resolves within 4–6 weeks, and persistent opacifications beyond that suggest inadequate pulmonary drainage, a chronic persistent problem, or the possibility of a congenital abnormality.

What are the radiographic manifestations of thoracic infections?

The most common radiographic manifestations of respiratory infection are foci of consolidation, bronchopneumonia, ground-glass opacities, or reticulonodular opacities. Alveolar air-space disease with consolidation and air bronchograms characterizes lobar pneumonia. This is the commonest radiographic manifestation of pneumonia in the vast majority of cases (Figure 12.2). The infection may be limited initially to a lobe or segment and initially appear radiographically as a subsegmental consolidation or 'round'

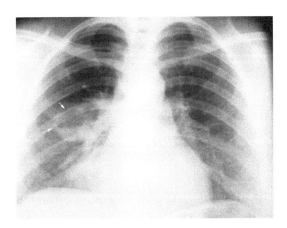

Figure 12.1
Staphyloccocal lung abscess. Posteroanterior chest radiograph in a 48-year-old alcoholic man shows an air-space consolidation in the right lower lobe. An abscess with an air-fluid level is also present (arrows).

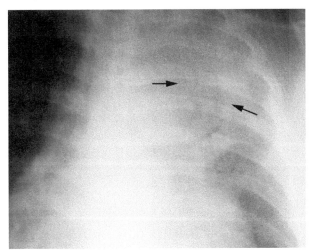

Figure 12.2
Lobar pneumonia. Posteroanterior chest radiograph shows extensive area of air-space consolidation in the left lobe. Air bronchogram is nicely seen within the consolidation (arrows).

pneumonia. Bronchopneumonia results from infection of the airways with an infectious agent, with subsequent airway obstruction and spread to air spaces; this pattern may not be distinguished from air-space disease if the radiograph is obtained later in the course. On the chest radiograph there is a prominence of the bronchovascular markings and, later, multiple ill-defined nodular opacities coalescing to air-space consolidation. Interstitial pneumonias may present radiographically with septal thickening and reticular densities resulting from the 'summation' of linear interstitial lines. This pattern is seen in viral infections and atypical bacteria such as *Mycoplasma pneumoniae* and *Chlamydia pneumoniae.*

Other less common radiographic findings include hilar and mediastinal lymphadenopathy, pleural effusion, cavitation, and chest wall invasion. These findings are not specific and may be seen in other conditions. Furthermore, any given organism may result in a variety of different patterns of presentation. For example, *Pneumocystis jiroveci* may result in bilateral ground-glass opacities or consolidation, or, less commonly, focal consolidation, nodules, miliary pattern, or reticulation.[19] In up to 10% of patients with proven pneumocystis pneumonia the chest radiograph is normal.[22]

What is the role of computed tomography in the diagnosis and follow-up of thoracic infections?

CT is a useful adjunct to conventional radiography and should be used in unresolved cases or when complications of pneumonia are suspected.[23–26] Chest CT reveals more thoracic disease than can be appreciated on chest radiograph and there is a large amount of literature indicating that CT is a sensitive method capable of imaging the lung with excellent spatial resolution and providing anatomical detail similar to that seen by gross pathological examination. Differences in tissue attenuation and parenchymal changes caused by an acute inflammatory process can be seen readily on CT.[23,26] CT can also be helpful in the detection, differential diagnosis, and management of patients with pulmonary complications. Radiological distinction from different infectious processes is difficult to establish and is largely made on the basis of the clinical setting and associated ancillary CT findings.

What are the computed tomography manifestations of thoracic infections?

Optimal assessment of the parenchyma is obtained with the use of high-resolution CT (HRCT) which allows assessment of the pattern and distribution of abnormalities

down to the level of the secondary pulmonary lobule.[23] The findings of air-space disease, including air-space nodules, ground-glass opacities, consolidation, air bronchograms, and centrilobular or perilobular distribution are seen better at CT than at conventional radiography.[22,23] Air-space nodules measure 6–10 mm in diameter and usually reflect the presence of peribronchiolar consolidation, and therefore are centrilobular in distribution. They are best appreciated in early disease and best seen at the edge of the pathological process where consolidation is incomplete. In some circumstances, nodules may be associated with a 'halo' of ground-glass attenuation (Figure 12.3). In severely neutropenic patients this 'halo' sign is highly suggestive of angioinvasive aspergillosis.[27] However, a similar appearance has been described in other conditions including infection by non-tuberculous mycobacteria, *Mucorales* spp., *Candida* spp., herpes simplex virus, and cytomegalovirus, and in Wegener's granulomatosis, Kaposi's sarcoma, and hemorrhagic metastases.[28]

Ground-glass opacity is defined as hazy increased lung opacity that does not obscure the underlying vascular structures (see Figure 12.3). Ground-glass opacities are a common but non-specific HRCT finding that may result from a variety of interstitial and air-space diseases. Infections that typically present with bilateral ground-glass opacities are pneumocystis and cytomegalovirus pneumonia (Figure 12.4). In AIDS patients the presence of extensive bilateral ground-glass opacities is highly suggestive of PCP. In immunocompromised non-AIDS patients the differential diagnosis includes cytomegalovirus pneumonia, drug-induced lung disease, pulmonary hemorrhage, and organizing pneumonia.[29]

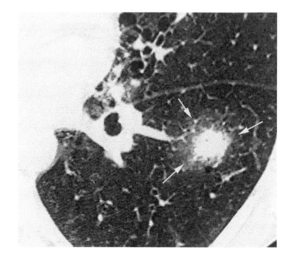

Figure 12.3
Angioinvasive aspergillosis. High-resolution CT scan (1.0-mm collimation) at the level of left pulmonary vein shows a nodule in the left lower lobe surrounded by a halo of ground-glass attenuation ('halo sign') (arrows). The patient was a 68-year-old man with severe neutropenia.

A 'tree-in-bud' pattern is a characteristic HRCT manifestation of infectious bronchiolitis. It consists of centrilobular branching tubular and nodular structures and reflects the presence of bronchiolar inflammation and filling of the lumen by inflammatory material or mucus.[30] This pattern may be seen in a variety of bacterial, mycobacterial, fungal, and viral infections (Figure 12.5).[30,31]

Air-space consolidation, defined as a localized increase in lung attenuation that obscures the underlying vascular structures, may be seen in association with bacterial, fungal, and viral infections (Figure 12.6). Focal areas of consolidation secondary to infection in immunocompromised AIDS and non-AIDS patients are most commonly due to bacterial pneumonia.[32] Fungal infection needs to be considered particularly in neutropenic patients with hematological malignancies.[29] Parenchymal disease in mycobacterial infection may also appear as patchy nodular areas of consolidation, with or without cavitation.[33]

The CT features of pyogenic pulmonary infection are variable and include lobar consolidation, nodules, infiltrates with pleural effusions, round infiltrates, and pleural effusions alone.[1,3]

Integrating clinical and imaging findings

Importance of clinicoradiological work-up

Imaging examinations should always be interpreted with awareness of the clinical findings including duration of symptoms, presence of fever, cough, dyspnea, and presence or absence of leukocytosis.[34] Knowledge of whether the patient has community-acquired or nosocomial pneumonia, as well as knowledge of the immune status of the patient, are most helpful in the differential diagnosis and determination of the most likely causative organisms.[34,35] Clinical information can greatly enhance the accuracy of the radiographic diagnosis. For example, the AIDS patient with an acute air-space process who has chills, fever, and purulent sputum probably has pyogenic rather than a pneumocystis pneumonia. In the absence of clinical information, radiologists cannot reliably distinguish between pneumonia and other pulmonary processes.[25] Unfortunately, the clinical data and radiographic findings often fail to lead to a definitive diagnosis of pneumonia because there are an extensive

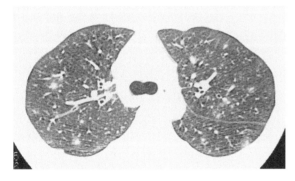

Figure 12.4
Cytomegalovirus pneumonitis. HRCT scan (1-mm collimation) at the level of the carina in a 25-year-old man with acute myeloid leukemia and bone marrow transplant shows multiple poorly defined nodules surrounded by a halo of ground-glass attenuation.

(a)

(b)

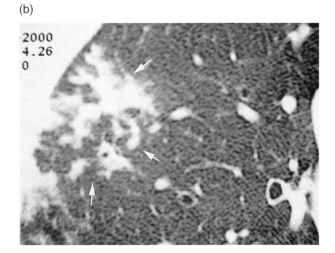

Figure 12.5
Tuberculosis. (a) View of the right lung from a posteroanterior chest radiograph in a 45-year-old smoker shows focal ill-defined opacity in the right upper lobe. (b) View from HRCT image (2-mm collimation) shows multiple rounded and branching opacities ('tree-in-bud') in a centrilobular distribution (arrows). Sputum cultures grew *Mycobacterium tuberculosis*.

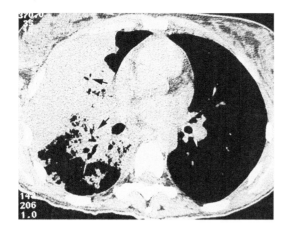

Figure 12.6
Pneumoccocal pneumonia. CT image (5-mm collimation) in a 53-year-old man shows a focal area of homogeneous consolidation in the right upper lobe. Note the presence of air bronchogram within the consolidation (arrow). Sputum culture produced a heavy growth of *Streptococcus pneumoniae*.

number of non-infectious processes associated with febrile pneumonitis, including drug-induced pulmonary disease, acute eosinophilic pneumonia, organizing pneumonia (bronchiolitis obliterans organizing pneumonia, BOOP), and pulmonary vasculitis, that may mimic pulmonary infection.[32]

Distinction of localized pneumonia from other pulmonary processes cannot be made with certainty on radiological grounds.[34,32] Localized pulmonary disease of a lobar or segmental distribution can be produced not only by pneumonia but also by obstructive pneumonitis, hemorrhage, or aspiration of sterile gastric contents. Diagnosis is equally difficult when pneumonia appears as a diffuse pulmonary abnormality. Extensive bilateral abnormalities may be due to bronchopneumonia or due to hydrostatic pulmonary edema, acute respiratory distress syndrome (ARDS), or diffuse pulmonary hemorrhage.[36–38]

Community-acquired pneumonia

CAP is a major health care problem due to its considerable incidence and mortality.[39] It is estimated that there are 2–4 million cases per year of CAP in the US[40] and 5–11 cases per 1000 population per year in Europe.[41,42] Hospital admission rates of pneumonia episodes vary from 22 to 51% of patients with CAP.[4] Between 485 000 and 1 million patients each year are hospitalized in the US for treatment of CAP. The costs of inpatient care exceed outpatient care and comprise the majority of the estimated $8.4 billion spent annually for care the patients with pneumonia.[4,6,41,43] Mortality is estimated to be approximately 14% becoming the sixth most common cause of death in the US.[44] The mortality is higher in less-developed countries, as well as in young and elderly patients.

The spectrum of causative pathogens of CAP includes Gram-positive bacteria (*Streptococcus pneumoniae*, *Staphylococcus aureus*), Gram-negative bacteria (*Haemophilus influenzae*), atypical bacteria (*Mycoplasma pneumoniae*, *Chlamydia pneumoniae*, *Legionella pneumophila*), oral anaerobes, and viral agents (adenoviruses, influenza viruses, severe acute respiratory syndrome).[45]

CAP is suspected in any patient with acute respiratory symptoms (cough, sputum production, and/or dyspnea), especially if accompanied by fever and auscultatory findings of abnormal breath sound and crackles, although these symptoms are not always present, especially in a patient with an inadequate immune response or advanced age.[46] In some cases CAP may be difficult to distinguish clinically and radiologically from other entities such as congestive heart failure, pulmonary embolism, and aspiration pneumonia.[1,47] When the diagnosis of CAP is considered, chest radiography plays a pivotal role in confirming or excluding pneumonia. Although the definitive diagnosis is completed with the results of cultures, the early diagnosis with a chest radiograph is essential to start empirical antibiotic therapy as soon as possible. Chest radiograph is not only important in diagnosis of CAP, but it also gives an excellent help in the differential diagnosis, in etiological work-up, in detecting CAP complications, in the follow-up procedure, and in improving the efficacy of invasive techniques.

What is the role of radiology in diagnosing community-acquired pneumonia?

Conventional chest radiography and CT are the imaging techniques commonly used in the diagnosis of pneumonia. In every patient with the suspicion of CAP, the chest radiograph is the initial imaging method, whereas CT is reserved for unclear cases.

The American Thoracic Society guidelines recommend that a chest radiograph should be obtained whenever pneumonia is suspected.[46] For the purpose of excluding or confirming pneumonia, this simple imaging method is both sensitive and specific,[48] and it is also relatively available and with a reasonable low cost and low radiation burden. However, chest X-ray it is not always available, especially in certain outpatient settings. Radiological infiltrates usually appear 12 hours after the onset of clinical symptoms.[45] The experience of the radiologist is very important for the radiological diagnosis of CAP. The interobserver agreement is quite fair in well experienced radiologist, but poor to fair if the interpretation of the radiograph is done by a resident or an inexperienced radiologist.[49,50] Written reports are another important part in the radiological evaluation of CAP. Interpretation of whether findings support the diagnosis of pneumonia (in reports with pneumonia-related observations), short sentences, and the redundancy of the pneumonia-related observations are the three variables independently associated with an unambiguous report.[51]

How reliable is chest radiography in establishing the diagnosis of pneumonia?

Radiographically, lobar pneumonia typically appears initially in the lung periphery abutting against the pleura and spreads towards the core portions of the lung. Round pneumonia occurs more frequently in children than adults and is most commonly caused by *Strep. pneumoniae*[20,52] (Figure 12.7). In children, active tuberculous and fungal infection also may present with nodular or mass-like opacities.[52] Bacterial infections may produce multiple rounded pulmonary nodules or masses, with or without cavitation. This may occur as a result of *Nocardia* spp., *Aspergillus* spp., *Legionella pneumophila*, Q fever, or *Mycobacterium tuberculosis* infection.[52–54]

Bronchopneumonia, which is most commonly caused by *Staph. aureus* and *H. influenzae*, occurs when infectious organisms, deposited on the epithelium of the bronchi, produce acute bronchial inflammation with epithelial ulcerations and fibrinopurulent exudate formation. As a consequence, the inflammatory reaction rapidly spreads through the airway walls and into the contiguous pulmonary lobules. Radiographically, these inflammatory aggregates cause a typical pattern of multifocal unilateral or bilateral areas of consolidation. Abscess formation may occur particularly in bronchopneumonia due to *Staph. aureus* or

anaerobes (Figure 12.8). Thin walled cavities (pneumatoceles), bronchopleural fistulas, and empyema also develop in the context of *Staph. aureus* infections. Cavitation and pneumatocele formation may also occur in Gram-negative infection and *Strep. pneumoniae* type 3 (Figures 12.9 and 12.10).

Pneumoccocal pneumonia in childhood usually presents as a distinct clinical syndrome characterized by acute onset and fever. Clinically, the spectrum of pneumoccocal pneumonia can vary from a very mild course managed in an ambulatory setting to a severe complicated pneumonia associated with pulmonary necrosis

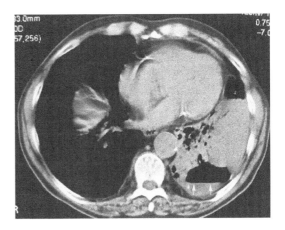

Figure 12.8

Necrotizing pneumonia. CT image (5-mm collimation) at the level of inferior pulmonary veins shows a lobar area of consolidation containing visible air bronchogram. An abscess with an air–fluid level also is present (arrows). The patient was a middle-aged woman. Culture grew mixed anaerobic organisms.

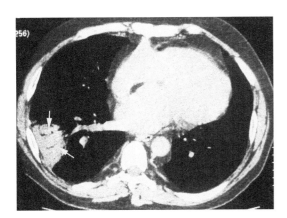

Figure 12.7

Rounded pneumonia. CT image (5-mm collimation) shows a dense mass-like consolidation in the right-lower lobe with visible air bronchogram (arrows). The patient was a middle-aged man.

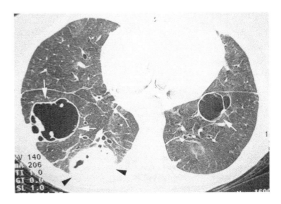

Figure 12.9

Pneumatoceles. CT image (2-mm collimation) in a 35-year-old female with persistent productive cough and fever shows bilateral thin-walled pneumatoceles in lower lobes. A dense mass-like consolidation in the right-lower lobe with visible air bubbles (arrows) is also seen. Immunofluorescence microscopy of sputum revealed *Micoplasma pneumoniae* organisms.

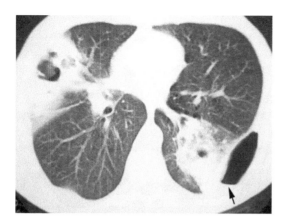

Figure 12.10
Pneumoccocal pneumonia: abcess formation. CT scan (5-mm collimation) at the level of the inferior pulmonary veins in a 56-year-old man shows bilateral segmental areas of consolidation with associated cavitation. A left hydro-pneumothorax secondary to a peripheral broncho-pleural fistula is present (arrow). Sputum culture produced a heavy growth of *Strep pneumoniae*.

(cavitation) and pleural effusion often requiring chest tube placement.

Pneumonia that is caused by pathogens of the *Chlamydia* species, together with *Mycoplasma pneumoniae*, is known as atypical pneumonia, which is clinically characterized by a non-productive cough or a mildly elevated or normal white blood cell count. Atypical pneumonia requires a different treatment strategy than usual bacterial pneumonia, such as streptococcal pneumonia, and therefore the correct diagnosis of atypical pneumonia is clinically important.[55] *Chlamydia pneumoniae* pneumonia has a wide spectrum of CT findings that consist of consolidation, ground-glass opacities, bronchovascular bundle thickening, and nodules in a different proportion.[56]

In the diagnosis of pneumonia, four radiographic patterns can be identified: localized air-space disease (lobar pneumonia), lobular pneumonia (bronchopneumonia), interstitial pneumonia, and nodular lesions.[45] Lobar pneumonia and bronchopneumonia are the most typical features in CAP. Lobar pneumonia is characterized by a homogeneous consolidation of lung parenchyma due to the damage directly produced to alveoli by the microorganism. It is common in Gram-positive, Gram-negative, and atypical bacteria, although it may also be seen in viral infections. Lobular pneumonia is typical in CAP caused by *Staph. aureus* and *Pseudomonas aeruginosa*. In this type of pneumonia, the microorganism directly damages the peripheral airways, so in early stages the presence of air-space nodules, lobular consolidation, and confluent focal areas of consolidation is typical. Interstitial pneumonia is rare in CAP, but when it is

observed in healthy outpatients, it is commonly associated with the respiratory syncytial virus (RVS).

Radiologically, interstitial or mixed interstitial and air-space opacities are typically due to viruses, *Chlamydia* species, or *Mycoplasma pneumoniae*.[57–61] Up to 30% of all pneumonias in the general population are caused by *Mycoplasma pneumoniae*.[25] During infection, the initial damage is directed towards the mucosa of the bronchioles, and later the peribronchial tissue and interlobular septa become edematous and infiltrated with inflammatory cells. Nodular lesions are very rare in CAP.

The described chest X-ray patterns generally correspond to those seen at CT. The tree-in-bud sign is a CT feature more specific of infection.[31,62] This phenomenon is observed when there are inflammatory changes in the small peripheral bronchioles with secretions in the lumen of the airways, wall thickening, and peribronchiolar inflammation. When this sign appears in the CT, it is suggestive of infectious bronchiolitis. *Mycoplasma pneumoniae* and viruses are the most frequent etiological agents, although it is also typical in mycobacterial infections.[31,62]

Although these patterns could be of assistance in the management of CAP, their value is limited in bacterial CAP because different patterns may overlap and a single organism may produce different patterns. Further patterns are influenced by the immunological status of the host and may be altered by other coexisting lung diseases.[45] Thus, in clinical practice it is not recommended to select the empirical antibiotic therapy based on radiological patterns.[39,46]

What is the role of radiology in the follow-up of community-acquired pneumonia?

It is advisable to monitor the resolution of pulmonary infiltrates in the clinical course of CAP whenever possible. The majority of pulmonary infiltrates in CAP are resolved within 21 days. However, in one-third of the patients the complete clearance of lung infiltrates could take up to 6 months.[63] It is important to differentiate these patients with slow improvement of CAP from those who do not have a favorable therapy response. There are many causes of non-responding pneumonia, the most frequent cause being the inadequate initial antibiotic therapy.[64] When the clinical and radiological course of CAP is atypical, differential diagnosis must also be done with other non-infectious diseases that may mimic pneumonia such as cryptogenic organizing pneumonia (COP), eosinophilic pneumonia, acute alveolar sarcoid, lupus pneumonitis, or malignant tumors, especially carcinoma, bronchogenic carcinoma with postobstructive pneumonitis and lymphoma. In those patients with slow response, CT and bronchoscopy may be useful in differentiating these pathologies from CAP.

What is the role of radiology in optimizing interventional diagnostic procedures?

Several invasive diagnostic techniques have been described in the diagnosis of CAP, although their use is limited to selected patients and they are not currently recommended as routine in CAP. The most commonly used procedures are bronchoscopy with a protected brush catheter and bronchoalveolar lavage, and direct percutaneous fine needle aspiration of the lung. With the exception of bronchoscopy these procedures are now infrequently performed because of concern about adverse effects and the lack of specialists skilled in these techniques.[39] In addition, retrospective studies have shown that in severe illness, outcome is not improved by establishing the etiological agent.[65] Bronchoscopy is recommended in patients with a fulminant course, who require admission to an intensive care unit (ICU) or have non-responding pneumonia despite correct empirical antibiotic therapy.[39] In all these techniques, radiography and CT are used for guidance of these methods to obtain samples from areas of maximum disease, improving the efficacy of the invasive method.

CAP is a major health care problem because of associated morbidity and mortality.[4,6]

Pulmonary opacities are usually evident on the radiograph within 12 hours of the onset of symptoms. Although the radiographic findings do not allow a specific etiological diagnosis, the radiograph may be helpful in narrowing down the differential diagnosis. In CAP, diagnosis and disease management most frequently involve chest radiography and, generally, do not require the use of other imaging modalities.[66]

The spectrum of causative organisms of CAP includes Gram-positive bacteria such as *Strep. pneumoniae* (pneumoccocus), *H. influenzae*, and *Staph. aureus*, as well as atypical organisms such as *Mycoplasma pneumoniae*, *Chlamydia pneumoniae*, or *Legionella pneumophila* and viral agents such as influenza A virus and respiratory syncytial viruses. *Strep. pneumoniae* is by far the most common cause of complete lobar consolidation.[67–69] Other causative agents that produce complete lobar consolidation include *Klebsiella pneumoniae* and other Gram-negative bacilli, *Legionella pneumophila*, *H. influenzae*, and occasionally *Mycoplasma pneumoniae*.[67–70]

A clinical diagnosis of pneumonia can usually be readily established on the basis of clinical signs and symptoms and the radiographic findings.

HOSPITAL-ACQUIRED (NOSOCOMIAL) PNEUMONIA

HAP is defined as pneumonia that occurs 48 hours or more after admission, which was not incubating at the time of admission. HAP is the leading cause of mortality from hospital-acquired infections. It occurs most commonly among intensive care unit (ICU) patients, predominately in individuals requiring mechanical ventilation.[71] When it refers to pneumonia that arises more than 48–72 hours after endotracheal intubation it is termed ventilator-associated pneumonia (VAP).[72]

The estimated prevalence of nosocomial pneumonia within the ICU setting ranges from 10 to 65%, with case fatality rates of 20–55% in most reported series.[70,71,73] In patients with ARDS, as many as 55% have secondary pneumonia, and this complication may adversely affect survival.[70]

In the hospitalized patient, the spectrum of pathogens associated with HAP is dominated by Gram-negative infections such *P. aeruginosa*, *Kebsiella* species, *Enterobacteriaceae*, *Escherichia coli*, *Serratia marcescens*, and *Proteus* species. In addition to these pathogens, Gram-positive cocci (*Strep. pneumoniae*, *Staph. aureus*), atypical bacterial (*Legionella* species), and viruses may be the etiological agent of HAP.[72] In most cases, the clinical course is not so clear compared with CAP, and pneumonias do not always present with characteristic symptoms. For this reason, radiology can be valuable in differentiating HAP from other causes of pulmonary infiltrates. Respiratory syncytial virus, influenza A and B, and parainfluenza are responsible for more than 70% of nosocomial viral diseases.[74]

What is the role of radiology in diagnosing hospital-acquired pneumonia?

In contrast with CAP, the appearance of pulmonary infiltrates may be delayed in HAP, particularly in patients with neutropenia,[50] and also in individuals with functional defects of granulocytes due to diabetes, alcoholism, and uremia. As the radiological manifestation of HAP may be atypical, CT can be valuable in the initial diagnosis particularly in mechanically ventilated patients.

In mechanically ventilated patients with suspected diagnosis of pneumonia, the interpretation of chest X-rays may be difficult because most patients present underlying chronic pulmonary diseases or processes that may mimic the radiological appearance of a pneumonia. In addition, portable chest X-rays performed at bedside are often of not very good quality and difficult to interpret. In patients with ARDS undergoing mechanical ventilation, it may be difficult to differentiate VAP from infiltrates secondary to ARDS. In the diagnosis of pneumonia, chest radiography in mechanically ventilated patients gives an overall accuracy of 52%, but when there is a coexistent ARDS, this accuracy decreases importantly.[75] Pugin et al.[76] developed the clinical pulmonary infection score (CPIS) which combines clinical, radiological, physiological (Pa_{O_2}/FI_{O_2}), and microbiological variables to obtain a single number. When this score is higher than 6, the diagnosis of VAP is very probable. Therefore, radiological findings in CPIS are just another item for the calculation of the score, unlike CAP, when radiology provides in most patients the definitive diagnosis of pneumonia.

Aspiration pneumonia

Aspiration pneumonia is particularly common in patients with decreased consciousness, chronic debilitating disease, and with oropharyngeal or airway instrumentation (e.g. patients on tube feeding or on mechanical ventilation). The aspirated material may include sterile gastric secretions, gastric content, or bacteria-laden oropharyngeal secretions (Figure 12.11). Aspiration of infected oropharyngeal secretions is more common than generally appreciated. The majority of bacterial pneumonias result from aspiration of infected material from the oropharynx into the lower respiratory tract.[47,77,78] Alcoholic patients and those with poor oral hygiene are prone to develop pulmonary infections after aspiration. Approximately 90% of infected aspiration pneumonias are caused by anaerobic organisms.[79] Anaerobic infections usually take the form of subacute or chronic constitutional and pulmonary symptoms. Anaerobes typically cause cavitary lesions (lung abscess), necrotizing pneumonia, or empyema.

In hospitalized patients who are colonized with highly virulent organisms, aspirations may overwhelm lung defenses, resulting in the development of pneumonia.[4,80] In the hospitalized patient, the stomach may become colonized with Gram-negative bacteria.[80] In these patients, intubation and mechanical ventilation may increase the incidence and size of aspirations, with resultant increase in

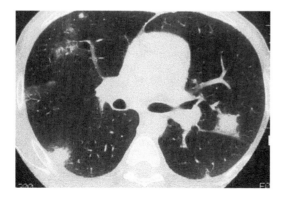

Figure 12.11
Periodontal aspiration. HRCT scan (2-mm collimation) at the level of the carina shows multiple nodules surrounded by a 'halo' of ground-glass attenuation. Findings are similar to those seen in angioinvasive aspergillosis. The patient was a 42-year-old alcoholic man with fever, putrid sputum, and pyorrhea.

the development of pneumonia.[77,80] The location of pneumonia depends on the position of the patient when aspiration occurs.

The radiographic manifestations usually consist of bilateral patchy areas of consolidation involving mainly the dependent regions. Since aspiration typically occurs with the patient supine the areas of consolidation tend to involve mainly the posterior and lateral basal segments of the lower lobes, superior segments of the lower lobes, and posterior segments of the upper lobes. The radiographic manifestations vary somewhat among the various species of Gram-negative bacilli. *P. aeruginosa* infection typically results in patchy unilateral or bilateral areas of consolidation (bronchopneumonia); lobar consolidation is uncommon.[80] Prolonged clinical course or large aspirations may result in severe necrotizing bronchopneumonia (Figure 12.12). An air–fluid level strongly suggests anaerobic disease. Although Gram-negative bacilli and *Staph. aureus* have similar radiographic findings, anaerobic infections have a more indolent clinical course.

Patients with advanced periodontal disease are at particular risk for development of aspiration pneumonia.[79] Radiographic findings include focal or patchy ill-defined areas of consolidation and progressive abscess formation. The opacities are usually unilateral but may involve both lungs.

A distinct form of infection is caused by *Actinomyces israelii*, a low-virulence anaerobic bacteria, that is normally found in the mouth of patients with poor oral hygiene.[4] Aspiration of infected material results in a localized or segmental pneumonia, usually in the dependent portions of the lung. If untreated, actinomycosis may invade the chest wall, the mediastinum, or the diaphragm. Radiographically, the disease starts as a localized subsegmental or segmental consolidation. Over a period of weeks to months after the aspiration event, cavitation and pleural effusion (empyema) may occur.

Septic pulmonary embolism

Septic pulmonary embolism generally presents with insidious onset of fever, cough, and pulmonary opacities.[81] It is seen most commonly in patients with indwelling catheters and in intravenous drug users; less common causes include pelvic thrombophlebitis and suppurative processes in the head and neck.[81] The radiographic manifestations usually consist of bilateral nodular opacities, which are frequently cavitated (Figure 12.13). The nodules may be circumscribed or poorly defined and may be associated with patchy areas of consolidation. CT is an important modality for confirming the presence of pulmonary septic emboli even when conventional chest radiographs remain negative.[82] CT findings include bilateral nodules most numerous in the peripheral lung regions and lower zones. The nodules may be well circumscribed or poorly defined and may

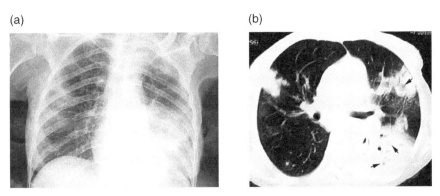

Figure 12.12
Aspiration pneumonia. (a) Anteroposterior radiograph shows bilateral ill-defined air-space consolidations in the right upper and left lower lobes. (b) CT scan (5.0-mm collimation) at the level of the carina shows hypodense areas within the consolidation representing necrosis (arrows). The patient was a 35-year-old female with pneumonia. *Staphylococcus aureus* was cultured from a bronchoscopic specimen.

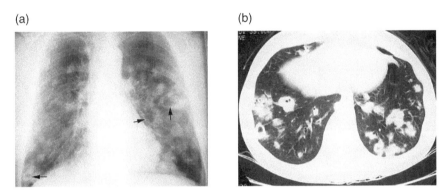

Figure 12.13
Septic pulmonary embolism. (a) Anteroposterior chest radiograph shows multiple bilateral nodular opacities some of which are cavitated (arrows). (b) HRCT scan (1.0-mm collimation) at the level of lung bases confirms the presence of multiple cavitated nodules. The patient was a 36-year-old male intravenous drug abuser with AIDS.

frequently cavitate.[81,83] Another common finding on CT is the presence of wedge-shaped pleural based areas of consolidation that may be homogenous or heterogenous and that may cavitate. The diagnosis of septic pulmonary embolism should be suggested by the presence of a predisposing factor, febrile illness, and CT findings of multiple, nodular lung infiltrates peripherally, with or without cavitation.[81]

Respiratory infections in the immuncompromised patient

The most common pulmonary complication of immunocompromised patients is respiratory infection, becoming a significant cause of morbidity and mortality. In the AIDS epidemic, a large number of respiratory pathogens have worsened the prognosis of the disease. In addition, the development of the treatment of cancer, organ transplantation, and immunosuppressive therapy, have resulted in the appearance of infections secondary to the alteration of the immune system.

Pulmonary infections represent at least 65% of all AIDS-defining illness. The etiological agents mainly associated with HIV-infected patients are *Pneumocystis jiroveci*, *Mycobacterium tuberculosis* and *Mycobacterium avium* complex, in addition to the common Gram-positive and Gram-negative bacteria.[84] In AIDS patients, CD4 lymphocyte count is a valuable measure for assessing the degree of impairment of the immune system. Opportunistic lung infections usually occur in patients with CD4 counts below 200 cells/mm³, meanwhile typical bacterial pneumonia is more associated with CD4 counts above 500 cells/mm³. So it is important to know the CD4 count for the correct interpretation of clinical and radiological findings.[84] In the past decade the prevalence of opportunistic infections has decreased with the introduction of highly active antiretroviral therapy (HAART).

The number of non-AIDS immunocompromised patients has significantly increased over recent years, mainly due to the increase of bone marrow or organ transplants, advances in the treatment of cancer and immunosuppressive therapy. In bone marrow transplantation (BMT), fungi (mainly *Aspergillus* species) are the common cause of pulmonary infection during the neutropenic phase of BMT (up to 3 weeks after transplantation), meanwhile cytomegalovirus (CMV) pneumonia is typical 3 weeks to 100 days after transplantation.[85] In solid organ transplantation, bacterial pneumonia is the most common respiratory infectious complication; CMV infection usually occurs within the first 3 months after transplantation.[59]

Whenever respiratory infection is suspected in immunocompromised patients, posteroanterior (and lateral when possible) chest radiography should be obtained. If the diagnosis is not clear, CT may be useful in narrowing the differential diagnosis. The most usual patterns seen at CT are nodules, tree-in-bud appearance, ground-glass attenuation, and consolidation.[84]

What is the role of imaging in the different pulmonary infectious diseases in the immunocompromised patient?

Pulmonary infections associated with immunocompromised patients include a wide range of infections including bacteria, mycobacteria, virus, and fungi, with different radiographic patterns depending on the state and type of immunosuppression associated.

Bacterial infections

The most common etiology of pulmonary infection in AIDS patients is bacterial pneumonia,[86] usually caused by typical agents as *Strep. pneumoniae, H. influenzae, P. aeruginosa* and *Staph. aureus*. Less frequently, *Bartonella henselae* (*formerly henselae*) *Rochamilacea* and *Rhodococcus equi* may be the cause of bacterial infection, usually seen as pneumonia associated with cavitation.[87] The classic radiological presentation is as single or multiple areas of focal distribution, although differentiation from the atypical patterns associated with opportunistic infections may be difficult on the basis of radiographic images, and it is necessary to perform more invasive techniques to obtain an etiological diagnosis.[84]

In the neutropenic phase of BMT, bacteremia is the most common bacterial infection, although in some cases focal or multifocal areas of consolidation may appear.[88] In solid organ transplants, bacterial pneumonias do not differ from pneumonias developed in immunocompetent patients.[85]

Mycobacterial infections

The increased prevalence of AIDS has been important in the re-emergence of tuberculosis in recent decades. Its risk is 200–500 times higher in AIDS patients than in the general population.[89] Mycobacterial infections are not only caused by *Mycobacterium tuberculosis*, but also non-tuberculous (atypical) mycobacteria such as *Mycobacterium avium* and *Mycobactenium intracellulare* (MAI) are frequently causes of opportunistic infections in AIDS. The immunosuppressed state associated with AIDS predisposes to the reactivation of latent tuberculosis, meanwhile MAI infection occurs in advanced stages of AIDS, when the CD4 count is lower than 50 cells/mm^3.[90] Radiological findings in tuberculosis are very similar to those in immunocompetent patients (see below), although mediastinal lymph node and bronchogenic spread forms occur more frequently in HIV-infected patients (Figure 12.14).[89] In non-HIV immunocompromised patients, depending on the state of immunosuppression, the risk of mycobacterial infection is increased; however, it is uncommon in BMT.[91]

Viral infections

CMV infection is commonly seen in immunocompromised patients. In AIDS, CMV pneumonia usually occurs in patients with a CD4 count below 50 cells/mm^3. The radiographic findings are unpredictable and may consist of a reticular or reticulonodular pattern, ground-glass opacities, air-space consolidation, or a combination of these findings.[92,93] Consolidation and masses are more typical of

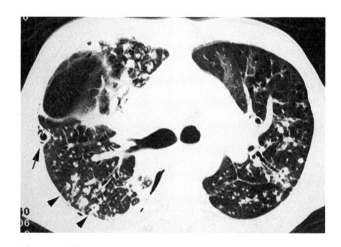

Figure 12.14
Endobronchial spread of tuberculosis. HRCT image (1.0-mm collimation) at the level of the carina shows diffuse bilateral branching linear opacities combined with centrilobular nodules (black arrowheads). The combination of branching linear opacities and centrilobular nodules gives the characteristic 'tree-in-bud' appearance. A right pneumothorax treated with a chest tube is seen (arrow). The patient was a 45-year-old HIV-positive male.

(a)

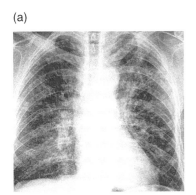

(b)

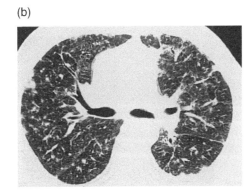

Figure 12.15
Acute bronchiolitis caused by CMV.
(a) Posteroanterior chest radiograph
shows numerous ill-defined nodules.
(b) HRCT scan (1-mm collimation) at the
level of the carina shows multiple
bilateral ill-defined small nodules. The
patient was a 38-year-old man after
allogeneic hematopoietic stem cell
transplantation.

AIDS patients compared with immunocompromised non-AIDS patients.[94,95]

CMV pneumonia has been reported particularly in BMT during the post-engraftment period (30–100 days after transplantation). Although mortality is high (85%), the main determinant of prognosis is the early diagnosis. The most typical radiographic findings consist of pulmonary consolidation and multiple nodules smaller than 55 mm in diameter[88] (Figure 12.15). In solid organ transplantation, CMV pneumonia is usually seen with a normal chest radiograph, although in some cases may demonstrate alveolar or interstitial infiltrates, necessitating the use of thin-section CT to clarify the radiological diagnosis.

Fungal infections

Pneumocystis jiroveci pneumonia is typical in AIDS patients with CD4 counts below 100 cells/mm^3. In 90% of patients with PCP chest radiograph abnormalities, have been reported, mainly the classical findings of diffuse bilateral interstitial infiltrates in a perihilar distribution, although normal radiographs do not exclude the diagnosis.[84] In these patients, CT may be helpful in confirming the diagnosis of PCP when clinical suspicion is high, showing typical images including perihilar ground-glass opacity, in a patchy or geographical distribution.[25] In AIDS patients receiving prophylaxis with aerosolized pentamidine and trimethroprim/sulfamethoxazole, a cystic form of PCP has been reported, associated with increased risk of spontaneous pneumothorax (Figure 12.16).

The risk of *Pneumocystis jiroveci* infection has substantially lowered in recent years in transplant patients due to the prophylactic use of trimethroprim/sulfamethoxazole.

Aspergillosis is a fungal disease caused by *Aspergillus* species, usually *A. fumigatus*. There are different patterns of aspergillosis including angioinvasive aspergillosis, bronchial invasive aspergillosis, pseudomembranous necrotizing tracheobronchial aspergillosis, obstructing bronchial aspergillosis, and chronic cavitary forms. Bronchial invasive aspergillosis is associated with patients with severe neutropenia and in patients with AIDS. The clinical and radiological manifestations include acute tracheobronchitis,

bronchiolitis, and bronchopneumonia.[84] Obstructing bronchopulmonary aspergillosis (OBA) is a non-invasive form of aspergillosis characterized by massive intraluminal overgrowth of *Aspergillus* species. The characteristic CT findings consist of bilateral bronchial and bronchiolar dilatations, large mucoid impactions, and postobstructive atelectasis.[96] Angioinvasive aspergillosis is almost exclusively seen in patients with severe neutropenia.[29] This form is characterized by invasion and occlusion of small to medium pulmonary arteries, developing necrotic hemorrhagic nodules or infarcts. The most common pattern seen in CT consists of multiple nodules surrounded by a halo of ground-glass attenuation (halo sign) or pleural-based wedge-shaped areas of consolidation (Figure 12.17). In mildly immunocompromised patients, such as those with chronic illness, diabetes mellitus, malnutrition, alcoholism, advanced age, prolonged corticosteroid administration, and chronic obstructive disease, an aspergillosis form termed semi-invasive or chronic necrotizing aspergillosis has been described. Radiological findings consist of unilateral or bilateral segmental areas of consolidation with or without cavitation and/or adjacent pleural thickening and multiple nodular opacities.[97]

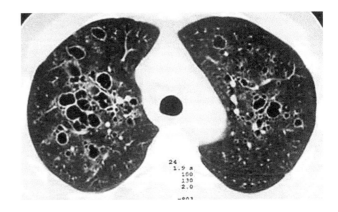

Figure 12.16
Pneumocystis jiroveci pneumonia cyst formation. HRCT at the level of the upper lobes (2.0-mm collimation) shows subtle areas of ground-glass attenuation and numerous thin-walled cystic lesions. The patient was a 43-year-old man with AIDS.

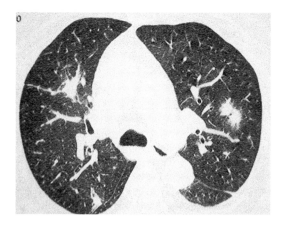

Figure 12.17
Angioinvasive aspergillosis. HRCT scan (2-mm collimation) at the level of the carina shows multiple bilateral nodules with a surrounding halo of ground-glass attenuation. These findings correspond to nodular areas of infarction surrounded by hemorrhage. The patient was a 47-year-old woman after allogeneic bone marrow transplantation.

In conclusion, aspergillosis may be presented in several forms of disease and radiological techniques are necessary to clarify the differential diagnosis. When *Aspergillus* species are isolated in cultures from respiratory samples, the clinical data and the interpretation of radiological findings will be helpful in defining which pattern of aspergillosis is present in the patients.

Cryptococcal pneumonia (*Cryptococcus neoformans*) is a common pulmonary infection in AIDS patients with a CD4 count below 100 cells/mm³. The most typical radiographic manifestation consists of reticular or reticulonodular interstitial pattern.[98]

Histoplasmosis (*Histoplasma capsulatum*) is an endemic infection of areas such as Ohio, Mississippi, and St Lawrence river valleys (North America). The most common radiographic findings are diffuse nodular opacities of 3 mm or less in diameter, nodules greater than 3 mm in diameter, small linear opacities, and focal or patchy areas of consolidation, although these findings are not seen in chest radiographs in approximately 40% of patients with pulmonary histoplasmosis, therefore CT imaging is valuable.[99]

Nocardiosis

Although nocardiosis (mainly caused by *Nocardia asteroides*) is an infrequent cause of pulmonary infection in AIDS patients, it is relatively common in solid organ transplants, patients with hematological diseases, and patients with systemic lupus erythematosus receiving high-dose corticosteroids. Radiological findings are solitary or multiple masses or areas of nodular air-space consolidations, usually homogeneous and non-segmental.[100]

Tuberculosis and non-tuberculous mycobacterial infection

As mentioned above, mycobacterial infections have increased in prevalence as a result of the AIDS epidemic. The spectrum of radiographic findings in tuberculosis and non-tuberculous infections is so variable that diagnosis may be difficult, so it is fundamental for the radiologist to know the different forms of thoracic mycobacterial infections.

The manifestations of pulmonary tuberculosis differ to a large extent between primary tuberculosis and postprimary tuberculosis. Primary tuberculosis occurs when the host immune response initially fails to overcome *Mycobacterium tuberculosis*. The reactivation of a dormant primary infection is called postprimary tuberculosis and it is usually associated with a reduction in immunocompetence, as occurs in poor nutrition, neoplasia, infections, or increasing age. In a minority of cases, post-primary tuberculosis represents the continuation of primary tuberculosis.

Radiographic manifestations of tuberculosis
Primary tuberculosis

Primary tuberculosis represents about 23–34% of all adult cases of tuberculosis.[101] Although primary tuberculosis typically presents with radiographic manifestations, chest radiograph may be normal in 15% of cases.[101] The most frequent manifestations of primary tuberculosis are parenchymal disease, lymphadenopathy, pleural effusion, miliary disease, or atelectasis.[102] Parenchymal disease usually presents with consolidation, most commonly in the middle and lower lobes,[103] associated with lymphadenopathy. The differential diagnosis may be difficult, especially with metastases and histoplasmosis in endemic areas. On CT imaging, the presence of centrilobular nodules and a 'tree-in-bud' appearance in the area near to the consolidation is typical of pulmonary tuberculosis. Indeed, lymph nodes characteristically present with a low attenuation, necrotic or caseous center, and a hypervascularized periphery that enhances following intravenous contrast.[104] Although cavitary lesions are present in up to 29% of patients with primary tuberculosis, they are more frequently associated with postprimary tuberculosis.[103]

Postprimary tuberculosis

The radiological features of postprimary tuberculosis can be classified as parenchymal affection, airway involvement, pleural disease, and other complications. In relation with parenchymal disease, the radiological manifestations may overlap with those of primary tuberculosis, but the absence of lymphadenopathy, more frequent cavitation and a predilection for the upper lobes, are more typical of postprimary tuberculosis.[105] Cavitation indicates active disease; communication with bronchi enables the expectoration of tubercle bacilli and endobronchial spread, leading to the appearance of the typical images of 'tree-in-bud' (Figure 12.18). If left untreated, the disease progresses to lobar or complete destruction of the lung. In most patients, the initial parenchymal lesions may evolve into clearly reticular and nodular opacified areas (fibroproliferative disease), finally resulting in upper lobe volume loss with cicatricial atelectasis, architectural distortion, and traction bronchiectasis.

What are the characteristic radiographic features of thoracic sequelae and complications of tuberculosis?

The course of tuberculosis depends to a large extent on the interaction between the host response and the virulence of the pathogen. When organisms overcome host defenses, the infection progresses, either locally or in other parts of the lung or body, after spread of bacteria via the airways, lymphatic vessels, or bloodstream.[106] Sequelae and complications may present in pulmonary or extrapulmonary portions of the thorax, as a consequence of the progression of pulmonary tuberculosis. These manifestations of tuberculosis usually affect parenchyma, airways, mediastinum, pleura, and chest wall.

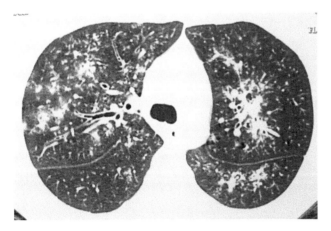

Figure 12.18
Endobronchial spread of tuberculosis. HRCT image (1.0-mm collimation) at the level of the carina shows numerous centrilobular nodules in a centrilobular distribution bilaterally affecting both upper lobes. An endobronchial spread of tuberculosis was proved by bronchoalveolar lavage. The patient was a 53-year-old man.

Parenchymal lesions

Tuberculoma and thin-walled cavity Tuberculoma is a round or oval granuloma caused by acid-fast bacilli with a wall lined by granulomatous inflammatory tissue or encapsulated by connective tissue, with a central area of caseation necrosis. The distribution may be as solitary or multiples nodules from 0.5 to 4.0 cm or more in diameter. Satellite lesions are seen in up to 80% and calcification in 20–30% of tuberculomas.[107] In areas of high prevalence of tuberculosis, the differential diagnosis with malignant nodules may be difficult, especially if the nodule is small and without calcification. In this case, the radiological follow-up of the nodule will be helpful in distinguishing between tuberculous and malignant nodules.

Residual thin-walled cavities may be present in both active and inactive disease. After antituberculous treatment, cavities may disappear, but occasionally, the wall becomes paper thin and air-filled cystic space remains.[108] Differential diagnosis with bullae, cysts, or pneumatoceles may be difficult.

Cicatrization and destruction of the lung Up to 40% of patient present, after infection, with cicatrization atelectasis of upper lobe, retraction of the hilum, compensatory lower lobe hyperinflation, and mediastinal shift toward the fibrotic lung. Complete destruction of the lung or a major part of it is frequently associated with the final stages of tuberculosis, with association of secondary pyogenic or fungal infection.[107] In such cases, the activity of tuberculosis is difficult to assess with radiographic studies.

Aspergilloma Aspergilloma consists of masses of fungal hyphae admixed with mucus and cellular debris, usually located in a cavity or ectatic bronchus.[109] The association with chronic tuberculosis has been reported to be 11%.[108] The classical radiological presentation consists of a rounded, mobile mass surrounded by a crescentic air shadow inside a lung cavity (air-crescent sign).

Bronchogenic carcinoma Tuberculosis may favor the development of bronchogenic carcinoma by local mechanisms (scar cancer) or may be coincidentally associated. When it occurs, the diagnosis can be difficult. As we previously referred, the radiological follow-up will be definitive and, any predominant or growing nodule, should be suspicious for coexisting lung cancer.

Airway lesions

Bronchiectasis, tracheobronchial stenosis, and broncholithiasis are typical lesions present in bronchial tree after tuberculosis. Bronchiectasis may appear as a complication of tuberculosis infection of the bronchial wall and subsequent fibrosis. Bronchiectasis located in upper lobes are highly suggestive of tuberculosis origin.[108]

Tracheobronchial stenosis after tuberculosis can be the result of direct extension from tuberculosis lymph nodes, endobronchial spread of infection, or lymphatic dissemination to the airway.[110] The clinical manifestation of bronchial stenosis may be as persistent segmental or lobar collapse, lobar hyperinflation, obstructive pneumonia, or mucoid impaction. The common findings on CT are irregular luminal narrowing with wall thickening, enhancement, and enlarged adjacent mediastinal nodes in active tuberculosis. When it occurs in a fibrotic stage, the CT features are concentric narrowing of the lumen, uniform thickening of the wall and involvement of a long bronchial segment. Although these radiographic manifestations are suggestive of tuberculous origin, bronchoscopy may be required to discard stenosis of cancer origin.[108]

Broncholithiasis is an uncommon complication of pulmonary tuberculosis and is defined as the presence of calcified or ossified material within the lumen of the tracheobronchial tree (Figure 12.19). The most common clinical manifestations are cough, hemoptysis, wheezing, or evidence of recurrent pneumonia.[111]

Mediastinal lesions

Tuberculous mediastinal lymphadenitis is a common manifestation of primary tuberculosis, especially in pubertal and young adult women, the elderly, and HIV-patients[112] (Figure 12.20). Extranodal extension may occur into adjacent structures such as the bronchus (see above), pericardium, and esophagus.

Esophageal affection by tuberculosis usually presents secondary to esophagomediastinal fistula due to the extranodal extension of the infection. The typical localization is the subcarinal region mainly because of the proximity of the esophagus to diseased lymph nodes in this area. The common radiological manifestation consists of localized gaseous collection in the mediastinum.[113]

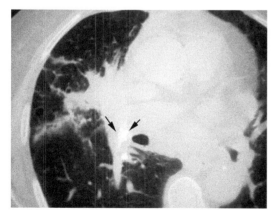

Figure 12.19
Post-tuberculosis broncholithiasis. Broncholithiasis due to granulomatous calcification in a 53-year-old man who had previous tuberculosis. CT scan shows calcified material in the middle lobe bronchus (arrows) with partial atelectasis of the right middle lobe.

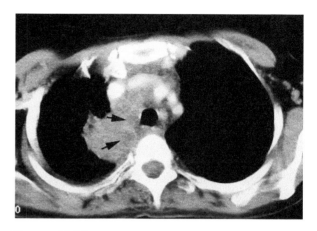

Figure 12.20
Tuberculous lymphadenitis. Multiple mediastinal lymph nodes are visible on contrast-enhanced CT. Lymph nodes show typical central low attenuation and a rim enhancement after intravenous contrast administration (arrows). The patient was a 42-year-old man with AIDS.

Fibrosing mediastinitis is a rare complication of tuberculosis and consists of the presence of excessive fibrosis in the mediastinum. CT manifestations consists of mediastinal or hilar mass, calcification in the mass, tracheobronchial narrowing, pulmonary vessel encasement, superior vena cava obstruction, and pulmonary infiltrates.[114]

Pleural lesions

Chronic tuberculous empyema and fibrothorax   The most common cause of tuberculous pleural infection is because of the rupture of a subpleural caseous focus into the pleural space. Afterwards, tuberculous pleurisy progresses to become chronic tuberculous empyema, which may be defined as persistent, glossly purulent fluid containing tubercle bacilli. Typical CT features include focal fluid collection with pleural thickening and calcification, with or without extrapleural fat proliferation. When fibrothorax appears (diffuse pleural thickening but without effusion) suggests inactivity.[108]

Bronchopleural fistula   Tuberculous bronchopleural fistula usually occurs after trauma or a surgical procedure, but can also present spontaneously. The diagnosis is suspected with increase of sputum production, air in the pleural space, a changing air–fluid level and contralateral spread of pneumonic infiltration.[108] Bronchopleural fistula associates high mortality.[115]

Pneumothorax   Pneumothorax secondary to tuberculosis usually presents in the course of the infection when the pulmonary involvement is extensive at the onset of bronchopleural fistula and empyema, mainly in patients with severe cavitary disease. Tube drainage is the treatment of choice, although in some cases the lung may be re-expanded spontaneously with chemotherapy.[108]

Chest wall tuberculosis

Chest wall lesions secondary to tuberculosis may occur by direct extension from a pleuropulmonary tuberculous lesion or by hematogenous spread from a distant focus. On CT imaging chest wall tuberculosis presents with bone or costal cartilage destruction and soft tissue masses that may show calcification of rim enhancement with or without evidence of underlying lung or pleural disease.[108] Empyema necessitatis may occur with spontaneous discharge of empyema through the parietal pleura into the chest wall, forming a subcutaneous abcess.

Pulmonary non-tuberculous mycobacterial infections

Pulmonary non-tuberculous mycobacteria (NTMB) infection is progressively increasing in prevalence, mainly due to *Mycobacterium avium, Mycobacterium intracellulare* and *Mycobacterium kansasii.* NTMB are classified into four groups as defined by Runyon.[116] The severity of disease depends on the presence of underlying lung disease and the status of immunocompetence. Diagnosis is often difficult because isolation of the pathogen from sputum or bronchoalveolar lavage fluid may represent colonization, not infection.[117] The combination of clinical signs, radiological findings, and subsequent isolations of NTMB from respiratory cultures, will be definitive to settle the diagnosis and begin antibiotic therapy.

What are the characteristic radiographic features of non-tuberculous mycobacterial infection?

In relation to radiology, the manifestations of NTMB infection are divided into five forms: classic infection, non-classic infection, nodules in asymptomatic patients, infection in patients with achalasia, and infection in immunocompromised patients (see above).

Classic infection is the most typical form of pulmonary NTMB infection and is frequently associated with elderly men with underlying lung disease. Radiological manifestations are very similar to postprimary tuberculosis, although in NTMB infection the progression is slower than in tuberculosis. Miliary disease is rare in immunocompetent hosts, and adenopathy and pleural effusion are uncommon.[117] Non-classic infection is the second most common form of pulmonary NTMB infection and mainly affects elderly white women without underlying lung disease. Radiological findings consists of mild to moderate cylindrical bronchiectasis and multiple 1–3 mm diameter centrilobular nodules.[118,119] Cavitation, ground-glass areas, volume loss, and adenopathy do not usually present in non-classic infection. In some cases, infection presents with solitary or multiple nodules, which are usually incidentally detected in asymptomatic patients and may represent the initial manifestation of pulmonary infection.[119] Patients with repeated aspiration, such as those with esophageal achalasia or gastric outlet obstruction, are predisposed to NTMB infection, usually with *Mycobacterium fortuitum* and *Mycobacteruim chelonae*, which present with the radiographic appearance of aspiration pneumonia.[120]

Non-resolving and recurrent pneumonia

Non-resolving or slowly resolving pulmonary infiltrates are a clinical diagnostic challenge for physicians. Non-resolving pneumonia is defined as focal radiographic infiltrates with clinical signs of pulmonary infection that have failed to resolve or resolve atypically.[121] When the radiograph has failed to resolve by 50% in 2 weeks or completely in 4 weeks, the pneumonia should be considered to be non-resolving or slowly resolving.[122]

What is the appropriate management of non-resolving or recurrent pneumonia?

In addition to chest radiographs, CT should be performed when appropriate and may even be the test of first choice in the evaluation of non-resolving or recurrent pulmonary infiltrates. It is extremely useful and particularly sensitive for the diagnosis of tracheobronchial abnormalities and congenital pulmonary disorders.

Different causes of non-resolving pneumonia need to be considered and the possible etiologies can be divided into four categories: complicated infections (abscess, empyema); other infections (anaerobes, tuberculosis, fungi); poor bronchial clearance (bronchiectais, foreign body); and inherent non-infectious disease of the pulmonary parenchyma. In adults, non-infectious mimics of pneumonia include neoplasms (e.g. bronchogenic carcinoma, bronchoalveolar cell carcinoma, and lymphoma), immunological disorders (e.g. Wegener's granulomatosis, bronchocentric granulomatosis, and organizing pneumonia), drug-induced lung diseases, thromboembolism, broncholithiasis, and aspirated foreign bodies.[122–126]

Recurrent pneumonia represents distinct episodes of pneumonia with fever, infiltrates, and leukocytosis, occurring in the same patient at least twice within 1 year. A complete resolution of the infiltrate for at least 1 month is required between recurrences.[127]

Causes and patterns of recurrent pneumonia will depend on the nature of the underlying predisposition. Recurrent pneumonias may involve either a single or multiple areas of lung parenchyma. This anatomical distribution is extremely helpful in establishing a diffential diagnosis. In infants, inhalational conditions (e.g. foreign body, lipid) and congenital malformations (congenital adenomatoid cystic malformation, bronchogenic cyst, and pulmonary sequestration) should be strongly considered when the recurrence appears in the same lobe; in the pediatric patients, multilobar recurrent pneumonia is associated with asthma, immunodeficiency syndromes, cystic fibrosis, and primary ciliary dyskinesias.

In adults, bronchial obstruction secondary to bronchogenic carcinoma is the leading cause of recurrent pneumonia; other causes are foreign bodies, broncholithiasis, and aspiration. Multilobar recurrent pneumonia suggests a broader differential diagnosis. Aspiration is the most common cause of recurrent bilateral pneumonia. Other causes are structural abnormalities of the tracheobronchial tree and non-infectious illnesses such as cryptogenic organizing pneumonia and chronic eosinophilic pneumonia. Wegener's granulomatosis and other pulmonary vasculitides may also present with recurrent pulmonary infiltrates.

Interventional procedures in patients with pneumonia

The only definitive way to reach a specific diagnosis is through demonstration of the organism, i.e. by examination of stained smears of sputum, pleural fluid, or other biological material, by culture of respiratory secretions and blood, or by other interventional procedures such transthoracic fine needle aspiration or biopsy under fluoroscopy or CT guidance.

However, in most large series of pneumonia a causative organism cannot be identified in 33–45% of patients, even when extensive diagnostic tests are undertaken. Previously healthly patients who are mildly ill due to pneumonia are managed in an empiric fashion. However, in certain circumstances, the lack of specific organism requires a more aggressive approach in order to obtain histopathological and cultural identification of the cause of the pulmonary infection.

There has been much debate on the diagnostic accuracy of specimens obtained for culture with various techniques. Material obtained from the sputum or nasopharyngeal secretions have limited diagnostic value because of the presence of normal flora and variable results obtained for the detection of anaerobic infection.[128]

Flexible fiberoptic bronchoscopy with lung biopsy

Fiberoptic bronchoscopy with bronchoalveolar lavage utilizing a protected brush is a well-established technique in the diagnosis of pulmonary infection.[129]

Although this technique may play an important role in the diagnosis of pulmonary infection, the yield of bronchoalveolar lavage is variable and sometimes the diagnosis of a pulmonary infection cannot be established.[128–130] This method has proved particularly useful in the diagnosis of pneumocystis pneumonia in AIDS patients providing an etiological diagnosis in about 95% of cases. In the specific setting of a serious pulmonary process and lack of definable cause with non-invasive methods, fiberoptic bronchoscopy in conjunction with transbronchial lung biopsy is indicated (Figure 12.21).

Transthoracic needle aspiration

Although the reported results in the diagnosis of pulmonary infection are variable, percutaneous fine needle aspiration is an alternative method used to identify causative pathogens

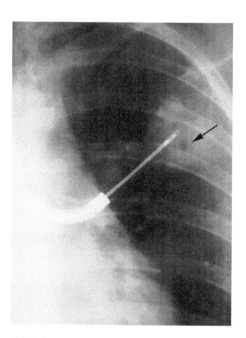

Figure 12.21
Imaging-guided bronchoscopy. Magnified view of the left upper lobe from an anteroposterior chest radiograph shows cavitary consolidation (arrow). Material for culture was obtained through fiberoptic bronchoscopy. Cultures grew *Mycobacterium tuberculosis*. Although this case illustrates a radiograph-guided bronchoscopy, it is most commonly performed under fluoroscopic guidance. With permission from Franquet.[1]

in selected patients with pneumonia.[131–134] Transthoracic needle aspiration should be considered for patients who have not responded to initial therapy, patients who may have nosocomial superinfection, who are immunocompromised, or in whom tuberculosis is suspected but has not been confirmed by examination of the sputum or gastric lavage. It is not clear whether use of transthoracic needle aspiration results in a reduction in mortality and morbidity in a cost-effective fashion, compared with a less invasive approach.[128] The specificity and positive predictive value of a positive culture have been reported to be as high as 100%, whereas the sensitivity and negative predictive value are 61% and 34%, respectively.[135]

Summary for optimal imaging evaluation of suspected pneumonia

Chest radiography is recommended in all patients with suspected pulmonary infection in order to confirm or exclude the presence of pulmonary abnormalities. Although the chest radiograph does not allow a specific diagnosis it is helpful in detecting alternative diagnosis or associated conditions, assessing the severity of pneumonia and providing guidance for subsequent diagnostic studies.

In patients with community-acquired pneumonia, diagnosis and disease management most frequently rely on chest radiographs and seldom require further diagnostic procedures such as CT, bronchoscopy, or biopsy. In the community setting, over 90% of patients who develop a segmental or lobar consolidation have either pneumococcal pneumonia or an atypical pneumonia caused by *Mycoplasma* species or a virus. In nosocomial pulmonary infection, patchy bronchopneumonia is the most common finding and most probably is caused by one of the Gram-negative organisms, particularly *Pseudomonas* species or *Klebsiella* species. In this particular setting, aspiration pneumonia is always an alternative diagnosis and should be suspected if pneumonia is present bilaterally in the dependent portions of the lungs.[1]

Effusions and empyema can complicate lower respiratory tract infections.[136, 137] CT of the chest is far more sensitive than plain film for detecting pleural abnormalities and should be considered as a valuable imaging technique to evaluate complicated pneumonias.[138] Although the value of CT is sometimes limited in establishing the cause of an undiagnosed pleural effusion, it can help to distinguish between transudates and exudates, and may influence therapeutic decisions.[138] Parietal pleural thickening at contrast-enhanced CT almost always indicates the presence of a pleural exudate.[139] A pleural exudate in the absence of pleural thickening occurs most frequently in patients with malignancy or uncomplicated parapneumonic effusion.[139] Accurate management of parapneumonic effusions is mandatory.[137] Delay of an appropriate treatment is likely to lead to a prolonged hospital course and the eventual need for thoracotomy.

In the ICU patients, there are few studies regarding the accuracy and efficacy of conventional chest radiographs. The overall incidence of abnormalities found on chest films

Fig. 12.22

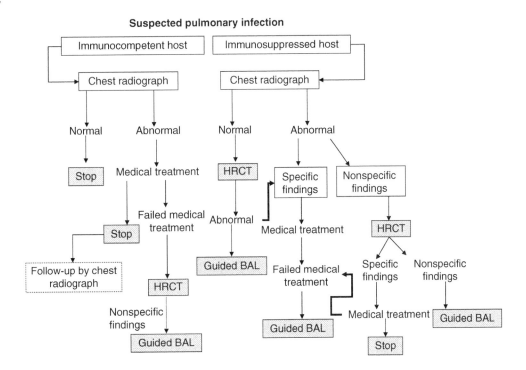

in the medical ICU has been reported to be as high as 57% in pulmonary and unstable cardiac patients.[140,141] Similar results were obtained in a study of patients in the medical ICU, where 43% of routine chest radiographs showed unexpected findings which influenced therapy.[141] Future studies on management and outcome efficacy as well as overall cost are necessary to evaluate the role of the routine chest radiograph in ICU patients. CT and invasive diagnostic procedures should be reserved only for complicated cases.

Conversely, management of immunocompromised patients is challenging and difficult because of the diversity of causative organisms. In this group of patients, HRCT and invasive procedures are commonly required. HRCT can be useful in patients who have respiratory symptoms but normal or questionable radiographic findings, depicting abnormalities not evident on the radiograph and the presence of complications and concurrent parenchymal, mediastinal, or pleural disease. In addition, HRCT is helpful in differentiating infectious from non-infectious acute parenchymal lung disease.[26]

Diagnostic information may also be obtained by means of bronchoalveolar lavage and transbronchial needle aspiration. Under these circumstances, CT is useful as a guide to direct fiberoptic bronchoscopy toward the region most likely to yield the diagnosis. The algorithm for evaluation of patients suspected of having pulmonary infection is shown in Fig. 12.22.

References

1. Franquet T. Imaging of pneumonia: trends and algorithms. Eur Respir J 2001; 18: 196–208.
2. Vilar J, Domingo ML, Soto C et al. Radiology of bacterial pneumonia. Eur J Radiol 2004; 51: 102–3.
3. Gharib AM, Stern EJ. Radiology of pneumonia. Med Clin North Am 2001; 85: 1461–91, x.
4. Niederman MS, McCombs JS, Unger AN et al. The cost of treating community-acquired pneumonia. Clin Ther 1998; 20: 820–37.
5. Vincent JL, Bihari DJ, Suter PM et al. The prevalence of nosocomial infection in intensive care units in Europe. Results of the European Prevalence of Infection in Intensive Care (EPIC) Study. EPIC International Advisory Committee. JAMA 1995; 274: 639–44.
6. Garibaldi RA. Epidemiology of community-acquired respiratory tract infections in adults. Incidence, etiology, and impact. Am J Med 1985; 78: 32–7.
7. Bouza E, Munoz P. Introduction: infections caused by emerging resistant pathogens. Clin Microbiol Infect 2005; 11: iv.
8. Schwartz DA, Bryan RT, Hughes JM. Pathology and emerging infections – quo vadimus? Am J Pathol 1995; 147: 1525–33.
9. Cheney PR. Update on emerging infections from the Centers for Disease Control and Prevention. Hantavirus pulmonary syndrome – Colorado and New Mexico, 1998. Ann Emerg Med 1999; 33: 121–3.
10. Hammel JM, Chiang WK. Update on emerging infections: news from the Centers for Disease Control and Prevention. Outbreaks of avian influenza A (H5N1) in Asia and interim recommendations for evaluation and reporting of suspected cases – United States, 2004. Ann Emerg Med 2005; 45: 88–92.
11. Cameron PA, Rainer TH. Update on emerging infections: news from the Centers for Disease Control and Prevention. Update: Outbreak of severe acute respiratory syndrome – worldwide, 2003. Ann Emerg Med 2003; 42: 110–2.
12. Franquet T, Rodriguez S, Martino R et al. Human metapneumovirus infection in hematopoietic stem cell transplant recipients: high-resolution computed tomography findings. J Comput Assist Tomogr 2005; 29: 223–7.
13. Hamelin ME, Abed Y, Boivin G. Human metapneumovirus: a new player among respiratory viruses. Clin Infect Dis 2004; 38: 983–90.
14. Madhi SA, Ludewick H, Abed Y, Klugman KP, Boivin G. Human metapneumovirus-associated lower respiratory tract infections among hospitalized human immunodeficiency virus type 1 (HIV-1)-infected and HIV-1-uninfected African infants. Clin Infect Dis 2003; 37: 1705–10.
15. Moe AA, Hardy WD. *Pneumocystis carinii* infection in the HIV-seropositive patient. Infect Dis Clin North Am 1994; 8: 331–64.
16. Murray JF, Mills J. Pulmonary infectious complications of human immunodeficiency virus infection. Part II. Am Rev Respir Dis 1990; 141: 1582–98.
17. Murray JF, Mills J. Pulmonary infectious complications of human immunodeficiency virus infection. Part I. Am Rev Respir Dis 1990; 141: 1356–72.
18. Lyon R, Haque AK, Asmuth DM, Woods GL. Changing patterns of infections in patients with AIDS: a study of 279 autopsies of prison inmates and nonincarcerated patients at a university hospital in eastern Texas, 1984–1993. Clin Infect Dis 1996; 23: 241–7.
19. Boiselle PM, Crans CA Jr, Kaplan MA. The changing face of *Pneumocystis carinii* pneumonia in AIDS patients. AJR Am J Roentgenol 1999; 172: 1301–9.
20. Tarver RD, Teague SD, Heitkamp DE, Conces DJ, Jr. Radiology of community-acquired pneumonia. Radiol Clin North Am 2005; 43: 497–512, viii.
21. Marrie TJ, Majumdar SR. Management of community-acquired pneumonia in the emergency room. Respir Care Clin North Am 2005; 11: 15–24.
22. Gruden JF, Huang L, Turner J et al. High-resolution CT in the evaluation of clinically suspected *Pneumocystis carinii* pneumonia in AIDS patients with normal, equivocal, or nonspecific radiographic findings. AJR Am J Roentgenol 1997; 169: 967–75.
23. Brown MJ, Miller RR, Muller NL. Acute lung disease in the immunocompromised host: CT and pathologic examination findings. Radiology 1994; 190: 247–54.
24. Janzen DL, Padley SP, Adler BD, Muller NL. Acute pulmonary complications in immunocompromised non-AIDS patients: comparison of diagnostic accuracy of CT and chest radiography. Clin Radiol 1993; 47: 159–65.
25. Primack SL, Muller NL. High-resolution computed tomography in acute diffuse lung disease in the immunocompromised patient. Radiol Clin North Am 1994; 32: 731–44.

26. Tomiyama N, Muller NL, Johkoh T et al. Acute parenchymal lung disease in immunocompetent patients: diagnostic accuracy of high-resolution CT. AJR Am J Roentgenol 2000; 174: 1745–50.

27. Kuhlman JE, Fishman EK, Siegelman SS. Invasive pulmonary aspergillosis in acute leukemia: characteristic findings on CT, the CT halo sign, and the role of CT in early diagnosis. Radiology 1985; 157: 611–4.

28. Primack SL, Hartman TE, Lee KS, Muller NL. Pulmonary nodules and the CT halo sign. Radiology 1994; 190: 513–5.

29. Worthy SA, Flint JD, Muller NL. Pulmonary complications after bone marrow transplantation: high-resolution CT and pathologic findings. Radiographics 1997; 17: 1359–71.

30. Im JG, Itoh H, Lee KS, Han MC. CT-pathology correlation of pulmonary tuberculosis. Crit Rev Diagn Imaging 1995; 36: 227–85.

31. Aquino SL, Gamsu G, Webb WR, Kee ST. Tree-in-bud pattern: frequency and significance on thin section CT. J Comput Assist Tomogr 1996; 20: 594–9.

32. Boiselle PM, Tocino I, Hooley RJ et al. Chest radiograph interpretation of *Pneumocystis carinii* pneumonia, bacterial pneumonia, and pulmonary tuberculosis in HIV-positive patients: accuracy, distinguishing features, and mimics. J Thorac Imaging 1997; 12: 47–53.

33. Primack SL, Logan PM, Hartman TE, Lee KS, Muller NL. Pulmonary tuberculosis and *Mycobacterium avium-intracellulare*: a comparison of CT findings. Radiology 1995; 194: 413–7.

34. Shah RM, Kaji AV, Ostrum BJ, Friedman AC. Interpretation of chest radiographs in AIDS patients: usefulness of CD4 lymphocyte counts. Radiographics 1997; 17: 47–58; discussion 59–61.

35. Hanson DL, Chu SY, Farizo KM, Ward JW. Distribution of CD4+ T lymphocytes at diagnosis of acquired immunodeficiency syndrome-defining and other human immunodeficiency virus-related illnesses. The Adult and Adolescent Spectrum of HIV Disease Project Group. Arch Intern Med 1995; 155: 1537–42.

36. Chastre J, Trouillet JL, Vuagnat A et al. Nosocomial pneumonia in patients with acute respiratory distress syndrome. Am J Respir Crit Care Med 1998; 157: 1165–72.

37. Niederman MS, Fein AM. Sepsis syndrome, the adult respiratory distress syndrome, and nosocomial pneumonia. A common clinical sequence. Clin Chest Med 1990; 11: 633–56.

38. Seidenfeld JJ, Pohl DF, Bell RC, Harris GD, Johanson WG, Jr. Incidence, site, and outcome of infections in patients with the adult respiratory distress syndrome. Am Rev Respir Dis 1986; 134: 12–6.

39. Bartlett JG, Dowell SF, Mandell LA et al. Practice guidelines for the management of community-acquired pneumonia in adults. Infectious Diseases Society of America. Clin Infect Dis 2000; 31: 347–82.

40. Halm EA, Teirstein AS. Clinical practice. Management of community-acquired pneumonia. N Engl J Med 2002; 347: 2039–45.

41. Jokinen C, Heiskanen L, Juvonen H et al. Incidence of community-acquired pneumonia in the population of four municipalities in eastern Finland. Am J Epidemiol 1993; 137: 977–88.

42. Woodhead MA, Macfarlane JT, McCracken JS, Rose DH, Finch RG. Prospective study of the aetiology and outcome of pneumonia in the community. Lancet 1987; 1: 671–4.

43. Finch RG, Woodhead MA. Practical considerations and guidelines for the management of community-acquired pneumonia. Drugs 1998; 55: 31–45.

44. Fine MJ, Smith MA, Carson CA et al. Prognosis and outcomes of patients with community-acquired pneumonia. A meta-analysis. JAMA 1996; 275: 134–41.

45. Herold CJ, Sailer JG. Community-acquired and nosocomial pneumonia. Eur Radiol 2004; 14 (Suppl 3): E2–20.

46. Niederman MS, Mandell LA, Anzueto A et al. Guidelines for the management of adults with community-acquired pneumonia. Diagnosis, assessment of severity, antimicrobial therapy, and prevention. Am J Respir Crit Care Med 2001; 163: 1730–54.

47. Franquet T, Gimenez A, Roson N et al. Aspiration diseases: findings, pitfalls, and differential diagnosis. Radiographics 2000; 20: 673–85.

48. Levy M, Dromer F, Brion N, Leturdu F, Carbon C. Community-acquired pneumonia. Importance of initial noninvasive bacteriologic and radiographic investigations. Chest 1988; 93: 43–8.

49. Melbye H, Dale K. Interobserver variability in the radiographic diagnosis of adult outpatient pneumonia. Acta Radiol 1992; 33: 79–81.

50. Zornoza J, Goldman AM, Wallace S, Valdivieso M, Bodey GP. Radiologic features of gram-negative pneumonias in the neutropenic patient. AJR Am J Roentgenol 1976; 127: 989–96.

51. Chapman WW, Fiszman M, Frederick PR, Chapman BE, Haug PJ. Quantifying the characteristics of unambiguous chest radiography reports in the context of pneumonia. Acad Radiol 2001; 8: 57–66.

52. Eggli KD, Newman B. Nodules, masses, and pseudomasses in the pediatric lung. Radiol Clin North Am 1993; 31: 651–66.

53. Kwong JS, Muller NL, Godwin JD, Aberle D, Grymaloski MR. Thoracic actinomycosis: CT findings in eight patients. Radiology 1992; 183: 189–92.

54. Quagliano PV, Das Narla L. Legionella pneumonia causing multiple cavitating pulmonary nodules in a 7-month-old infant. AJR Am J Roentgenol 1993; 161: 367–8.

55. McConnell CT Jr, Plouffe JF, File TM et al. Radiographic appearance of *Chlamydia pneumoniae* (TWAR strain) respiratory infections. CBPIS Study Group. Community-based Pneumonia Incidence Study. Radiology 1994; 192: 819–24.

56. Nambu A, Saito A, Araki T et al. *Chlamydia pneumoniae*: comparison with findings of *Mycoplasma pneumoniae* and *Streptococcus pneumoniae* at thin-section CT. Radiology 2006; 238: 330–8.

57. Ettinger NA, Trulock EP. Pulmonary considerations of organ transplantation. Part I. Am Rev Respir Dis 1991; 143: 1386–405.

58. Ettinger NA, Trulock EP. Pulmonary considerations of organ transplantation. Part 3. Am Rev Respir Dis 1991; 144: 433–51.

59. Ettinger NA, Trulock EP. Pulmonary considerations of organ transplantation. Part 2. Am Rev Respir Dis 1991; 144: 213–23.

60. Lee I, Kim TS, Yoon HK. *Mycoplasma pneumoniae* pneumonia: CT features in 16 patients. Eur Radiol 2006; 16: 719–25.

61. Reittner P, Muller NL, Heyneman L et al. *Mycoplasma pneumoniae* pneumonia: radiographic and high-resolution CT features in 28 patients. AJR Am J Roentgenol 2000; 174: 37–41.

62. Eisenhuber E. The tree-in-bud sign. Radiology 2002; 222: 771–2.

63. Mittl RL Jr, Schwab RJ, Duchin JS et al. Radiographic resolution of community-acquired pneumonia. Am J Respir Crit Care Med 1994; 149: 630–5.

64. Ioanas M, Ferrer M, Cavalcanti M et al. Causes and predictors of nonresponse to treatment of intensive care unit-acquired pneumonia. Crit Care Med 2004; 32: 938–45.

65. Leroy O, Santre C, Beuscart C et al. A five-year study of severe community-acquired pneumonia with emphasis on prognosis in patients admitted to an intensive care unit. Intensive Care Med 1995; 21: 24–31.

66. Tanaka N, Matsumoto T, Kuramitsu T et al. High resolution CT findings in community-acquired pneumonia. J Comput Assist Tomogr 1996; 20: 600–8.

67. Cameron DC, Borthwick RN, Philp T. The radiographic patterns of acute mycoplasma pneumonitis. Clin Radiol 1977; 28: 173–80.

68. Dietrich PA, Johnson RD, Fairbank JT, Walke JS. The chest radiograph in legionnaires' disease. Radiology 1978; 127: 577–82.

69. Kantor HG. The many radiologic facies of pneumococcal pneumonia. AJR Am J Roentgenol 1981; 137: 1213–20.

70. Hospital-acquired pneumonia in adults: diagnosis, assessment of severity, initial antimicrobial therapy, and preventive strategies. A consensus statement, American Thoracic Society, November 1995. Am J Respir Crit Care Med 1996; 153: 1711–25.

71. Ibrahim EH, Ward S, Sherman G, Kollef MH. A comparative analysis of patients with early-onset vs late-onset nosocomial pneumonia in the ICU setting. Chest 2000; 117: 1434–42.

72. Guidelines for the management of adults with hospital-acquired, ventilator-associated, and healthcare-associated pneumonia. Am J Respir Crit Care Med 2005; 171: 388–416.

73. Kollef MH. The prevention of ventilator-associated pneumonia. N Engl J Med 1999; 340: 627–34.

74. Taylor GD, Buchanan-Chell M, Kirkland T, McKenzie M, Wiens R. Bacteremic nosocomial pneumonia. A 7-year experience in one institution. Chest 1995; 108: 786–8.

75. Winer-Muram HT, Rubin SA, Ellis JV et al. Pneumonia and ARDS in patients receiving mechanical ventilation: diagnostic accuracy of chest radiography. Radiology 1993; 188: 479–85.

76. Pugin J, Auckenthaler R, Mili N et al. Diagnosis of ventilator-associated pneumonia by bacteriologic analysis of bronchoscopic and nonbronchoscopic "blind" bronchoalveolar lavage fluid. Am Rev Respir Dis 1991; 143: 1121–9.

77. DePaso WJ. Aspiration pneumonia. Clin Chest Med 1991; 12: 269–84.

78. Marom EM, McAdams HP, Erasmus JJ, Goodman PC. The many faces of pulmonary aspiration. AJR Am J Roentgenol 1999; 172: 121–8.

79. Bartlett JG, Finegold SM. Anaerobic infections of the lung and pleural space. Am Rev Respir Dis 1974; 110: 56–77.

80. Unger JD, Rose HD, Unger GF. Gram-negative pneumonia. Radiology 1973; 107: 283–91.

81. Cook RJ, Ashton RW, Aughenbaugh GL, Ryu JH. Septic pulmonary embolism: presenting features and clinical course of 14 patients. Chest 2005; 128: 162–6.

82. Kuhlman JE, Fishman EK, Teigen C. Pulmonary septic emboli: diagnosis with CT. Radiology 1990; 174: 211–3.

83. Iwasaki Y, Nagata K, Nakanishi M et al. Spiral CT findings in septic pulmonary emboli. Eur J Radiol 2001; 37: 190–4.

84. Franquet T. Respiratory infection in the AIDS and immunocompromised patient. Eur Radiol 2004; 14 (Suppl 3): E21–33.

85. Sable CA, Donowitz GR. Infections in bone marrow transplant recipients. Clin Infect Dis 1994; 18: 273–81; quiz 282-274.

86. Hirschtick RE, Glassroth J, Jordan MC et al. Bacterial pneumonia in persons infected with the human immunodeficiency virus. Pulmonary Complications of HIV Infection Study Group. N Engl J Med 1995; 333: 845–51.

87. Padley SP, King LJ. Computed tomography of the thorax in HIV disease. Eur Radiol 1999; 9: 1556–69.

88. Leung AN, Gosselin MV, Napper CH et al. Pulmonary infections after bone marrow transplantation: clinical and radiographic findings. Radiology 1999; 210: 699–710.

89. Leung AN. Pulmonary tuberculosis: the essentials. Radiology 1999; 210: 307–22.

90. Kotloff RM. Infection caused by nontuberculous mycobacteria: clinical aspects. Semin Roentgenol 1993; 28: 131–8.

91. Martino R, Martinez C, Brunet S et al. Tuberculosis in bone marrow transplant recipients: report of two cases and review of the literature. Bone Marrow Transplant 1996; 18: 809–12.

92. Olliff JF, Williams MP. Radiological appearances of cytomegalovirus infections. Clin Radiol 1989; 40: 463–7.

93. Schulman LL. Cytomegalovirus pneumonitis and lobar consolidation. Chest 1987; 91: 558–61.

94. Franquet T, Lee KS, Muller NL. Thin-section CT findings in 32 immunocompromised patients with cytomegalovirus pneumonia who do not have AIDS. AJR Am J Roentgenol 2003; 181: 1059–63.

95. Moon JH, Kim EA, Lee KS et al. Cytomegalovirus pneumonia: high-resolution CT findings in ten non-AIDS immunocompromised patients. Korean J Radiol 2000; 1: 73–8.

96. Franquet T, Muller NL, Oikonomou A, Flint JD. Aspergillus infection of the airways: computed tomography and pathologic findings. J Comput Assist Tomogr 2004; 28: 10–6.

97. Franquet T, Muller NL, Gimenez A et al. Semiinvasive pulmonary aspergillosis in chronic obstructive pulmonary disease: radiologic and pathologic findings in nine patients. AJR Am J Roentgenol 2000; 174: 51–6.

98. Stansell JD. Fungal disease in HIV-infected persons: cryptococcosis, histoplasmosis, and coccidioidomycosis. J Thorac Imaging 1991; 6: 28–35.

99. Conces DJ, Jr., Stockberger SM, Tarver RD, Wheat LJ. Disseminated histoplasmosis in AIDS: findings on chest radiographs. AJR Am J Roentgenol 1993; 160: 15–9.

100. Yoon HK, Im JG, Ahn JM, Han MC. Pulmonary nocardiosis: CT findings. J Comput Assist Tomogr 1995; 19: 52–5.

101. Miller WT, Miller WT, Jr. Tuberculosis in the normal host: radiological findings. Semin Roentgenol 1993; 28: 109–18.

102. Harisinghani MG, McLoud TC, Shepard JA et al. Tuberculosis from head to toe. Radiographics 2000; 20: 449–70; quiz 528–9, 532.

103. Choyke PL, Sostman HD, Curtis AM et al. Adult-onset pulmonary tuberculosis. Radiology 1983; 148: 357–62.

104. Im JG, Song KS, Kang HS et al. Mediastinal tuberculous lymphadenitis: CT manifestations. Radiology 1987; 164: 115–9.

105. Ellis SM. The spectrum of tuberculosis and non-tuberculous mycobacterial infection. Eur Radiol 2004; 14 (Suppl 3): E34–42.

106. Ellner JJ. Review: the immune response in human tuberculosis – implications for tuberculosis control. J Infect Dis 1997; 176: 1351–9.

107. Lee KS, Song KS, Lim TH et al. Adult-onset pulmonary tuberculosis: findings on chest radiographs and CT scans. AJR Am J Roentgenol 1993; 160: 753–8.

108. Kim HY, Song KS, Goo JM et al. Thoracic sequelae and complications of tuberculosis. Radiographics 2001; 21: 839–58; discussion 859–60.

109. Logan PM, Muller NL. CT manifestations of pulmonary aspergillosis. Crit Rev Diagn Imaging 1996; 37: 1–37.

110. Smith LS, Schillaci RF, Sarlin RF. Endobronchial tuberculosis. Serial fiberoptic bronchoscopy and natural history. Chest 1987; 91: 644–7.

111. Galdermans D, Verhaert J, Van Meerbeeck J, de Backer W, Vermeire P. Broncholithiasis: present clinical spectrum. Respir Med 1990; 84: 155–6.

112. Hopewell PC. A clinical view of tuberculosis. Radiol Clin North Am 1995; 33: 641–53.

113. Im JG, Kim JH, Han MC, Kim CW. Computed tomography of esophagomediastinal fistula in tuberculous mediastinal lymphadenitis. J Comput Assist Tomogr 1990; 14: 89–92.

114. Lee JY, Kim Y, Lee KS, Chung MP. Tuberculous fibrosing mediastinitis: radiologic findings. AJR Am J Roentgenol 1996; 167: 1598–9.

115. Johnson TM, McCann W, Davey WN. Tuberculous bronchopleural fistula. Am Rev Respir Dis 1973; 107: 30–41.

116. Runyon EH. Anonymous mycobacteria in pulmonary disease. Med Clin North Am 1959; 43: 273–90.

117. Woodring JH, Vandiviere HM. Pulmonary disease caused by nontuberculous mycobacteria. J Thorac Imaging 1990; 5: 64–76.

118. Hartman TE, Swensen SJ, Williams DE. *Mycobacterium avium-intracellulare* complex: evaluation with CT. Radiology 1993; 187: 23–6.

119. Miller WT, Jr. Spectrum of pulmonary nontuberculous mycobacterial infection. Radiology 1994; 191: 343–50.

120. Miller WT, Jr, Miller WT. Pulmonary infections with atypical mycobacteria in the normal host. Semin Roentgenol 1993; 28: 139–49.

121. Kirtland SH, Winterbauer RH. Slowly resolving, chronic, and recurrent pneumonia. Clin Chest Med 1991; 12: 303–18.

122. Rome L, Murali G, Lippmann M. Nonresolving pneumonia and mimics of pneumonia. Med Clin North Am 2001; 85: 1511–30, xi.

123. Muller NL, Staples CA, Miller RR. Bronchiolitis obliterans organizing pneumonia: CT features in 14 patients. AJR Am J Roentgenol 1990; 154: 983–87.

124. Wright BA, Jeffrey PH. Lipoid pneumonia. Semin Respir Infect 1990; 5: 314–21.

125. Zissin R, Shapiro-Feinberg M, Rozenman J et al. CT findings of the chest in adults with aspirated foreign bodies. Eur Radiol 2001; 11: 606–11.

126. Seo JB, Song KS, Lee JS et al. Broncholithiasis: review of the causes with radiologic-pathologic correlation. Radiographics 2002; 22 Spec No: S199–213.

127. Fein AM, Feinsilver SH, Niederman MS, Fiel S, Pai PB. "When the pneumonia doesn't get better". Clin Chest Med 1987; 8: 529–41.

128. Sanchez-Nieto JM, Torres A, Garcia-Cordoba F et al. Impact of invasive and noninvasive quantitative culture sampling on outcome of ventilator-associated pneumonia: a pilot study. Am J Respir Crit Care Med 1998; 157: 371–6.

129. Jolis R, Castella J, Puzo C, Coll P, Abeledo C. Diagnostic value of protected BAL in diagnosing pulmonary infections in immunocompromised patients. Chest 1996; 109: 601–7.

130. Castellino RA, Blank N. Etiologic diagnosis of focal pulmonary infection in immunocompromised patients by fluoroscopically guided percutaneous needle aspiration. Radiology 1979; 132: 563–7.

131. Haverkos HW, Dowling JN, Pasculle AW et al. Diagnosis of pneumonitis in immunocompromised patients by open lung biopsy. Cancer 1983; 52: 1093–7.

132. Hwang SS, Kim HH, Park SH, Jung JI, Jang HS. The value of CT-guided percutaneous needle aspiration in immunocompromised patients with suspected pulmonary infection. AJR Am J Roentgenol 2000; 175: 235–8.

133. Johnston WW. Percutaneous fine needle aspiration biopsy of the lung. A study of 1,015 patients. Acta Cytol 1984; 28: 218–24.

134. Perlmutt LM, Johnston WW, Dunnick NR. Percutaneous transthoracic needle aspiration: a review. AJR Am J Roentgenol 1989; 152: 451–5.

135. Dorca J, Manresa F, Esteban L et al. Efficacy, safety, and therapeutic relevance of transthoracic aspiration with ultrathin needle in nonventilated nosocomial pneumonia. Am J Respir Crit Care Med 1995; 151: 1491–6.

136. Light RW, Macgregor MI, Luchsinger PC, Ball WC, Jr. Pleural effusions: the diagnostic separation of transudates and exudates. Ann Intern Med 1972; 77: 507–13.

137. Sahn SA. Management of complicated parapneumonic effusions. Am Rev Respir Dis 1993; 148: 813–7.

138. Waite RJ, Carbonneau RJ, Balikian JP et al. Parietal pleural changes in empyema: appearances at CT. Radiology 1990; 175: 145–50.

139. Aquino SL, Webb WR, Gushiken BJ. Pleural exudates and transudates: diagnosis with contrast-enhanced CT. Radiology 1994; 192: 803–8.

140. Strain DS, Kinasewitz GT, Vereen LE, George RB. Value of routine daily chest x-rays in the medical intensive care unit. Crit Care Med 1985; 13: 534–6.

141. Greenbaum DM, Marschall KE. The value of routine daily chest x-rays in intubated patients in the medical intensive care unit. Crit Care Med 1982; 10: 29–30.

13

Chronic obstructive pulmonary disease

Sanjay Kalra and David L Levin

Introduction

Chronic obstructive pulmonary disease (COPD) has been variously defined, but it includes the common thread of (expiratory) airflow limitation that is progressive and only partly, if at all, reversible. It is characterized by abnormal airway inflammation, may be accompanied by airway hyperreactivity, and encompasses both, primarily clinically defined, chronic bronchitis and, the more pathologically or radiographically evident, emphysema.[1]

Chronic bronchitis is defined as chronic productive cough for at least 3 months in 2 consecutive years and emphysema is defined pathologically as the presence of permanent enlargement of the air spaces distal to the terminal bronchioles, accompanied by destruction of their walls and without significant fibrosis. There are sufficient clinical and radiological surrogates for the pathological changes that define emphysema to make routine lung biopsies unnecessary for diagnosis. The two components often coexist and, particularly in North America, the term emphysema is used more generically to refer to all COPD.[2]

Although cigarette smoking appears finally to be in decline, the consequences of current and past use will continue to be major health concerns for at least the first half of this century. The primary pulmonary complications of smoking are lung cancer and COPD. The latter is the only one of the current leading causes of mortality that still shows a rising trend in the developed world, reflecting both its chronicity and relative irreversibility. Its impact on the developing world, where data continue to show alarmingly high smoking patterns, is not only currently immense but also potentially even longer lasting.

Estimates for the US suggest that 6% of the adult population (~10 million) have COPD, resulting in 14 million ambulatory visits to hospitals and clinics, and 650 000 hospitalizations annually. An additional 2.5 million patients have COPD as a significant co-morbid disease contributing to hospital admission every year. In patients above the age of 65, COPD accounts for nearly 20% of all hospitalizations.

Over 100 000 deaths occur annually due to COPD. Within this is a changing gender pattern with women showing a progressive increase in death rates between 1995 and 1998 from 29.3 to 32.1 per 100 000 population while those in men have remained constant. Data from the developing world are incomplete but, based on smoking patterns, are likely to be even worse.[3]

Cigarette smoking is by far the leading risk factor for the development of COPD. Occupational and other exposures are recognized as contributors with an estimated 31% of COPD in non-smokers being attributable to work-related factors. Socioeconomic status and race also have an influence. Especially notable is the increasing recognition that women may be at greater risk than men, partly because of body size differences that magnify the effects of tobacco use, and partly because of disproportionate exposure to biomass and other cooking fuels in many parts of the world. Alpha-1-antitrypsin (AAT) deficiency is the only well-characterized genetic predisposition to emphysema but it is likely there are others that may explain differences in individual susceptibility to tobacco smoke and other exposures.[2]

How can chronic obstructive pulmonary disease be diagnosed?

COPD should always be considered in adult smokers complaining of cough, sputum production, or dyspnea (see Table 13.1 for differential diagnosis). It is also an important consideration in the non-smoker with other relevant exposures, often occupational, and perhaps even worth at least passing thought in those exposed passively to cigarette smoke. A family history of COPD, or a new diagnosis made in patients under 45 years old, should prompt testing for AAT deficiency. Sputum production is often prominent and change in volume and color often herald exacerbations.

Dyspnea is usually exertional and may be accompanied by wheezing. Hemoptysis, generally streaky and minor, does occur but should always be viewed with suspicion. Its presence frequently leads to additional evaluation to ensure that it is not due to other conditions such as bronchiectasis or lung cancer.

The physical examination is often normal, especially in those without severe disease. A number of patients will show evidence of weight loss, but, in general, body habitus parallels the unfortunately excessive weights of our modern times. Signs of hyperinflation secondary to airflow obstruction-related air trapping may range from subtle to the overtly barrel-shaped chest (due to an increasing anteroposterior (AP) diameter that approaches or exceeds the usually greater transverse dimension), reduced chest movements and inspiratory expansion, low placed diaphragm with limited excursion as defined by observation and percussion, use of accessory strap muscles of the neck, and diminished

intensity of breath sounds accompanied by expiratory prolongation or even wheezes. These signs all support the presence of significant airflow limitation and often foreshadow a forced expiratory volume in 1 second (FEV1) of less than 40% predicted. Inspiratory crackles are common, but occasionally may represent additional processes such as heart failure or coexisting bronchiectasis or interstitial lung disease. Distant heart sounds are the norm in patients with advanced disease and the presence of signs of right-sided heart failure (peripheral edema and elevated jugular venous pressure) all point towards secondary pulmonary hypertension, although the hyperinflation often muffles the accentuated pulmonary component of the second heart sound and makes a right parasternal lift distinctly unusual. Cyanosis does occur in proportion to hypoxemia but clubbing should not be attributed to COPD.

The diagnosis of COPD requires confirmatory spirometry both to identify the presence of airflow obstruction and to assess its severity (Table 13.2). The presence of significant reversibility (defined as a 12% or greater improvement in the FEV1 and/or forced vital capacity (FVC), which is at least 200 ml, after bronchodilator) should raise the possibility of asthma although it is quite common to see some reversibility even in these diseases of 'fixed' airway obstruction.

Scales that combine clinical and physiological parameters to grade severity have been proposed and the BODE index appears the most robust.[4] This combines body mass index (BMI, B), airflow obstruction (O) assessed by the post-bronchodilator percentage predicted FEV1, dyspnea (D) using the Medical Research Council (MRC) dyspnea scale, and effort tolerance (E) determined by the 6 minute walk distance. Vital additional information may be obtained by measuring oxygenation (pulse oximetry at rest, during exercise, and while asleep, as well as arterial blood gas studies) and selected patients may need assessment of cardiac function looking especially for pulmonary hypertension ('cor pulmonale').

Table 13.1 Differential diagnosis of COPD

COPD
Asthma
Bronchiectasis including cystic fibrosis
Congestive heart failure
Tuberculosis and other chronic infections
Constrictive (obliterative) bronchiolitis
Diffuse panbronchiolitis
Others
   central airway tumors
   airway foreign bodies
   laryngeal/vocal cord diseases
   tracheo- and bronchomalacia
   vascular rings
   fibrosing mediastinitis
   airway stenoses

Table 13.2 Staging of COPD

Stage	Severity	Post-bd FEV1/FVC ratio	%Predicted FEV1
0	**At risk**		
	Patients who:		
	smoke or have exposure to pollutants		
	have cough, sputum, or dyspnea		
	have family history of respiratory disease	> 0.7	80
I	**Mild COPD**	≤0.7	80
II	**Moderate COPD**	≤0.7	50–80
III	**Severe COPD**	≤0.7	30–50
IV	**Very severe COPD**	≤0.7	< 30 or < 50% + chronic respiratory failure

BD, bronchodilator; FEV1, forced expiratory volume in one second; FVC, forced vital capacity.
Adapted from American Thoracic Society/European Respiratory Society Guidelines and Global Initiative for Chronic Obstructive Lung Disease (GOLD) classification.[2,3]

What are the imaging features of chronic obstructive pulmonary disease?

The radiographic features of COPD result from a mixture of the enlarged air spaces, thickened airways, and reduced blood flow. These structural changes may, however, be more or less apparent within a given individual.

Conventional radiographs

With conventional radiographs, the classic features of emphysema are hyperinflation, bullous changes, and oligemia (Figure 13.1). Hyperinflation results in a flattening of the hemidiaphragms, an increase in the width of the retrosternal space, and an increase in the overall AP diameter of the chest. These findings are best identified on the lateral radiograph. While the presence of hyperinflation is typically a subjective impression, specific criteria can be used to aid in identification.[5] Flattening is present when the dome of the hemidiaphragm does not rise more than 1.5 cm above a line between the anterior and posterior costophrenic sulci. An increased retrosternal space is present when the distance between the posterior margin of the sternum and the ascending aorta is greater than 2.5 cm. Bullous disease results in focal areas of lucency within the lung parenchyma. The reduction in pulmonary blood flow that accompanies emphysema primarily manifests as an overall reduction of vessel caliber with a more rapid tapering of the peripheral branches. This can be difficult to identify with conventional radiographs. In some individuals, airway thickening is a dominant feature, relating primarily to chronic bronchitis.[6] Of the radiographic features that might be present in a patient with obstructive pulmonary disease, hyperinflation is the most useful in the identification of emphysema.[7]

Computed tomography

Computed tomography (CT) allows for the direct identification of the enlarged distal air spaces found in emphysema (Figure 13.2).[8] While many of the early descriptions of emphysema made use of a high-resolution CT technique, the qualitative features of emphysema are similar regardless of the CT technique used – especially given the proliferation of multislice helical scanners. There are three basic patterns of emphysema that can be identified: centrilobular, panlobular, and paraseptal. Centrilobular emphysema is the most common form and is strongly associated with cigarette smoking. With CT, centrilobular emphysema is characterized by focal regions of decreased attenuation, without definable walls, that are confined to the center of the secondary lobule. The disease is typically more pronounced within the upper lobes. Panlobular (panacinar) emphysema is most frequently associated with AAT (Figure 13.3). On CT imaging, it is characterized by larger regions of low attenuation leading to an apparent simplification of lung architecture. The changes of panlobular emphysema are most pronounced within the mid and lower lungs. Paraseptal emphysema is also commonly associated with smoking and is frequently seen as focal areas of lucency immediately adjacent to the pleura. However, these can also be seen in non-smokers.

CT can also be used to objectively score the amount of emphysema present.[9] CT imaging characterizes the density of tissue in terms of Hounsfield units (HU). This scale is defined with water having a value of 0 HU and air with a density of roughly −1000 HU. Tissues with a CT density

(a)

(b)

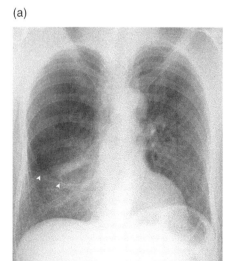
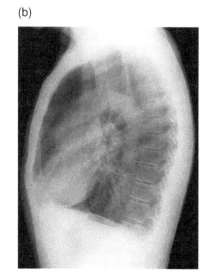

Figure 13.1

Frontal (a) and lateral (b) radiographs in a patient with emphysema. There is hyperinflation with flattening of the hemidiaphragms. Increased lucency is present, especially within the right upper lobe. Inferior displacement of the minor fissure (arrowheads) is also present.

greater than water, such as muscle or bone, will have positive HU values. The lung, which contains a large amount of air, primarily consists of voxels with negative HU values. As discussed, emphysema results in regions of decreased attenuation within the lung parenchyma. In terms of the CT density of lung, emphysema will result in an overall decrease in HU values. Figure 13.4 shows the distribution of HU values for the lungs of two individuals: a healthy subject (a) and a patient with emphysema (b). In the healthy subject, there is a distribution of HU values with a peak at −867 HU. In the patient with emphysema, this peak is centered at −935 HU. This reduction is related to the greater amount of air relative to tissue present within the lung. There are many ways to quantify this change in CT density. One of the simplest is to define the volume of the lung with a density below a given cut-off. For a slice thickness of 10 mm, a threshold value of −910 HU is commonly used.[9] In Figure 13.4, the healthy subject has only 3.6% of total voxels below this cut-off, while the patient with emphysema has 56.3% below this value. From the histogram, however, it is clear that there could be many possible measures used to define emphysema. In addition to using a standardized cut-off value, one can define a HU value which identifies a specific centile of the histogram. For example, the HU value that defines the 15th centile has been proposed as a measure of emphysema.[10] The lower (more negative) this value, the greater the amount of

emphysema present. While these methods have been used in investigational studies, they are not widely used in a clinical setting.

Magnetic resonance imaging

Magnetic resonance (MR) imaging is typically not used in the evaluation of suspected pulmonary parenchymal disease. Conventional MR imaging relies on the signal from protons in hydrogen (primarily water) to generate clinical images. The lung presents several challenges in this respect: there is a very low proton density and the numerous air/soft tissue interfaces lead to magnetic susceptibility artifacts that further reduce MR signal. Additionally, the spatial resolution of MR imaging is typically substantially less than that of CT, which further limits the evaluation of parenchymal disease.

Some of the newer MR techniques make use of hyperpolarized noble gases to overcome many of these limitations. In these techniques, hyperpolarized non-radioactive isotopes of helium or xenon gas are used as inhaled contrast agents. The nuclear spins of these hyperpolarized gases can be imaged directly using MR. Hyperpolarized gas imaging can be used in a variety of ways. One of the most promising techniques for the evaluation of emphysema is diffusion imaging. This technique is sensitive to the motion of

(a)
(b)

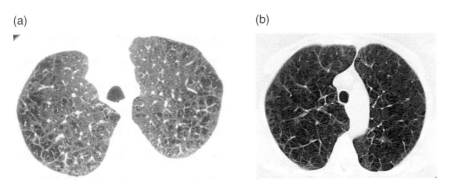

Figure 13.2
Axial CT images through the upper lobes in two patients with moderate (a) and severe (b) centrilobular emphysema demonstrate multiple foci of lucency within the lung parenchyma.

(a)
(b)

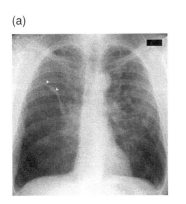
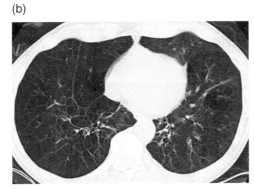

Figure 13.3
Frontal radiograph (a) and axial CT image (b) from a patient with alpha-1-antitrypsin emphysema. The radiograph demonstrates severe hyperinflation with increased lucency primarily involving the lung bases. There is superior displacement of the minor fissure (arrowheads) reflecting the uneven hyperinflation. Increased lucency is present in a relatively uniform fashion throughout the lungs on the CT image.

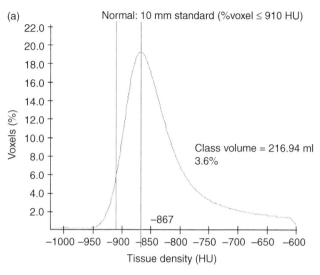
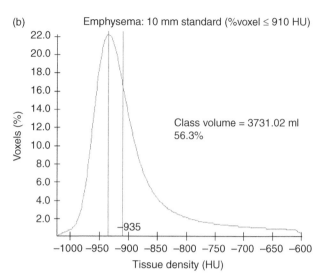

Figure 13.4

Quantitative evaluation of the lung parenchyma in a healthy subject (a) and a patient with emphysema (b). The histogram plots demonstrate the density distribution of voxels within the lung. In the healthy subject, the mean density for the lung is −867 HU and only 3.6% of all voxels have a density less than −910 HU. In the patient with emphysema, the mean lung density decreases to −935 HU and the percentage of lung voxels below −910 HU has increased to 56.3%.

hyperpolarized gas atoms within the air spaces and it can be used to determine an apparent diffusion coefficient (ADC). Normal alveoli restrict the motion of gas within the lung. As the distal airspaces increase in size, there is a reduction in this restriction to gas movement. This leads to an increase in the measured ADC.[11,12] ADC has been shown to be elevated in patients with severe emphysema when compared with healthy subjects.[13] The ability to detect changes in ADC in otherwise healthy smokers has not been fully evaluated.

Hyperpolarized imaging has, so far, been confined almost exclusively to use in a research setting. These techniques require significant modifications to conventional MR scanners and the equipment used to produce hyperpolarized gas is quite expensive. If and when these costs become less prohibitive, this technique is likely to have a significant impact on the clinical evaluation of COPD.

What are the treatment options for chronic obstructive pulmonary disease?

Smoking cessation

Several large and well-controlled studies have already demonstrated the central role of cigarette smoking in the pathogenesis of COPD as well as its continued progression.[3] In the relatively asymptomatic patient with early or mild disease, smoking cessation may be the only active intervention required and no opportunity to achieve this should be overlooked. Smoking status should be assessed at every clinical encounter. Pharmacotherapy may be of major value.

Prevention of infection

The use of prophylactic antibiotics to prevent acute COPD exacerbations has not been shown to be effective and has little to commend it. However, immunizations against influenza[14] and pneumococcal pneumonia[15] have been established as useful preventative measures. The former is used annually, preferably as the inactivated virus vaccine, just before the start of the 'flu season' (autumn in the Northern hemisphere), and the latter is recommended as one dose of the polyvalent vaccine with a booster dose after a minimum gap of 5 years.

Pharmacotherapy

Bronchodilators: β-agonists, anticholinergics, and others

Bronchodilator therapy is the linchpin of the treatment of symptomatic COPD (Table 13.3).[16] These agents come in two major types, the β₂-agonists (albuterol, formoterol, and salmeterol) and the anticholinergics (ipratropium and tiotropium). They are most commonly prescribed in the inhaled form, often in combination, and both types are available in rapid-onset, short-acting as well as delayed-onset, long-acting forms.[17–19] One exception, formoterol, is

Table 13.3

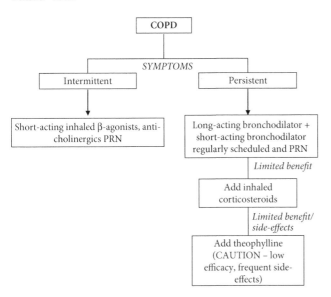

a β_2-agonist with a rapid onset of action but a prolonged duration of effect. Some β_2-agonists are available in oral and parenteral form but are infrequently administered through these routes. Side-effects are uncommon but include anxiety type symptoms, tachyarrhythmias, tremors and, for the anticholinergic agents, a small risk of precipitating acute closed angle glaucoma and urinary retention. There have been questions about a link between β_2-agonist use and an increased risk of death, primarily in asthmatics. Current data do not convincingly establish a causal connection and it is likely that increased use of these drugs is a marker of severe disease.

Methylxanthine agents (aminophylline derivatives) suffer from unpredictable efficacy and a narrow therapeutic window. Side-effects including cardiac arrhythmias, seizures, and even death have been attributed to these drugs. They tend to interact with multiple other medications and their metabolism is also affected by cigarette smoking. Their use has progressively declined, largely as other safer and more effective bronchodilators have emerged.

Corticosteroids: inhaled, systemic

Inhaled corticosteroids (beclomethasone, flunisolide, fluticasone, budesonide, and triamcinolone) are frequently used and there are data to suggest a modest benefit in both post-bronchodilator FEV1 measurements as well as airway hyperreactivity. Neither of these effects appears to produce measurable clinical improvement and several large trials have failed to support the routine use of inhaled corticosteroids in stable disease. The best available evidence suggests a small role in reducing both the frequency and severity of exacerbations in patients with severe disease.[20–22] Although there is little evidence to recommend the use of systemic corticosteroids in stable COPD, there are data to support their use in acute exacerbations.[23]

Others: mucolytics and AAT replacement

Several mucolytic agents have been used with limited, largely symptomatic, benefit. The best studied is *N*-acetylcysteine, which has additional antioxidant effect, and may reduce the number of acute exacerbations. Overall its value is unclear and, at best, its role should be considered marginal. Other agents, including guafenesin, are even less supported by available data.[24]

The presence of AAT deficiency associated emphysema often leads to consideration of replacement therapy. Observational data suggest patients with a FEV1 < 80% predicted and an abnormal phenotype combined with a serum AAT level < 11 mmol/l may show slower FEV1 decline with replacement therapy but no controlled studies have been performed. The limited benefit must be balanced against the high cost of this therapy that is administered by intravenous infusion every 2–4 weeks.[25]

Long-term oxygen therapy

Long-term oxygen therapy (LTOT) has been validated in two landmark randomized studies. The British MRC study showed a significant reduction in mortality with 15 h/day use of supplemental oxygen[26] and the Nocturnal Oxygen Treatment Trial established the added advantage of continuous (average 19 h/day) oxygen use.[27] Benefits, other than improved survival, include improvements in exercise tolerance, cognitive function, quality of life, and a reduction in both polycythemia and pulmonary hypertension severity.[28] Conventional criteria for use of LTOT require the demonstration of hypoxemia (Sp_{O_2} = 88% or Pa_{O_2} = 55 torr) although these can be less stringent if polycythemia or pulmonary hypertension is present. The benefits of oxygen supplementation for exercise or sleep associated hypoxemia (without hypoxemia at rest) are less clear and probably limited to improvements in exercise tolerance and perhaps daytime cognitive function.[29]

Pulmonary rehabilitation

Rehabilitation in the patient with pulmonary disease achieves improvements in the performance of the activities of daily living, exercise tolerance, and quality of life. No improvement in pulmonary function is expected or observed as a consequence of such therapy. It has also not been shown to unequivocally impact survival but there are data that suggest a reduction in health care utilization.[30]

Acute exacerbations

The majority of acute COPD exacerbations are related to infection (viral and/or bacterial) and are characterized by a combination of increasing dyspnea, cough, and increasing sputum production, often with associated purulence.[31] Some episodes are attributable to irritant/environmental airborne exposures and exacerbations may be mimicked by heart failure and pulmonary emboli. Exacerbations are important contributors to both morbidity and mortality and, despite treatment, are associated with a significant 2–4 week relapse rate of 15–30%.[32,33]

What interventional options are available for chronic obstructive pulmonary disease?

Surgical treatment: bullectomy, lung volume reduction surgery, non-surgical lung volume reduction procedures, and lung transplantation

The dominant abnormality in emphysema is the presence of hyperinflation. It has been suggested that reversal of this may improve function and this hypothesis has been tested in several ways. The most comprehensive such information comes from the National Emphysema Treatment Trial (NETT) in which patients were randomized to receive either lung volume reduction surgery (LVRS) or aggressive medical therapy. NETT identified a subset of patients (non-homogenous emphysema and low exercise capacity despite pulmonary rehabilitation) in whom LVRS produced both improvement in function and survival.[34] However, the NETT also defined another group (FEV1 = 20%, Dlco = 20% predicted) that showed a marked increase in mortality with the procedure.[35] The demand for this procedure peaked several years ago and it is now offered only to the highly selected group of patients that was defined by NETT as likely to benefit. The situation may be clearer in the occasional patient who shows large/giant bullae (>30% of hemithoracic volume) where surgical bullectomy may allow improvement in overall function.

Non-surgical volume reduction procedures using a variety of bronchoscopic techniques are currently being evaluated and appear to be technically feasible. Their benefits have not yet been defined and the various devices under study must be considered experimental at present.

Lung transplantation is established therapy for patients with advanced-stage disease.[36] The benefits in COPD translate more into improved exercise tolerance and quality of life rather than prolongation of life as the expected 5 year 50–60% survival is not significantly different from the disease course in the non-transplant severe COPD population. The large numbers of eligible patients has elevated this disease to the most frequent lung transplant indication in the US.

What complications are associated with chronic obstructive pulmonary disease?

Respiratory infections

The course of COPD is often punctuated by superimposed respiratory events. Dominant amongst these are acute infections, bronchial or pulmonary parenchymal ('pneumonia'). Offending organisms are usually common respiratory pathogens, bacterial and viral, but the disease course is often more severe, especially in patients with severe COPD. In these cases, acute respiratory failure, with all its attendant needs, often ensues and usually requires progressive intensification of respiratory support (see Acute exacerbations section).

Occasionally more chronic infections may occur and amongst these the best described include chronic fibro-cavitary histoplasmosis and atypical mycobacterial infections (especially with *Mycobacterium kansasii*, *M. avium–intracellulare* complex). Less commonly seen are manifestations of disease caused by fungi, especially *Aspergillus* species. These include invasive forms, both acute and chronic, as well as localized mycetoma formation ('aspergilloma') within bullous cavities. The latter has a propensity to cause hemoptysis, potentially massive, and may even be an indication for prophylactic resection if the patient's respiratory and general condition permits.

Pneumonia in patients with underlying COPD can manifest as a focus of parenchymal consolidation or as airway wall thickening. Given the underlying parenchymal destruction, regions of consolidation are often inhomogeneous and ill-defined at their margins. Because of the risk of malignancy, these opacities need to be followed to document resolution (Figure 13.5).

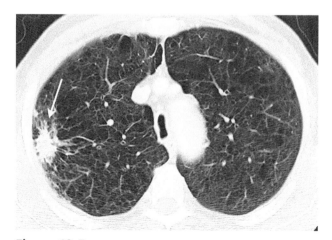

Figure 13.5
Lung carcinoma in a patient with emphysema. An irregular, spiculated mass (arrow) is present within the right upper lobe.

Extra-alveolar gas: pneumothorax, pneumomediastinum, and subcutaneous emphysema

The anatomical changes in the lungs of patients with COPD, especially the combination of thin walled blebs/bullae and airway obstruction, significantly increase the likelihood of developing an air leak. This risk is further magnified during acute exacerbations, especially in those where positive pressure ventilation forms part of the treatment. Occasionally the air leak, especially in the form of a pneumothorax, is the proximate cause for the worsening symptoms and not all exacerbations should be automatically attributed to infection.

Pneumomediastinum (Figure 13.6) is usually asymptomatic and rarely occurs alone, being more common as a supplementary finding with the clinically more important pneumothorax. Auscultation may provide a clue to the presence of the pneumomediastinum by identifying a crunching sound synchronous with the heartbeat. Subcutaneous emphysema can be dramatic in appearance, though it is more often a radiographic finding, and like pneumomediastinum, is usually less important than the commonly coexisting pneumothorax. Therapy is directed at the latter and, especially in the symptomatic patient, typically requires intercostal drainage. Recurrent episodes may require more definitive surgical management.

In general, the hallmark of extra-alveolar gas is focal lucency within the mediastinum, pleural space, or soft tissues. Pneumomediastinum is characterized primarily by linear lucency outlining the mediastinal structures. While these areas of lucency might be subtle on conventional radiographs, they are typically readily identified on CT as focal air collections lying medial to the mediastinal pleura. Subcutaneous emphysema is similarly identified as focal lucency within the soft tissues. Again, this is typically well demonstrated using CT.

Pneumothorax is diagnosed by identifying air separating the visceral and parietal pleural surfaces. On occasion, it can be difficult to distinguish between a loculated pneumothorax and bullous disease. In these cases, the wall of a focal bullous lesion can mimic the visceral pleural surface. Findings that favor a pneumothorax in this setting include compression of the adjacent lung parenchyma, the presence of air outlining both sides of the wall of a bulla, and lucency that is not confined to a single lobe.[37]

Congestive heart failure

COPD and heart disease, especially coronary artery disease, often coexist because of shared risk and demographic factors, and problems with distinguishing congestive heart failure from a COPD exacerbation are not an uncommon clinical dilemma. The radiographic features of congestive heart failure can be quite subtle when superimposed on a background of moderate to severe emphysema. In these patients, the pulmonary vasculature is typically attenuated. In the presence of early failure, the pulmonary vessels may dilate but will remain within normal limits for overall size. This change will be noticeable only with a direct comparison to prior studies. The presence of interlobular septal thickening seen either on conventional radiographs or CT, especially when new, is suggestive of superimposed failure. It can take a combination of clinical assessment, pulmonary function testing, radiography, echocardiography, and even invasive cardiac testing, to make an accurate attribution in patients with both heart disease and COPD.

Other cardiac abnormalities commonly associated with COPD include atrial arrhythmias (such as multifocal atrial tachycardia), pulmonary hypertension ('cor pulmonale') with or without heart failure,[38,39] and a somewhat increased risk of pulmonary thromboembolic events.

Conclusion

In summary, COPD is a widely prevalent disease with a high morbidity, mortality, and economic burden. Radiological imaging and pulmonary function testing are central to diagnosis, with the former being of great value in the recognition of complications. The chronic course of the disease is often punctuated by acute events, primarily infective exacerbations that may be compounded by respiratory failure. Although the obstructive component is largely irreversible, symptoms and complications can be ameliorated with preventive interventions as well as pharmacotherapy. The elimination of cigarette smoking by education and legislation should be the foundation of public health policy in controlling this global epidemic.

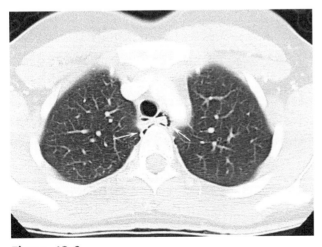

Figure 13.6
Pneumomediastinum. Focal lucencies (arrows) are present within the mediastinum.

References

1. American Thoracic Society. Chronic bronchitis, asthma and pulmonary emphysema: a statement by the Committee on Diagnostic Standards for Nontuberculous Respiratory Diseases. Am Rev Respir Dis 1962; 85: 762–8.

2. American Thoracic Society/European Respiratory Society Task Force. Standards for the Diagnosis and Management of Patients with COPD Internet. Version 1.2. New York: American Thoracic Society; 2004 (updated 2005 September 8). Available from http://www-test.thoracic.org/copd/.

3. Pauwels R, Buist A, Calverley P, Jerkins C, Hurd S. Global strategy for the diagnosis, management and prevention of chronic obstructive pulmonary disease. NHLBI/WHO Global Initiative for Chronic Obstructive Lung Disease (GOLD) Workshop summary. Am J Respir Crit Care Med 2001; 163: 1256–76.

4. Celli BR, Cote CG, Marin JM et al. The body-mass index, airflow obstruction, dyspnea, and exercise capacity index in chronic obstructive pulmonary disease. N Engl J Med 2004; 350: 1005–12.

5. Reich SB, Weinshelbaum A, Yee J. Correlation of radiographic measurements and pulmonary function tests in chronic obstructive pulmonary disease. AJR Am J Roentgenol 1985; 144: 695–9.

6. Friedman PJ. Radiology of the airways with emphasis on the small airways. J Thorac Imaging 1986; 1: 7–22.

7. Pratt PC. Role of conventional chest radiology in diagnosis and exclusion of emphysema. Am J Med 1987; 82: 998–1006.

8. Bergin CJ, Müller NL, Nichols DM et al. The diagnosis of emphysema: a computed tomographic pathological correlation. Am Rev Respir Dis 1986; 133: 541–6.

9. Müller NL, Staples CA, Miller RR et al. "Density mask": an objective method to quantitate emphysema using computed tomography. Chest 1988; 94: 782–7.

10. Newell JD, Hogg JC, Snider GL. Report of a workshop: quantitative computed tomography scanning in longitudinal studies of emphysema. Eur Respir J 2004; 23: 769–75.

11. Chen XJ, Hedlund LW, Moller HE et al. Detection of emphysema in rat lungs by using magnetic resonance measurements of 3He diffusion. Proc Natl Acad Sci U S A 2000; 97: 11478–81.

12. Yablonskiy DA, Sukstanskii AL, Leawoods JC et al. Quantitative in vivo assessment of lung microstructure at the alveolar level with hyperpolarized 3He diffusion MRI. Proc Natl Acad Sci U S A 2002; 99: 3111–6.

13. Saam BT, Yablonskiy DA, Kodibagkar VD et al. MR imaging of diffusion of 3He gas in healthy and diseased lungs. Magn Reson Med 2000; 44: 174–9.

14. Nichol KL, Baken L, Nelson A. Relation between influenza vaccination and outpatient visits, hospitalization, and mortality in elderly persons with chronic lung disease. Ann Intern Med 1999; 130: 397–403.

15. Nichol KL, Baken L, Wuorenma J, Nelson A. The health and economic benefits associated with pneumococcal vaccinations of elderly persons with chronic lung disease. Arch Int Med 1999; 159: 2437–47.

16. Hay JG, Stone P, Carter J et al. Bronchodilator reversibility, exercise performance and breathlessness in stable chronic obstructive pulmonary disease. Eur Respir J 1992; 5: 659–64.

17. Mahler DA, Donohue JF, Barbee RA et al. Efficacy of salmeterol xinafoate in the treatment of COPD. Chest 1999; 115: 957–65.

18. Van Noord JA, de Munck DR, Bantje TA et al. Long-term treatment of chronic obstructive pulmonary disease with salmeterol and the additive effect of ipratropium. Eur Respir J 2000; 15: 878–85.

19. Casaburi R, Mahler DA, Jones PW et al. A long-term evaluation of once-daily inhaled tiotropium in chronic obstructive pulmonary disease. Eur Respir J 2002; 19: 217–24.

20. Pauwels RA, Lofdahl CG, Laitinen LA et al. Long-term treatment with inhaled budesonide in persons with mild chronic obstructive pulmonary disease who continue smoking. N Engl J Med 1999; 340: 1948–53.

21. The Lung Health Study Research Group. Effect of inhaled triamcinolone on the decline in pulmonary function in chronic obstructive pulmonary disease. N Engl J Med 2000; 343: 1902–9.

22. Calverley P, Pauwels R, Vestbo J et al. Combined salmeterol and fluticasone in the treatment of chronic obstructive pulmonary disease: a randomised controlled trial. Lancet 2003; 361: 449–56.

23. Niewhoehner DE, Erbland ML, Deupree RH et al. Effect of systemic glucocorticoids on exacerbations of chronic obstructive pulmonary disease. Department of Veterans Affairs Cooperative Study Group. N Engl J Med 1999; 340: 1941–7.

24. Poole PJ, Black PN. Mucolytic agents for chronic bronchitis or chronic obstructive pulmonary disease. Cochrane Database Syst Rev 2000; 2: CD001287.

25. Dirksen A, Dijkman JH, Madsen F et al. A randomized clinical trial of a(1)-antitrypsin augmentation therapy. Am J Respir Crit Care Med 1999; 160: 1468–72.

26. Report of the Medical Research Council Working Party. Long-term domiciliary oxygen therapy in chronic hypoxic cor pulmonale complicating chronic bronchitis and emphysema. Lancet 1981; 1: 681–5.

27. Nocturnal Oxygen Therapy Trial Group. Continuous or nocturnal oxygen therapy in hypoxemic chronic obstructive lung disease. Ann Intern Med 1980; 93: 391–8.

28. Zielinski J. Effects of long-term oxygen therapy in patients with chronic obstructive pulmonary disease. Curr Opin Pulm Med 1999; 5: 81–7.

29. Petty TL, Casaburi R. Recommendations of the Fifth Oxygen Consensus Conference. Writing and organizing committees. Respir Care 2000; 45: 957–61.

30. American Thoracic Society/European Respiratory Society Statement on Pulmonary Rehabilitation. Am J Respir Crit Care Med 2006; 173: 1390–413.

31. Anthonisen NR, Manfreda J, Warren CPW et al. Antibiotic therapy in exacerbations of chronic obstructive pulmonary disease. Ann Intern Med 1987; 106: 196–204.

32. Connors AF Jr, Dawson NV, Tomas C et al. Outcomes following acute exacerbation of severe chronic obstructive lung disease. The SUPPORT investigators (Study to Understand Prognoses and Preferences for Outcomes and Risks of Treatment). Am J Respir Crit Care Med 1996; 154: 959–67.

33. Miravitlles M. Epidemiology of chronic obstructive pulmonary disease exacerbations. Clin Pulm Med 2002; 9: 191–7.

34. National Emphysema Treatment Trial Research Group. A randomized trial comparing lung-volume-reduction

surgery with medical therapy for severe emphysema. N Engl J Med 2003; 348: 2059–73.

35. National Emphysema Treatment Trial Research Group. Patients at high risk of death after lung-volume-reduction surgery. N Engl J Med 2001; 345: 1075–83.

36. Patterson GA, Maurer JR, Williams TJ et al. Comparison of outcomes of double and single lung transplantation for obstructive lung disease. The Toronto Lung Transplant Group. J Thorac Cardiovasc Surg 1991; 101: 623–31; discussion 631–2.

37. Waitches GM, Stern EJ, Dubinsky TJ. Usefullness of the double-wall sign in detecting pneumothorax in patients with giant bullous emphysema. AJR Am J Roentgenol 2000; 174: 1765–68.

38. MacNee W. Pathophysiology of cor pulmonale in chronic obstructive pulmonary disease. Part one. Am J Respir Crit Care Med 1994; 150: 833–52.

39. MacNee W. Pathophysiology of cor pulmonale in chronic obstructive pulmonary disease. Part two. Am J Respir Crit Care Med 1994; 150: 1158–68.

14

Hemoptysis

Jay H Ryu and Anne-Marie Sykes

Introduction

Hemoptysis is a symptom encountered frequently by clinicians. Hemoptysis is coughing up of blood originating from the airways or lung parenchyma. Bronchial arteries are generally a more important source of bleeding than the pulmonary circulation. Occasionally, the expectorated blood may involve an extrapulmonary source, e.g. aorto-pulmonary fistula.

Differential diagnosis of hemoptysis is broad. Hemoptysis is a manifestation of a variety of benign and malignant processes involving the tracheobronchial tree or the lung parenchyma. In some cases, the pathological process may originate in an extrathoracic site with secondary involvement of the respiratory structures, e.g. septic pulmonary embolism.

Evaluation of a patient with hemoptysis includes initial assessment of the rate of bleeding and clinical status, followed by localization of the site of bleeding and identification of the underlying cause. Although hemoptysis is modest in amount and self-limited in most cases, it can be massive and lethal.

Management of hemoptysis depends on the rate of bleeding, overall clinical status, site of bleeding, and the underlying cause for the hemoptysis.

What methods are available to localize the site of bleeding?

Initial evaluation of a patient with hemoptysis assesses the rate of bleeding and overall clinical status. Bleeding is more commonly from airway disease (including bronchogenic carcinoma) than parenchymal or vascular disorders. Indications for hospitalization include persistent hemoptysis in large volumes, respiratory distress, hypoxemia, or hemodynamic instability.

History and physical examination may sometimes yield clues to the site of bleeding. These clues include lateralizing chest pain or discomfort, and localized crackles or wheeze. Initial laboratory testing includes complete blood count, coagulation parameters, chemistry panel, and sputum examination (including stains and microbial cultures if the situation warrants). Ordering of other blood tests as well as urinalysis is dictated by the clinical circumstances and differential diagnosis.

Chest radiography is the initial imaging test used in the evaluation of a patient with hemoptysis. Chest radiography may sometimes reveal the location and the underlying cause of hemoptysis, e.g. lung cancer (Figure 14.1). Other diagnostic findings may include lung abscess, mycetoma, arteriovenous malformation, broncholithiasis, etc. Patchy alveolar infiltrates seen bilaterally may indicate diffuse pulmonary alveolar hemorrhage, as seen in Goodpasture's syndrome or pulmonary vasculitides (Figure 14.2). However, chest radiography may only reveal non-specific findings or no relevant abnormalities in 20–40% of patients with hemoptysis.[1] It may also show abnormalities in areas other than the actual site of bleeding and potentially mislead the clinician. For example, blood from an upper lobe lesion may extend to the lower lung, resulting in areas of parenchymal opacification in the lower lungs. The radiograph can also be used to help target bronchoscopy. However, the diagnostic yield of fiberoptic bronchoscopy for patients with hemoptysis and a normal or non-localizing chest radiograph is only 10–20%.

Computed tomography (CT) of the chest is a valuable procedure in the evaluation of hemoptysis. When the chest radiograph is normal, CT may provide lateralizing abnormalities (Figure 14.3), which will guide the bronchoscopist to the area of abnormality. The advantage of CT is that the anatomy of the airways, pulmonary parenchyma, and vascular structures are visualized in more detail. Therefore, CT can allow more specific diagnoses, such as bronchiectasis, mycetomas, mass lesions (including cancer), and vascular abnormalities such as arteriovenous malformations. In patients with non-massive hemoptysis, CT should generally be performed before bronchoscopy.

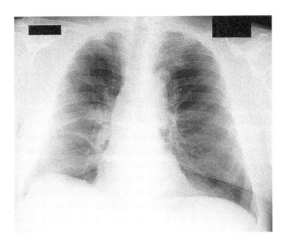

Figure 14.1
Posteroanterior (PA) chest radiograph in a 69-year-old man with a 3-day history of hemoptysis shows a mass near the right hilum which was subsequently shown to be a bronchogenic carcinoma. Incidentally noted is a focal aneurysm off the arch of the aorta.

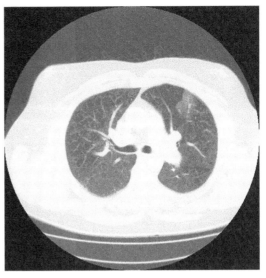

Figure 14.3
Fifty-one-year-old woman who presented with hemoptysis and a normal chest radiograph. CT image through the level of the carina shows a focal area of increased attenuation in the left upper lobe anteriorly compatible with hemorrhage. Subsequent work-up failed to demonstrate a localizing lesion and the hemoptysis was felt to be secondary to pulmonary arterial hypertension. Note the enlarged main pulmonary arteries.

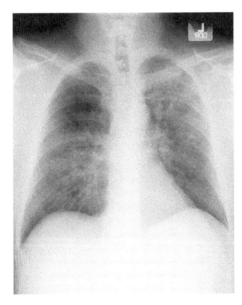

Figure 14.2
PA chest radiograph of a 55-year-old man with Wegener's granulomatosis who presented with hemoptysis. There are bilateral alveolar infiltrates which are compatible with diffuse alveolar hemorrhage.

Multidetector row helical CT angiography provides more precise depiction of bronchial and non-bronchial systemic arteries than does conventional angiography and may enable detection of the bronchial and non-bronchial arteries causing hemoptysis.[2,3]

How can imaging assist in the diagnosis of the underlying cause for the hemoptysis?

The major task in the diagnostic evaluation of a patient presenting with hemoptysis is to identify those with potentially serious underlying causes, e.g. lung cancer, and those at risk for massive hemoptysis, e.g. arteriovenous malformation.

Worldwide, tuberculosis is probably the most common cause of hemoptysis (Figure 14.4). In developed countries, the most common causes of hemoptysis include bronchitis, bronchiectasis (including cystic fibrosis), and lung cancer. There are many additional causes and these include pneumonia, pulmonary embolism, lung abscess, pulmonary hemorrhage syndromes, broncholithiasis (Figure 14.5), mycetoma, pulmonary vascular anomalies, trauma, and foreign body.

Hemoptysis is unusual in children; pneumonia and foreign body aspiration are the most common causes. Other causes in children include cystic fibrosis, congenital heart disease, and pulmonary–renal syndromes.

When no cause can be identified, it is referred to as cryptogenic or idiopathic hemoptysis. This accounts for 10–30% of patients with hemoptysis.[4]

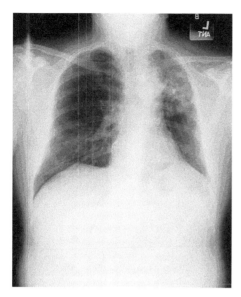

Figure 14.4
Forty-nine-year-old man who presented with hemoptysis. PA chest radiograph shows scarring and volume loss in the left upper lung from prior tuberculosis. Alveolar infiltrate in the left mid-lung is compatible with hemorrhage due to reactivation tuberculosis.

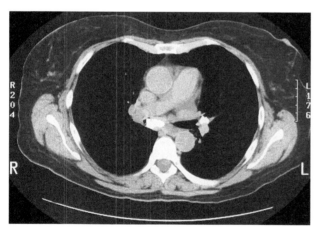

Figure 14.5
Sixty-year-old woman who presented with hemoptysis. CT scan at the level of the bronchus intermedius shows a calcified node eroding into the posterior wall of the bronchus intermedius compatible with broncholithiasis. This was confirmed at bronchoscopy.

History and physical examination provide the initial guide in prioritizing the list of diagnostic possibilities. These factors include age, sex, smoking history, antecedent events such as aspiration or trauma, medications, family history, and previous or chronic medical illnesses. Prior history of hemoptysis and respiratory diseases must be elicited.

Beyond localizing the site of the bleeding, CT may also allow a specific diagnosis to be made. High-resolution CT is particularly useful in the diagnosis of bronchiectasis and mycetomas (Figure 14.6).[5] Thin section CT of the airways (1–2 mm collimation through the central airways) can also detect other endobronchial abnormalities such as tumors or broncholithiasis. Contrast-enhanced chest CT can be helpful in detecting vascular abnormalities, such as arteriovenous malformations. In addition, bronchial and non-bronchial systemic feeder vessels can be detected at contrast-enhanced CT.[6]

In a stable patient with hemoptysis and a normal or non-localizing chest radiograph, CT should be performed before bronchoscopy because it has an overall higher diagnostic yield, and may allow localization of a lesion to guide bronchoscopy.[5,7–9] In such patients, CT of the chest can detect nearly all tumors identified by fiberoptic bronchoscopy and provide a specific diagnosis in 50% of patients with negative fiberoptic bronchoscopy, most often previously unrecognized bronchiectasis and occasionally tumors that were beyond bronchoscopic range.[5,7–9]

What are the options for managing massive or persistent hemoptysis?

There is no consensus on the definition of massive hemoptysis. Most commonly, massive hemoptysis is defined as

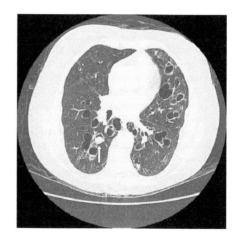

Figure 14.6
Twenty-two-year-old woman with cystic fibrosis who presented with hemoptysis. CT scan through the level of the bronchus intermedius shows cystic bronchiectasis bilaterally.
Additionally there is a soft tissue nodule in a right lower lobe bronchus (arrow) that was subsequently shown to be a mycetoma.

expectoration of 600 ml or more over 48 hours. Massive hemoptysis is relatively rare and accounts for less than 5% of patients with hemoptysis. In most cases, massive hemoptysis originates from the bronchial circulation.[10] However, non-bronchial systemic arteries can also be a source of massive hemoptysis and can be a cause of recurrent hemoptysis after successful bronchial artery embolization (BAE).[6]

Tuberculosis is probably the most common cause of massive hemoptysis, worldwide. In developed countries, the most common causes of massive hemoptysis include bronchiectasis/cystic fibrosis, lung cancer, and lung abscess.[11]

Most patients with massive hemoptysis need to be observed in the intensive care unit while undergoing initial management and diagnostic testing. Thoracic surgical consultation should be obtained early. Early bronchoscopy for diagnostic and therapeutic purposes or single-lumen endotracheal tube to protect the non-bleeding lung also needs to be considered.

Chest radiography is usually abnormal in patients with massive hemoptysis but may not identify the underlying cause of the bleeding. If the patient is clinically stable, CT scan of the chest before bronchoscopy is reasonable. CT scan of the chest may provide a likely diagnosis or localize the site of bleeding that helps guide subsequent bronchoscopy.

If the patient is clinically unstable, bronchoscopy is needed to further localize the bleeding site and to institute initial therapeutic measures such as endobronchial tamponade, topical application of vasoconstrictor agents or coagulants, or laser therapy.[11,12] However, some authors have suggested that CT be performed prior to bronchoscopy in all cases of massive hemoptysis.[6] Multidetector row CT allows for rapid scanning, making timely examination feasible even in critically ill patients. Bronchial and non-bronchial systemic arterial feeder vessels can be detected at contrast-enhanced CT, allowing for selection of vessels for potential embolization (Figure 14.7). CT angiography may also have a role in predicting recurrent hemoptysis as one study showed the total number of dilated bronchial and non-bronchial systemic arteries was a significant variable associated with recurrent hemoptysis.[13]

Technetium radionuclide-tagged red blood cell (RBC) scans have shown limited success in locating the area of hemorrhage.[14] The bleeding site can be localized in only a small minority of patients. A rapid rate of bleeding is required for this test to be useful and there can be false localization when the blood pools in dependent regions.

What is the role of interventional radiology in the treatment of hemoptysis?

Interventional radiology has a role in the treatment of hemoptysis, particularly massive hemoptysis. Bronchial

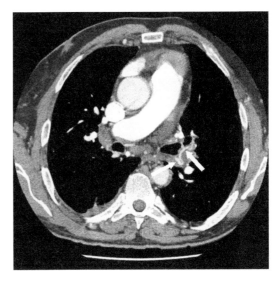

Figure 14.7
Sixty-year-old-man with chronic pulmonary emboli. Multidetector CT image with contrast at the level of the carina shows a dilated bronchial collateral coursing through the left hilum (arrows).

artery embolization (BAE) therapy is particularly useful for patients who are not candidates for surgical resection due to poor pulmonary reserve or non-pulmonary issues, e.g. unstable cardiac disease. BAE therapy may control bleeding in patients with massive or non-massive but persistent hemoptysis (Figure 14.8). It is a safe and effective non-surgical treatment. It may also allow for stabilization of the patient for elective surgery or continued medical therapy. Potential complications include transient chest pain and dysphagia. Rarely spinal cord ischemia can occur (1.4–6.5%), and is the most serious complication.[6] In massive hemoptysis, BAE is associated with a 75–90% success rate and a 10–20% recurrence rate.[11,15,16] Recurrent bleeding may occur due to incomplete embolization, recanalization of embolized vessels, collateral circulation or non-bronchial systemic arterial supply, and inadequate treatment or progression of the underlying disease (particularly in patients with chronic tuberculosis, aspergilloma, or neoplasm).

Contrast-enhanced chest CT and interventional radiology also play a role in diagnosis and management of patients with hemoptysis due to pulmonary arterial abnormalities, most commonly pulmonary arteriovenous malformations. Contrast enhanced spiral volumetric CT can reveal location, size, and number of the malformations as well as the configuration of the feeding and draining vessels. These lesions can also be defined with pulmonary angiography, where they can often be successfully embolized.[17]

(a)

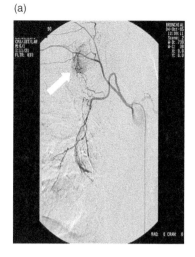

(b)

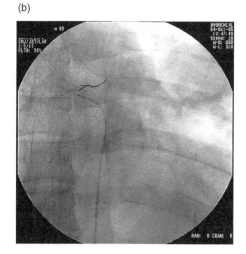

Figure 14.8
Twenty-seven-year-old man with hemoptysis secondary to metastatic melanoma to the lungs.
(a) Bronchial artery angiogram showing tumor blush of a metastatic lesion in the right upper lobe (arrows).
(b) Postembolization image showing coils in the bronchial artery.

Conclusion

Hemoptysis is commonly encountered by clinicians. The major task in the diagnostic evaluation of a patient presenting with hemoptysis is to identify those with potentially serious underlying causes and those at risk for massive hemoptysis. Imaging, particularly the chest radiograph and chest CT, plays an important role in localizing the site of bleeding and identifying the underlying cause of the bleeding. Imaging guided interventional procedures can play an important role in the management of patients with hemoptysis.

References

1. Marshall TJ, Flower CDR, Jackson JE. The role of radiology in the investigation and management of patients with haemoptysis. Clin Radiol 1996; 51: 391–400.
2. Remy-Jardin M, Bouaziz N, Dumont P et al. Bronchial and nonbronchial systemic arteries at multi-detector row CT angiography: comparison with conventional angiography. Radiology 2004; 233: 741–9.
3. Yoon YC, Lee KS, Jeong YJ et al. Hemoptysis: bronchial and nonbronchial systemic arteries at 16-detector row CT. Radiology 2005; 234: 292–8.
4. Corder R. Hemoptysis. Emerg Med Clin North Am 2003; 21: 421–35.
5. McGuiness G, Beacher JR, Harkin TJ et al. Hemoptysis: prospective high-resolution CT/bronchoscopic correlation. Chest 1994; 105: 1155–62.
6. Yoon W, Kim JK, Kim YH, Chung TW, Kang HK. Bronchial and nonbronchial systemic artery embolization for life-threatening hemoptysis: a comprehensive review. Radiographics 2002; 22: 1395–409.
7. Set PAK, Flower CDR, Smith IE et al. Hemoptysis: comparative study of the role of CT and fiberoptic bronchoscopy. Radiology 1993; 189: 677–80.
8. Millar AB, Boothroyd AE, Edwards D et al. The role of computed tomography in the investigation of unexplained hemoptysis. Respir Med 1992; 86: 39–44.
9. Naidich DP, Funt S, Ettenger NA et al. Hemoptysis: CT-bronchoscopic correlation in 59 cases. Radiology 1990; 177: 357–62.
10. Jean-Baptiste E. Clinical assessment and management of massive hemoptysis. Crit Care Med 2000; 28: 1642–7.
11. Lordan JL, Gascoigne A, Corris PA. The pulmonary physician in critical care. Illustrative case 7: assessment and management of massive haemoptysis. Thorax 2003; 58: 814–19.
12. Valipour A, Kreuzer A, Koller H, Koessler W, Burghuber OC. Bronchoscopy-guided topical hemostatic tamponade therapy for the management of life-threatening hemoptysis. Chest 2005; 127: 2113–18.
13. Jeong YJ, Kim CW, Kim KI et al. Prediction of recurrent hemoptysis with MDCT angiography. J Comput Assist Tomogr. 2006; 30: 662–8.
14. Winzelberg GG, Wholey MH, Jarmolowski CA et al. Patients with hemoptysis examined by Tc-99m sulfur colloid and Tc-99m-labeled red blood cells: a preliminary appraisal. Radiology 1984; 153: 523–6.
15. Swanson KL, Johnson M, Prakash UBS et al. Bronchial artery embolization: experience with 54 patients. Chest 2002; 121: 789–95.
16. Wong ML, Szkup PM, Hopley MJ. Percutaneous embolotherapy for life-threatening hemoptysis. Chest 2002; 121: 95–102.
17. Gossage JR, Kanj G. Pulmonary arteriovenous malformations, a state of the art review. Am J Respir Crit Care Med 1998; 158: 643–61.

15

Cough

Tomás Franquet and Antoni Torres

Introduction

Cough is a common manifestation of most respiratory disorders, and a natural defensive mechanism and protective reflex for clearing the upper and lower airways of large amounts of mucus due to excessive secretions or impaired mucociliary clearance, inhaled particles or foreign material, and infectious organisms. In the US, it is the most common symptom for which patients seek medical attention; it constitutes about 10–38% of the chest specialist's outpatient practice.

Cough may be indicative of trivial to very serious airway or parenchymal lung diseases, as well as of extrapulmonary processes. For clinical and differential diagnosis it is very useful to separate acute from chronic cough. The clinician confronted with a patient with cough needs specific knowledge of diverse lung disorders either limited to the lung or associated with systematic medical problems. Despite the importance of cough, its etiology often goes undiagnosed, untreated, or incorrectly treated.

After eliminating the most common causes of cough, the clinician's ability is directed toward a broad differential diagnosis. Diagnosis of many of the uncommon pulmonary disorders is difficult not only because of the lack of consideration of the disorder on the part of the clinician, but also because many of these entities do not readily exhibit specific or characteristic abnormalities on imaging procedures. This chapter attempts to consider the value of imaging tests in answering these potentially vexing clinical problems.

Mechanisms of cough

The mechanisms responsible for cough are complex, multifactorial, and incompletely understood. The cough reflex is subserved by vagal afferent pathways arising from the larynx and tracheobronchial tree. A great variety of stimuli and irritants can induce cough through the stimulation of multiple receptors located throughout the respiratory tract. These cough receptors belong to the group of rapidly adapting irritant nerve receptors (RARs).[1] The RARs found at the level of the larynx, trachea, and proximal bronchi are normally silent. When activated by mechanical or chemical stimuli, they cause rapidly adapting discharges with an irregular pattern that are conducted in phase-velocity vagal myelinated (Aδ) fibers.[1] Other afferent nerve endings of the tracheobronchial tree, such as slow-adapting pulmonary stretch receptors and pulmonary and bronchial C fibers, may also participate in cough.

The afferent pathways for cough are carried to the medulla oblongata in the brain stem; the motor outputs are in the nucleus retroambigualis, sending impulses via motor neurons to the respiratory muscles, and in the nucleus ambiguous, via motor neurons to the larynx and bronchial tree.[2,3] The cortical pathways controlling cough are also not well understood.

Useful clinical approach in the management of patients with cough: is cough acute, episodic, or chronic?

Although management of patients with cough can be challenging and difficult, identification of a potential cause of cough has been reported in 78–99% of patients presenting at a cough clinic.[4] The differential diagnosis is extensive and includes infections, inflammatory and neoplastic conditions, as well as many pulmonary and extrapulmonary conditions (Table 15.1).

A useful clinical approach that narrows the differential considerations is based on the duration of the cough and other presenting respiratory symptoms of the patient.

It is important to know whether the cough is acute, episodic, or chronic, and whether it is associated with a previously known illness. It is also essential to establish a lifetime exposure history including a complete list of

Table 15.1 Causes of cough

Airway causes

Tracheal diseases (non-tumoral)

Focal airway stenosis/strictures
   congenital
   postintubation
Diffuse tracheal thickening
   postinfectious tracheitis
   Saber sheath trachea
   tracheopathia osteochondroplastica
   relapsing polychondritis
   tracheobronchomegaly
   amyloidosis
   sarcoidosis
   Wegener's granulomatosis

Bronchial diseases (non-tumoral)

Bronchiectasis
   congenital: Williams–Campbell syndrome
   dyskinetic cilia syndrome and Kartagener's syndrome
   postinfectious bronchiectasis
Bronchiolitis
   exudative (cellular)
      infectious
   constrictive
      idiopathic
      secondary: toxic fumes, postinfectious, connective
      tissue disorders, etc.
Obstructive lung diseases
   chronic bronchitis
   asthma
      eosinophilic bronchitis

Tracheobronchial tumors and tumor-like conditions

Squamous cell carcinoma
Mucoepidermoid carcinoma
Adenoid cystic carcinoma
Carcinoid
Other tumors
   lipoma
   plasma-cell granuloma
   hamartoma
Foreign bodies and mucus plugs
Broncholithiasis

Parenchymal causes

Diffuse parenchymal diseases

Known cause
   drugs
   connective tissue disorders
   environmental exposure
   pulmonary edema
Granulomatous
   sarcoidosis, etc.
Rare with defined clinicopathological manifestations:
   lymphangioleiomyomatosis
   alveolar proteinosis, etc.
Idiopathic interstitial pneumonias
   usaual interstitial pneumonia
   non-specific interstitial pneumonia

Table 15.1 (Cont.)

   acute interstitial pneumonia
   cryptogenic organizing pneumonia
   desquamative interstitial pneumonia
   lymphocytic interstitial pneumonia
   respiratory bronchiolitis-interstitial lung disease
Smoking related interstitial lung disease
   respiratory bronchiolitis
   respiratory bronchiolitis-interstitial lung disease
   desquamative interstitial pneumonia
   Langerhans' cell histiocytosis

Gastroesophageal reflux

Postnasal drip syndrome

Other

Idiopathic chronic cough
Mediastinal masses
Thyroid disorders

occupations, drug use, hobbies, contact with pets, travel history, immunosuppression, and smoking and alcohol habits. Based on duration, cough can be divided into three categories as follows: acute, lasting 3 weeks; subacute, lasting between 3 and 8 weeks; and chronic, lasting more than 8 weeks.[4] Acute cough can persist and become a subacute or chronic problem.

Cough with sputum production usually points toward conditions such as chronic bronchitis and bronchiectasis, pneumonia, or other causes of excessive sputum production.[5] However, non-productive cough has been associated with disorders such as asthma, postnasal drip syndrome, and gastroesophageal reflux (GER).[6]

Acute cough

Acute cough in immunocompetent patients is common and usually attributed to upper respiratory infection, acute bronchitis, or acute sinusitis.[7] When there is no clinical or radiographic evidence of pneumonia, acute asthma, or an exacerbation of chronic obstructive pulmonary disease (COPD) for the cause of cough, acute bronchitis is the most frequent diagnosis.[8]

Other causes of acute cough include pneumonia, congestive cardiac failure, exacerbation of COPD, gastric aspiration, and pulmonary embolism.[9] Although, in these conditions, cough is usually associated with other symptoms such as shortness of breath and fever, it may be the predominant, or rarely the only, respiratory symptom.

Chronic cough

Chronic cough can be caused by many diseases. In approximately 95% of immunocompetent patients with chronic cough, the cough is caused by one of the following: postnasal drip syndrome from conditions of the nose and sinuses, asthma, gastroesophageal reflux disease, chronic bronchitis due to cigarette smoking or other irritants, bronchiectasis, eosinophilic bronchitis, or the use of an angiotensin-converting–enzyme inhibitor (ACE).[10] Other disorders causing cough include bronchogenic carcinoma, sarcoidosis, metastatic carcinoma, chronic aspiration, interstitial lung disease, and left ventricular failure. In the pediatric population, etiologies include congenital abnormalities (e.g. vascular rings, tracheobronchomalacia, pulmonary sequestration), mediastinal tumors, foreign bodies in the airway, and aspiration. More than one etiology can be present, or disease of one organ can affect others (e.g. systolic cardiac dysfunction can cause increased work of breathing through increased lung stiffness).

What is the role of imaging in the diagnosis of causes of cough?

Conventional chest radiographs

Imaging has an important role in assessing patients with cough. Although the chest radiograph remains an integral part of the examination of a patient with cough, it has shortcomings with respect to sensitivity and specificity. In patients with chronic cough, it is important to obtain previous chest radiographs for review. This allows the clinician to ascertain the onset, progression, chronicity, and/or stability of the patient's disease. In patients with chronic cough and a normal chest radiograph who are non-smokers and are not receiving therapy with an ACE inhibitor, the diagnostic approach should focus on the detection and treatment of upper airway cough syndrome, asthma, non-asthmatic eosinophilic bronchitis, or gastroesophageal reflux disease, alone or in combination.

When cough occurs in association with radiologically demonstrable pulmonary abnormalities, it is reasonable to assume that the two are related. In this setting, significant radiographic abnormalities, combined with the clinical history, is usually sufficient to limit the differential diagnosis.[11] Radiological findings may include focal consolidation, emphysema, diffuse parenchymal changes, atelectasis, and pleural effusion. A diffuse increase in pulmonary markings could represent atypical lung infection, interstitial lung disease, or a less common condition such as lymphangitic carcinomatosis.

There will be many patients for whom the chest radiograph is non-diagnostic. For example, overlying soft tissues may render diffuse lung diseases invisible on chest radiography, or in obese patients may give rise to a false impression of abnormal lung shadowing. Chest radiograph can also be normal in diseases for which abnormalities are typically present (e.g. COPD, asthma, interstitial lung disease, bronchiectasis).

Computed tomography scan

Chest computed tomography (CT) is not a first-line choice in the evaluation of a patient with cough but can be useful in patients who have respiratory symptoms but normal or questionable radiographic findings, depicting abnormalities not evident on the radiograph (e.g. emphysema, interstitial lung diseases, bronchiectasis), and the presence of complications and concurrent parenchymal, mediastinal, or pleural disease.[12–15]

It has also proved especially valuable in identification of occult airway pathology, evaluation of airway patency and identification of inflammatory airway disease, especially in the diagnosis of bronchiectasis. Expiratory CT is particularly accurate in detecting air trapping. CT can help further delineate the extent and distribution of disease and guide further diagnostic evaluation such as bronchoscopy and/or biopsy.[12,15] Finally, the value of CT is not limited to the pulmonary parenchyma and may also demonstrate a neck or mediastinal mass that produces airway obstruction or an occult lung mass.

How reliable is CT in establishing the etiology of cough?

After the development of helical CT in the 1990s, the ability of axial CT to image the normal and abnormal bronchial tree was well established. During recent years, the introduction of multidetector (MD) CT has provided a completely new radiological method for the assessment of thoracic diseases.[16,17]

Numerous reports comparing CT and fiberoptic bronchoscopy (FOB) have documented that CT is an extremely accurate modality for detecting pathological changes within the airways, caused by intrinsic or extrinsic mechanical narrowing, or by a functional abnormality.[17–19] In addition, CT is extremely useful in delineating the extent of peribronchial abnormalities, by defining the precise location and extent of disease surrounding the airways. In patients with central airway obstruction, especially those with associated collapse, CT allows distinction between central tumor and distal collapse, especially in cases in which intravenous contrast material has been administered. Relative to bronchoscopy, three-dimensional (3D) images have the additional advantage of assessing airways distal to an impassable stricture or mass.[19,20] Placement of metallic stents within narrowed airways has been shown to restore airway caliber and to relieve or diminish respiratory symptoms.

Diagnostic approach to the causes of cough

The patient with cough presents a formidable diagnostic challenge to physicians, and an organized approach is critical. The differential diagnosis of cough is extensive. The diagnostic approach includes diseases of the airways, pulmonary parenchymal diseases, gastroesophageal reflux, idiopathic cough, and miscellaneous disorders. More than one etiology can be present, or disease of one organ can affect others. Although there is some overlap, this section covers the entire spectrum of etiologies and highlights important but less common etiologies that often go unrecognized or misdiagnosed.

Airway causes of cough

Airway causes of cough result from focal or diffuse tracheobronchial disorders, including strictures after intubation or surgery, inflammatory diseases, extrinsic compression, tracheomalacia, trauma, and neoplasms.

Focal tracheal diseases

Obstructing tracheal disorders can result in cough, dyspnea, and stridor. Benign tracheal strictures may be congenital or acquired and can cause variable as well as fixed upper airway obstruction. The majority of acquired tracheal strictures occur as the result of intubation (Figure 15.1). They are a consequence of pressure necrosis, ischemia, and subsequent scarring.

Diseases producing focal thickening of the tracheal wall and narrowing of the tracheal lumen are difficult to diagnose on chest radiographs.[21] Both CT and magnetic resonance have proved reliable methods for assessing tracheobronchial strictures. On CT, tracheal stenosis may be seen as eccentric or concentric soft tissue thickening internal to normal-appearing tracheal cartilage. The outer tracheal wall has a normal appearance without evidence of deformity or narrowing. Expiratory CT shows little change in tracheal diameter.[22] It has been widely accepted that CT with multiplanar and 3D images provides more accurate assessment of the extent of tracheobronchial narrowing than axial images, with sensitivies of greater than 90% reported[18,23,24] (Figure 15.2).

Iatrogenic tracheomalacia associated with previous intubation or surgery may be the result of inflammation with subsequent thinning and weakening of the tracheal wall in the segment between the stoma and cuff, or caused by granulation tissue resulting from direct tracheal injury by the endotracheal or tracheostomy tube tip. Until recently, diagnosis was extremely difficult especially in determining the length of the segment of tracheomalacia. However, multislice CT scanning has revolutionized our ability to image structural changes in the central airways making it a feasible alternative to bronchoscopy for the diagnosis of suspected tracheomalacia.

Diffuse tracheal diseases

Diseases producing generalized thickening of the tracheal wall and narrowing of the tracheal lumen may be diagnosed on chest radiographs. Thickening of the tracheal wall is best diagnosed by the examination of the paratracheal stripes; a right paratracheal stripe measuring more than 4 mm in width is abnormal and, although a non-specific finding, must be investigated.[25]

Generalized thickening of the tracheal wall is usually associated with benign processes (e.g. tracheopathia osteochondroplastica, ulcerative colitis, amyloidosis, sarcoidosis, Wegener's granulomatosis, relapsing polychondritis, and various infections). Structural airway disorders such as saber sheath trachea and tracheobronchomegaly can also cause cough and dyspnea through expiratory tracheal collapse.

(a)

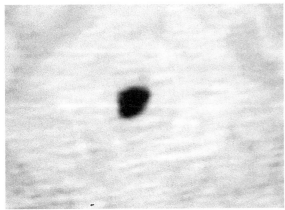

(b)

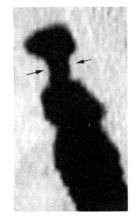

Figure 15.1
Postintubation subglottic tracheal stenosis. (a) Axial section at the level of the thoracic inlet shows markedly increased soft tissue density internal to the tracheal cartilage causing severe narrowing of the tracheal lumen. (b) Multiplanar coronal reconstruction shows a focal subglottic stenosis (arrows).

Saber sheath trachea is defined as a tracheal deformity in which the coronal tracheal diameter is equal to or less than one half the sagittal diameter measured 1 cm above the superior aspect of the aortic arch. It may be a useful sign of COPD[26] (Figure 15.3).

Tracheobronchomegaly (Mounier–Kuhn's syndrome) is thought to result from a congenital deficiency in the internal elastic membrane of the trachea and central bronchi. Tracheobronchomegaly has also been observed in patients with Ehlers–Danlos syndrome, generalized elastolysis, Marfanoid condition, or ankylosing spondylitis. Radiological manifestations include dilatation of trachea and main bronchi, and a corrugated appearance of airway walls due to mucosal herniation between adjacent cartilage rings (Figure 15.4). Expiratory collapse of the affected airway may be seen on dynamic CT.

Tracheobronchopathia osteochondroplastica (TO) is a rare benign disease characterized by the presence of osseous and cartilaginous submucosal nodules projecting into the tracheobronchial tree. The most common symptoms are cough, sinusitis, hemoptysis, hoarseness, dyspnea, and wheezing. It usually involves the lateral and anterior walls of the trachea and is associated with a variable degree of diffuse tracheal narrowing[27] (Figure 15.5).

Tracheomalacia, bronchomalacia, and tracheobronchomalacia result from an abnormal degree of compliance of the airways caused by structural weakness of the airway wall and its supporting cartilage. Cough and expiratory wheeze are the two common symptoms observed in almost all patients with airway malacia. For assessing the resultant airway flaccidity associated with tracheomalacia, paired end-inspiratory and end-expiratory sagittal two-dimensional images along the axis of the trachea are helpful for displaying the craniocaudad extent of excessive tracheal collapse during expiration[28,29] (Figure 15.6).

Relapsing polychondritis is a rare inflammatory disorder of cartilaginous and proteoglycan-rich tissues characterized by episodic inflammation and tissue destruction of the cartilaginous structures in the tracheobronchial tree, external

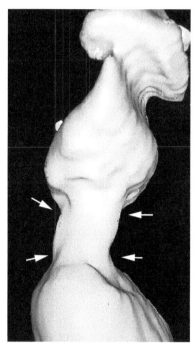

Figure 15.2
Postintubation tracheal stenosis. Multiplanar 3D surface rendered coronal reconstruction shows the true extent of the stricture (arrows).

(a) (b)

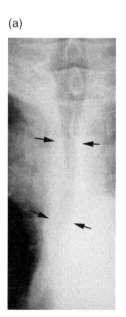 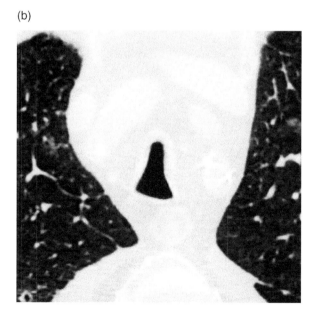

Figure 15.3
Saber sheath trachea. (a) Coned posteroanterior chest radiograph shows diffuse tracheal narrowing (arrows). (b) Axial CT section at the level of the supraaortic vessels shows a significant narrowing of the width of the trachea caused by deformity of the tracheal cartilage. The patient was a 54-year-old male smoker with chronic cough.

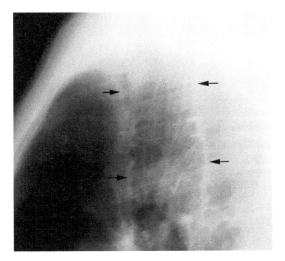

Figure 15.4
Tracheobronchomegaly (Mounier–Kuhn's syndrome). Coned view of a lateral chest radiograph shows marked dilatation of the trachea (arrows).

ear and nasal septum, as well as in a number of other organ systems. Laryngotracheal cartilage inflammation produces inspiratory obstruction and choking, cough, shortness of breath, and/or wheezing. Radiological manifestations include narrowing of the larynx, trachea, and main bronchi. On CT, abnormalities are characterized by tracheal wall thickening, expansion and calcification of cartilage, and luminal narrowing with a polygonal configuration.[30,31] Airway collapse and air trapping may be seen in expiratory CT in 50% of cases[32] (Figure 15.7).

Fiberoptic bronchoscopic balloon dilatation also referred to as balloon bronchoplasty can be safely performed in the management of non-malignant tracheobronchial obstruction such as saber sheath trachea, bronchial stenosis resulting from lung transplantation, sarcoidosis, Wegener's granulomatosis, and idiopathic stenosis.[33,34] It is also successful in the resolution of poststenotic lung abscesses, retention pneumonias, and atelectases.[33]

Bronchiectasis

Bronchiectasis is a condition that is characterized by the permanent dilatation of bronchi with destruction of elastic

(a)

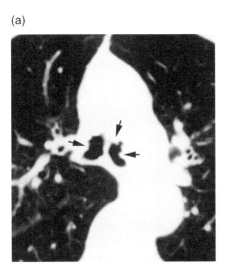

(b)

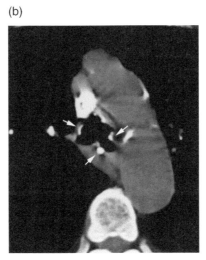

(c)

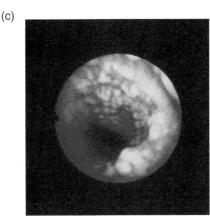

Figure 15.5
Tracheobronchopathia osteochondroplastica. Axial CT images at the level of the carina ((a) lung window; (b) mediastinal window) show characteristic appearance of submucosal calcified nodules, resulting in an irregular lumen narrowing the main bronchi lumen (arrows). (c) Bronchoscopic image shows irregular protrusions caused by multiple white griseous osteocartilaginous nodules, described as resembling a rock garden, on anterolateral wall of the trachea. The patient was a 67-year-old man.

(a)   (b)

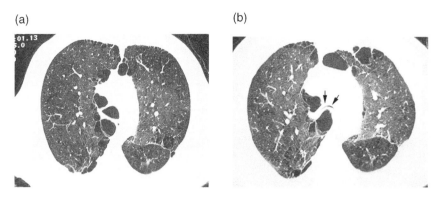

Figure 15.6
Tracheomalacia. (a) Axial high-resolution (HR) CT scan obtained at level of the aortic arch during inspiration shows normal caliber of the trachea. Note the presence of emphysema predominantly in a subpleural distribution. (b) HRCT scan at the same level during dynamic expiration shows crescent bowing of posterior membranous trachea and a marked narrowing of the tracheal lumen (arrows).

(a)   (b)

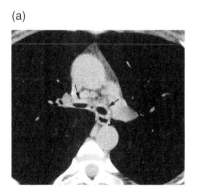   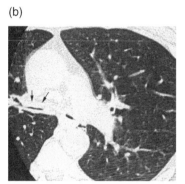

Figure 15.7
Relapsing polychondritis. (a) Axial thoracic CT displayed in soft tissue windows shows thickening of the wall of the main bronchi. (b) Axial CT, performed during dynamic expiration displayed in lung windows, shows extensive collapse of the main bronchi (arrows). The patient was a 50-year-old woman.

and muscular components of their walls, usually due to acute or chronic infection. A large percentage of patients have had a recognized episode of infection that resulted in the development of bronchiectasis, usually in early childhood. Once a common disorder, bronchiectasis is now a relatively infrequent medical problem that is diagnosed in approximately 4% of patients with chronic cough. However, in a patient with chronic productive cough, bronchiectasis should always be considered as a potential etiology. Although most cases of bronchiectasis in adults are idiopathic, a variety of causes, such as endobronchial abnormalities (e.g. tumors, tuberculosis, sarcoidosis, retained sutures, or broncholithiasis), isolated suppurative lower airway infection, habitual or psychogenic cough, or neuromuscular disorders, should be considered in the differential diagnosis.

The characteristic clinical findings of bronchiectasis are cough and purulent sputum production. Hemoptysis may occur in 50% of older patients. Patients with advanced cases may be complicated by the development of cor pulmonale and amyloidosis.

Chest radiograph must be the initial imaging examination in patients with suspected bronchiectasis. Although some authors have reported a high incidence of positive findings on conventional radiograph, in most instances the radiographic findings are either absent or non-specific.[35,36]

High-resolution (HR) CT scanning of the chest is the best test to establish this diagnosis with sensitivity and specificity exceeding 90%.[37] The diagnosis of bronchiectasis is generally established by recognition of characteristic signs, in particular the presence of signet rings (Figure 15.8). Bronchial wall thickness on thin-section CT scans should be evaluated with window centers between -250 and -700 HU and with window widths greater than 1000 HU. Other than window settings, notably window widths less than 1000 HU can lead to substantial artificial thickening of bronchial walls.[38]

Bronchial postinflammatory changes during or immediately after an episode of acute pneumonia may simulate bronchiectasis; these changes ('reversible bronchiectasis') revert to normal in 1–3 months.[39]

In patients for whom there is no obvious cause, a diagnostic evaluation for an underlying disorder causing bronchiectasis should be performed. Certain congenital diseases that cause defects in the supporting structures of the bronchi, abnormal secretions, or abnormal ciliary action definitely predispose to the development of bronchiectasis. The Kartagener's syndrome refers to the triad of situs inversus totalis, bronchiectasis, and either nasal polyps or recurrent sinusitis, occurring in approximately half of patients with primary ciliary dyskinesia (PCD) (Figure 15.9).

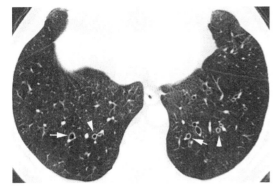

Figure 15.8
Bronchiectasis. HRCT scan (1-mm collimation) at the level of the lung bases in a 25-year-old man shows multiple dilated bronchi with increase in the bronchoarterial ratio. Note the presence of the typical signet-ring sign (white arrows) and bronchial wall thickening (arrowheads).

(a)

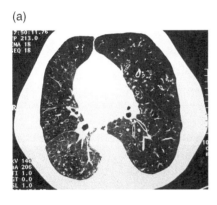

(b)

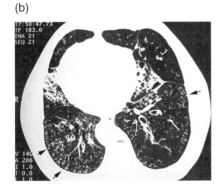

Figure 15.9
Kartagener's syndrome. (a) HRCT image (2-mm collimation) shows right sided aortic arch and bilateral cylindrical bronchiectasis. Note decreased attenuation and vascularity in the left lung suggesting the presence of obliterative bronchiolitis. (b) Bilateral cystic bronchiectasis in the middle lobe and lingula with associated lobar collapse. Multiple small branching opacities with a 'tree-in-bud' appearance are also visible in the right lower lobe (arrows).

Bronchiectasis related to allergic bronchopulmonary aspergillosis (ABPA) is seen most commonly in patients with long-standing bronchial asthma.[9] It is characterized pathologically by the presence of plugs of inspissated mucus containing *Aspergillus* organisms and eosinophils. Bronchiectasis tends to predominate centrally and in the upper lobes. When a similar disorder is caused by other *Aspergillus* species, different from *A. fumigatus*, or other fungi, the term allergic bronchopulmonary mycosis may be preferable.[40]

Acute clinical symptoms include recurrent wheezing, malaise with low-grade fever, cough, and sputum production. Patients with chronic ABPA may also have a history of recurrent pneumonia.

Radiological manifestations include homogeneous, tubular, finger-in-glove opacities in a bronchial distribution, usually involving predominantly or exclusively the upper lobes.[41] These shadows are related to plugging of airways by hyphal masses with distal mucous impaction and can migrate from one region to another. Occasionally, isolated lobar or segmental atelectasis may occur. A disparity between the extent of radiographic abnormality and the symptoms of the patient may occur. Extensive consolidation or multiple 'gloved-finger' opacities may be seen on the radiograph, yet the patient may be virtually asymptomatic.[41,42] The CT findings of ABPA consist principally of mucoid impaction and bronchiectasis involving predominantly the segmental and subsegmental bronchi of the upper lobes.[43] In approximately 30% of patients, mucoid impaction in these dilated, thick walled bronchi may be high in attenuation or calcified (Figure 15.10). Differential diagnoses include other causes of mucoid impaction such as endobronchial lesions, bronchial atresia, and bronchiectasis.

Adult patients with cystic fibrosis typically have panlobular bronchiectasis.[44] Mild reversible bronchial dilatation may be seen with severe chronic bronchitis as well as associated with acute pneumonia. Patients with an established diagnosis of cystic fibrosis may have significant worsening of respiratory symptoms with little visible radiographic changes.

Bronchiolitis

The term 'bronchiolitis' refers to a heterogeneous group of inflammatory disorders that are centered on small conducting airways. A variety of infectious and non-infectious diseases may affect the small airways causing either reversible or fixed bronchiolar obstruction. Although different classifications of bronchiolitis based on pathological, clinical, or radiological findings have been proposed, no one classification has been widely accepted.[45–47]

On the basis of a simple pathological classification, bronchiolitis can be divided into two types: constrictive (characterized by an irreversible scarring of the small airways), and exudative (characterized by a reversible exudative disease).

(a)
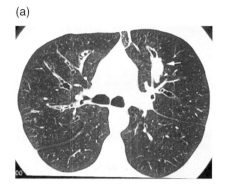

(b)
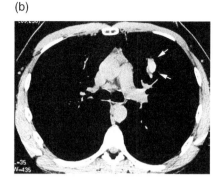

Figure 15.10
Allergic bronchopulmonary aspergillosis. (a) HRCT image (2-mm collimation) shows bilateral bronchiectasis and a mucus plug visible within dilated bronchus in the left upper lobe (arrow). (b) Mediastinal window image at the same level as (a) shows high attenuation mucus plug (arrows). The patient was a 25-year-old man with a history of asthma and chronic cough.

The CT features of bronchiolitis correlate closely with the findings seen on pathological specimens and can be divided into three broad categories: direct CT findings resulting from morphological changes in the airway wall or lumen (bronchiolar wall thickness and plugging of the lumen/'tree-in-bud' pattern), indirect CT findings reflecting regional abnormalities (mosaic attenuation pattern), and associated CT abnormalities within large airways.[46,48]

Bronchiolar wall thickening is a frequent but inconstant feature of bronchiolitis that occurs when inflammation, either acute or chronic, and fibrosis involve the bronchiolar wall. CT scan findings of mild bronchial wall thickening are not usually evident because the very small thickness increases are beyond the scanner resolution. Narrow lung window settings can mimic wall thickening due to 'blooming' artifact.

Mucoid impaction is often a prominent radiological finding in patients with bronchiolar diseases. The 'tree-in-bud' pattern, first described in diffuse panbronchiolitis (DPB) and endobronchial spread of tuberculosis, represents bronchioles filled with mucus or inflammatory material resulting in centrilobular tubular, branching, or nodular structures.[49–52] Additionally, peribronchiolar inflammation may result in poorly defined centrilobular opacities. When filled or impacted, CT scanning of dilated small airways shows subpleural nodules, in cross section, whereas when imaged lengthwise, branching subpleural structures of high attenuation are seen. This pattern is mostly associated with diseases associated with mucus stasis or infection.[50] It is the presence of bronchiolar wall thickening or plugging of the lumen that renders small airways visible in the lung periphery. Unfilled bronchiolar dilatation (bronchiolectasis) appears as subpleural tubular branching structures with well defined walls, or the classic 'signet ring' sign when seen in cross section.

Air trapping is a frequent indirect CT finding of constrictive bronchiolitis. Paired inspiratory/expiratory CT scans are being used increasingly because of increased sensitivity for early findings and greater specificity of diagnosis.[53,54]

In patients with cough and incomplete or irreversible airflow limitation, when direct or indirect signs of small airways disease are seen on HRCT scan, or purulent secretions are seen on bronchoscopy, non-bronchiectatic suppurative airways disease (cellular bronchiolitis) should be suspected as the primary cause.

Exudative bronchiolitis (cellular bronchiolitis)

A large number of bacterial, mycobacterial, fungal, and viral pathogens may cause exudative airway diseases. The characteristic pathological findings of exudative airway diseases include cellular bronchiolitis with inflammatory cells in the walls of the bronchioles and inflammatory exudate and mucus in the bronchiolar lumen. Bronchogenic dissemination of pyogenic bacteria and/or mycobacteria can result in dilatation and thickening of bronchiolar walls. Peripheral bronchioles may also be impacted by mucus or pus resulting in typical poorly defined centrilobular nodules and branching opacities, the so called non-specific 'tree-in-bud' appearance.[55,56]

In the healthy population, most cases of exudative airway diseases (cellular bronchiolitis) are due to viruses and mycoplasma. Bacterial bronchiolitis is more commonly seen in patients with impaired airway defenses.[55,56] Immunocompromised patients are highly susceptible to the more common Gram-positive (*Staphylococcus* species and, *Streptococcus* species) and Gram-negative (*Escherichia coli*, *Klebsiella* species, *Pseudomonas* species) bacteria. Most exudative airway diseases due to pyogenic infections are diagnosed by non-invasive means and do not require lung biopsy.

The cardinal CT feature in exudative (cellular) bronchiolitis is the 'tree-in-bud' pattern which reflects bronchioles impacted with inflammatory material[56] (Figure 15.11). Although the inflammatory changes are reversible in the majority of cases, recurrent and persistent infections may lead to bronchiolectasis.

A world-wide resurgence of tuberculosis is partly due to the high incidence of the disease in patients with AIDS. The most common route of dissemination in patients with postprimary (reactivation) tuberculosis is by bronchogenic spread from an area of cavitation. Airway involvement has been reported in 10–20% of all patients with pulmonary

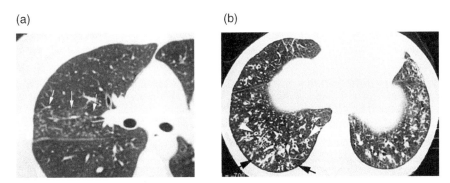

Figure 15.11

Exudative (cellular) bronchiolitis in two patients. (a) HRCT image (2-mm collimation) at the level of the carina shows centrilobular branching nodular and linear opacities resulting in a tree-in-bud appearance (arrows). The patient was a 20-year-old man with cough and recurrent respiratory infections. (b) Bronchiolitis due to *Streptococcus pneumoniae*. HRCT at the level of lung bases shows bilateral centrilobular nodules and branching opacities (tree-in-bud pattern) (arrows) and bronchial and bronchiolar wall thickening (arrowheads). The patient was a 45-year-old patient with AIDS.

tuberculosis.[51,57–59] Characteristic CT features include air-space consolidation, cavitation, scattered centriacinar nodules, and centrilobular branching structures in a 'tree-in-bud' appearance. Centrilobular nodules reflect the presence of intrabronchiolar caseous material, airway inflammation, and peribronchiolar inflammation. Coalescence of some acinar nodules may occur resulting in focal areas of bronchopneumonia. A combination of these CT findings, in an appropiate clinical setting, allows a specific diagnosis of endobronchial spread of tuberculosis in the majority of cases[51,57–59] (Figure 15.12).

Aspergillus infection has increased its frequency in immunocompromised patients and airway involvement occurs in up of 10% of cases with pulmonary aspergillosis.[60] Airway-invasive aspergillosis is diagnosed histologically on the basis of identification of organisms deep to the basement membrane.[60–62] The CT findings in pulmonary aspergillosis are variable, depending on the immunological status of the patient.[63,64] Thick-walled cavitary lesions are the most common radiological manifestations of invasive pulmonary aspergillosis in patients with AIDS, whereas consolidation and ill-defined nodules are frequently encountered in patients with hematological malignancies, and after bone marrow transplant. Invasive aspergillosis of the airways have been reported in immunocompromised patients.[63,64] The characteristic CT manifestations include lobar or peribronchiolar areas of consolidation, ground-glass opacity, centrilobular nodules less than 5 mm in diameter, and bronchiectasis.

Cytomegalovirus (CMV) bronchiolitis is a common complication following hematopoietic stem cell and lung transplantation. CMV bronchiolitis typically presents with fever, non-productive cough, dyspnea and hypoxemia. The CT findings of CMV-induced bronchiolitis are non-specific and include bronchial wall thickening, small branching

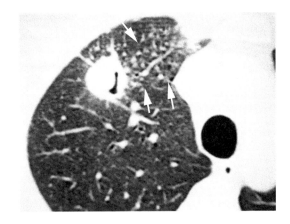

Figure 15.12

Endobronchial spread of tuberculosis. HRCT image (2-mm collimation) at the level of the aortic arch shows a nodule with central cavitation and adjacent multiple tree-in-bud opacities (arrows). These findings are highly suspicious of active tuberculosis with endobronchial spread. The patient was a middle-aged man with tuberculosis.

opacities, and centrilobular opacities. The diagnosis of CMV bronchiolitis is usually made by a combination of an appropriate clinical presentation, bronchoscopy with lavage and/or transbronchial biopsy, and a high-resolution CT of the lungs.

Approximately 20% of chest radiographs in patients with *Mycobacterium avium* complex (MAC)-related pulmonary disease are normal.[65] Radiological appearances of MAC-related pulmonary disease are similar to tuberculosis including multifocal patchy consolidation or ill-defined nodules that may cavitate.[66,67]

Diffuse panbronchiolitis (DPB) is characterized by chronic airflow limitation and airway inflammation with bronchiolar lesions.[68] In addition to progressive airway obstruction, patients with DPB develop episodic bacterial infection, often with *Pseudomonas aeruginosa*. The CT findings include centrilobular small rounded areas of attenuation, poorly defined centrilobular nodules and branching opacities ('tree-in-bud' pattern), dilated airways with thick walls, and a 'mosaic pattern of lung attenuation'. In these patients, an appropriate clinical setting and characteristic HRCT scan findings may obviate the need for invasive testing and a trial of macrolide therapy (erythromycin or other 14-member ring macrolides such as clarithromycin and roxithromycin) is appropriate.[68,69]

Obstructing bronchopulmonary aspergillosis is a descriptive term for the unusual pattern of a non-invasive form of aspergillosis characterized by the massive intraluminal overgrowth of *Aspergillus* species, usually *Aspergillus fumigatus*, in patients with AIDS[70,71] (Figure 15.13). Other fungal infections including *Histoplasma capsulatum* and *Coccidioides immitis* are seen in endemic areas.[72,73] The characteristic CT findings in obstructing bronchial aspergillosis mimic those of allergic bronchopulmonary aspergillosis (ABPA) consisting of bilateral bronchial and bronchiolar dilatations, mucoid impactions mainly in the lower lobes, and diffuse lower lobe consolidation caused by postobstructive atelectasis.

Constrictive bronchiolitis (obliterative bronchiolitis)

Constrictive or obliterative bronchiolitis is characterized by inflammation of the walls of membranous and res-

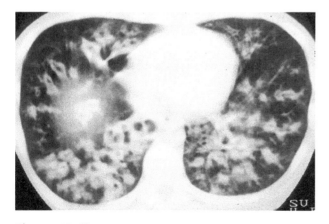

Figure 15.13
Obstructing bronchopulmonary aspergillosis. CT image (8.0-mm collimation) at the level of lower lung zones shows bilateral bifurcating tubular shadows caused by impacted mucous material within markedly dilated bronchi. Bronchoscopy revealed that the lumen was packed with inflammatory material. CT findings are similar to those of allergic bronchopulmonary aspergillosis. The patient was a 24-year-old man with AIDS.

piratory bronchioles leading to fibrosis with concentric narrowing or obliteration of the bronchiolar lumen.[45,47] The pathological changes in constrictive bronchiolitis are considered to be irreversible. A variety of different clinical syndromes and etiologies are associated with the similar histopathological abnormalities.[45,47] Conditions associated with constrictive bronchiolitis include mycoplasmal or viral infection, toxic-fume inhalation, lung or bone marrow transplantation, and collagen vascular diseases, especially rheumatoid arthritis.

Chest roentgenograms in cases of constrictive bronchiolitis are often normal or show only hyperinflation. CT scans, however, can be extremely helpful by showing a characteristic 'mosaic attenuation pattern' produced by reflex vasoconstriction secondary to hypoventilation of alveoli distal to bronchiolar obstruction and blood flow redistribution to adjacent normal lung parenchyma.

Swyer–James syndrome (McLeod syndrome) is secondary to an infectious insult to the small airways early in infancy and childhood that usually occurs prior to 8 years of age, before the total number of alveoli have fully developed. Adenovirus has been implicated as the primary agent. However, a wide variety of other organisms have been described, including measles, tuberculosis, pertussis, and *Mycoplasma pneumoniae*.

Although classically described and considered to affect one lung, CT has demonstrated that the disease may be multilobular in distribution and even bilateral. On HRCT, evidence of air trapping is extensive on the affected side and sometimes is also identified in the contralateral lung.[74,75] Other CT findings associated with air trapping are bronchiectasis and small foci of abnormal opacities representing residual scarring[74,75] (Figure 15.14). In the adult, differential diagnosis includes central obstruction from tumor, pulmonary embolism, and congenital hypoplasia or absence of a pulmonary artery. The last two conditions are not associated with air trapping at expiratory CT scanning.

Fume related bronchiolitis occurs after smoke inhalation. During a fire, a large number of potentially injurious chemicals can be released into the air. For example, wood and wood products release carbon monoxide (CO), oxides of nitrogen, acetaldehyde, and formaldehyde; plastics can release CO, hydrogen chloride (HCl), and phosgene. These fumes cause damage to the respiratory epithelium culminating in obliterative bronchiolitis with the associated clinical manifestations. Although the mechanism of disease varies with the inhaled product(s), the clinical manifestations and pathological reactions appear similar.[48,54,76] HRCT findings in patients with fume related bronchiolitis consist of patchy irregular areas of high and low attenuation in variable proportions ('mosaic pattern of lung attenuation'). These changes are accentuated on expiration (Figure 15.15).

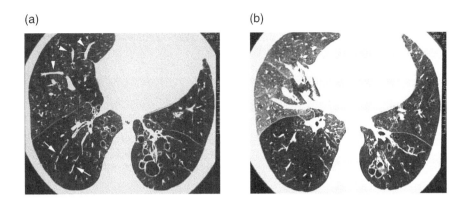

Figure 15.14
Constrictive bronchiolitis (Swyer–James syndrome). HRCT in a 45-year-old man with postinfectious obliterative bronchiolitis (Swyer–James syndrome). (a) Inspiratory CT scan shows bilateral patchy areas of lucency and bilateral bronchiectasis in the lower lobes. Note that the pulmonary vessels in the lucent-appearing lung (arrows) are smaller than vessels in the normal lung (arrowheads). In patients with obliterative bronchiolitis, bronchiectasis is commonly visible. (b) On expiratory CT, performed at the same level as (a), a significant degree of air trapping is clearly demonstrated. Note that bronchiectasis has also diminished in size.

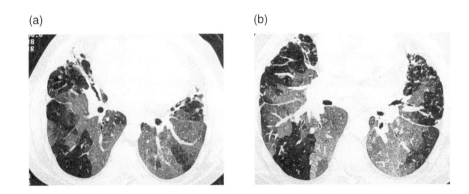

Figure 15.15
Fume related bronchiolitis (mosaic perfusion pattern). HRCT image (2.0-mm collimation) in a 52-year-old man after smoke inhalation. (a) An inspiratory scan shows patchy bilateral inhomogeneous lung attenuation consisting of ground-glass opacity and lobular areas of lucency due to mosaic perfusion. Note the relatively small size of pulmonary vessels in the lucent regions. (b) On expiration, there was no attenuation increase in the lucent areas. This finding suggests small airway obstruction and is consistent with obliterative bronchiolitis.

Obstructive lung disease

Obstructive lung diseases are characterized by progressive expiratory airway flow limitation and respiratory symptoms, including chronic cough, sputum production, and dyspnea. Although chest radiographs are clearly useful in the initial assessment of patients with obstructive lung diseases, the value of chest radiography in patients with acute exacerbations of their symptoms is less clear. In a study of 242 patients hospitalized with an exacerbation of COPD, only 35 (14%) had an abnormal chest radiograph, and in only 11 cases (4.5%) did radiographic findings result in management changes that were appropriate and clinically significant.[77]

Chronic bronchitis is one of the most common causes of lower airway disease and has been traditionally defined when cough and sputum expectoration occur on most days for at least 3 months of the year and for at least 2 consecutive years. In developed countries, cigarette smoking is responsible for 85–90% of cases of chronic bronchitis. Other airway diseases such as cystic fibrosis and asthma have clinical and histological features that overlap those of chronic bronchitis. The role of infection in chronic bronchitis remains unclear.

Asthma has been defined as a chronic inflammatory disorder of the airways that is associated with recruitment of inflammatory cells. It affects 5% of the US population and accounts for 2 million emergency department visits, 470 000 hospitalizations, and 4500 deaths annually.[78]

In a patient with chronic cough, asthma should always be considered as a potential etiology because asthma is a common condition with which cough is commonly associated. Different studies have shown that asthma is one of the most common etiologies of chronic cough (24–29%) in adult non-smokers.[4,6] Clinically, the patient experiences intermittent episodes of cough, dyspnea, and wheezing that may be associated to exposure to specific sensitizing substances (extrinsic asthma). Intrinsic asthma is characterized by the absence of atopy or specific external triggers of bronchoconstriction. Symptoms may reverse either spontaneously or as a result of treatment.

Conventional chest radiograph is rarely used to make a diagnosis of asthma. On chest radiography, increased lung volume, increased lung lucency, mild bronchial wall thickening, and mild prominence of hilar vasculature are the most common findings seen in adults with asthma. It is not surprising that the radiological changes, when present, are often slight and that the chest radiograph is commonly normal. The reported frequency of hyperinflation in adults with acute asthma varies between 20 and 70%. Moreover, chest radiographs are useful to exclude the presence of a number of complications and associations with asthma such as consolidation, atelectasis with mucoid impaction, pneumothorax, pneumomediastinum, and allergic bronchopulmonary aspergillosis. Consolidation in asthmatics is commonly infective but in some cases is due to eosinophilic consolidation.

CT is not usually indicated in the routine assessment of patients with asthma. However, the majority of symptomatic patients have an abnormal CT showing both bronchial and parenchymal abnormalities. The characteristic CT findings are bronchial dilatation, bronchial wall thickening, mucoid impaction, cylindrical bronchiectasis, centrilobular bronchiolar abnormalities such as tree-in-bud, patchy areas of mosaic perfusion and regional areas of air trapping on expiratory scans, and thick linear opacities representing discoid atelectasis[79,80] (Figure 15.16). When air trapping is severe, it can be seen on the inspiration scans.

In patients with severe asthma, a mosaic pattern of lung attenuation is indistinguishable from that seen in patients with constrictive bronchiolitis. In patients in whom bronchiolitis is suspected, a surgical lung biopsy should be performed when the combination of the clinical syndrome, physiology, and HRCT findings do not provide a confident diagnosis.

Improvements in CT scanning techniques together with faster quantitative algorithms to measure airway wall and lumen areas and to quantify and localize air trapping are being applied with increased frequency in research efforts to understand the changes in airways that occur in chronic obstructive lung diseases.

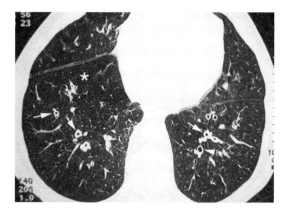

Figure 15.16
Asthma. HRCT image (2.0-mm collimation) in a 45-year-old man with chronic persistent asthma shows bronchial dilatation (arrowhead), bronchial wall thickening in both lungs (arrows), and patchy areas of air trapping (asterisk).

Emphysema is defined as 'a condition of the lung characterized by abnormal, permanent enlargement of air spaces distal to terminal bronchioles, accompanied by destruction of their walls, without obvious fibrosis'. Clinically, emphysema is characterized by irreversible airflow obstruction, pulmonary hyperinflation, and dyspnea on exertion.

Chest radiograph remains unreliable in the detection of emphysema, except in the advanced stage of the condition. The radiological appearances of emphysema may closely resemble those seen in severe asthma. In severe emphysema, the diaphragm is low and flat, the retrosternal space is increased, and the heart is small and vertical, all signs of overinflation. However, loss of peripheral vessels and diminution in the size of the mid-lung vessels in emphysema are not as uniform throughout the lung as in asthma.

CT is now widely used for evaluation of emphysema.[81] In terms of sensitivity, specificity, and assessment of disease extension, CT, and particularly MDCT, represents a significant advance over chest radiography. CT lung densitometry is more sensitive than the results of pulmonary function tests (PFTs) in detecting the progression of emphysema.[81] Longitudinal CT studies in emphysema have shown that quantitative analyses of low-attenuation clusters may be helpful for not only the elucidation of emphysema progression but also clarification of relation with risk factor such as smoking.[82]

Tumors and tumor-like conditions

A large variety of tumors, both benign or malignant, may arise within the trachea and large central bronchi. The symptoms of tracheal tumors are non-specific and can mimic a variety of diseases. Cough occurs in 33–85% of

(a)

(b)

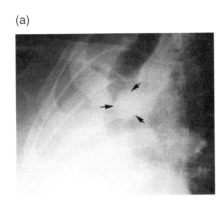
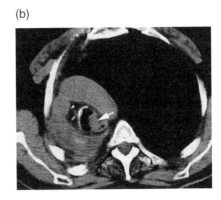

Figure 15.17
Squamous cell carcinoma. (a) Close-up view of a lateral chest radiograph shows a well circumscribed mass along the medial wall of the distal trachea (arrows). (b) Mediastinal window CT image (2-mm collimation) at the level of the aortic arch confirms the presence of the nodule. The patient was a 56-year-old male smoker with a previous right pneumectomy for a squamous cell carcinoma. Histologically, the nodule corresponded to a squamous cell carcinoma.

patients, hemoptysis in 27–66%, and dyspnea in 20–73%.[83] Chest radiograph is of limited value in the detection of tracheal tumors. The penetration of mediastinal structures on standard posteroanterior chest radiographs is often insufficient to allow adequate visualization of the tracheal lumen.[83] Moreover, endotracheal mass lesions visible on routine radiographs may be easily overlooked, if the entire trachea is not carefully examined (Figure 15.17). In a patient with cough who has risk factors for lung cancer or a known or suspected cancer in another site that may metastasize to the lungs, a chest radiograph should be obtained.

Primary tracheal tumors are rare, representing less than 1% of bronchial neoplasms.[84,85] The majority of tumors are malignant and most often arise in the posterior or lateral wall of the lower third of the trachea.[83] Squamous cell carcinoma and adenoid cystic carcinoma are the most common malignant tracheal tumors[86] (Figure 15.18). Direct extension into the mediastinum has been reported in squamous cell carcinomas.[87] Other primary malignant lesions are carcinoid and mucoepidermoid tumors (Figure 15.19). The trachea may be involved by direct invasion from tumors arising from thyroid, lung, or esophagus, or less commonly by hematogenous metastases resulting from renal and colonic neoplasms.

Whereas localized tracheal tumors appear radiographically as mass lesions of soft tissue density obscuring a portion of the tracheal air column, tracheal invasion from adjacent malignancies usually results in an asymmetric, irregular tracheal narrowing; an associated mediastinal mass is frequently seen (Figure 15.20).

The most common benign tracheal neoplasms are squamous cell papilloma; other benign tumors are hamartoma, plasma cell granuloma, and lipoma. On CT, they appear as polypoid intraluminal masses that may contain

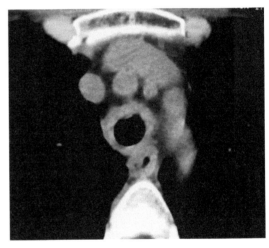

Figure 15.18
Adenoid cystic carcinoma. Mediastinal window CT image (2.0-mm collimation) at the level of the supraaortic vessels shows circumferential thickening of the tracheal mucosa. The patient was a 39-year-old man with an adenoid cystic carcinoma.

foci of calcification and fat or exclusively fat as occurs in lipoma (Figure 15.21).

Cough is present in 65% of patients at the time lung cancer is diagnosed, and productive cough is present in 25% of patients.[88,89] Co-morbid diseases such as obstructive chronic bronchitis, not just the tumor itself, may be independent or contributing causes to cough.[90] Obstructing primary bronchogenic carcinoma may lead to postobstructive pneumonia, which may accentuate the cough.[90]

The radiographic features of bronchogenic carcinoma are determined by the size of the lesion, its site of origin,

(a)
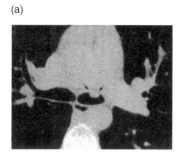

(b)
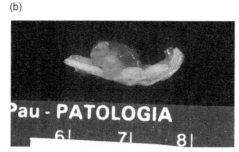

Figure 15.19
Mucoepidermoid carcinoma. (a) CT scan (2-mm collimation) at the level of the carina shows a well marginated nodule in left main bronchus. (b) Corresponding surgical specimen. The patient was an 18-year-old man with hemoptysis.

(a)
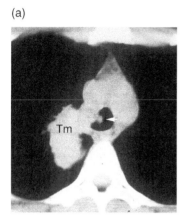

(b)
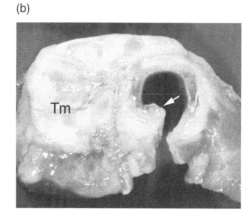

Figure 15.20
Bronchogenic carcinoma. (a) Non-enhanced CT scan (5-mm collimation) at the level of the aortic arch shows a right upper lobe lung cancer (Tm) invading the adjacent mediastinum and the lateral wall of the trachea (arrow). (b) Corresponding gross specimen obtained from autopsy confirms the mediastinal mass (Tm) and tracheal invasion (arrow).

(a)
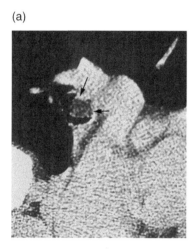

(b)
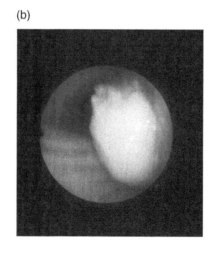

Figure 15.21
Intrabronchial lipoma. Mediastinal window CT scan (2.0-mm collimation) shows an endobronchial fatty mass (arrows) in the intermediate bronchus. (b) Fiberoptic bronchoscopy confirmed the lipomatous nature of the tumor. The patient was a 42-year-old man with persistent cough.

and its growth and dissemination. At the time of detection, most bronchogenic carcinomas are no longer amenable to surgical cure. Conventional radiographs show abnormal findings in approximately two-thirds of patients with bronchial tumors.[89] In half of these patients, a mass lesion can be visible; in the remainder, a partial or complete bronchial obstruction results in obstructive pneumonitis or lung collapse respectively (Figure 15.22). Occasionally, a central bronchogenic carcinoma may not cause a radiographic change in the contour of the hilar structures on the conventional chest radiograph but may give an increased density to the hilus.[89]

In patients with a suspicion of airway involvement by a malignancy (e.g. smokers with hemoptysis), even when the chest radiograph findings are normal, fiberoptic bronchoscopy is indicated.[89]

Bronchial carcinoid tumors are neuroendocrine neoplasms that arise within bronchial or bronchiolar epithelium. More than 80% of bronchial carcinoid tumors occur centrally, in the main or lobar bronchi, and appear as hilar masses on chest radiograph, or cause obstructive atelectasis and pneumonia. Carcinoid tumors may cause hyperinflation or air trapping in the distal lung parenchyma (Figure 15.23). Hyperlucency of the lung resulting from diminished blood within the vessels and parenchyma of the lung can be observed on radiographs obtained at full inspiration. The degree of hyperinflation is variable and radiographs obtained in expiration improve its visualization.

Because the extension of bronchial carcinoid beyond the bronchial wall occurs commonly, CT is extremely useful to provide additional information regarding extraluminal tumor extension. Usually, the intraluminal component may be relatively small compared with the bulk of the tumor and it represents only the 'tip of the iceberg'. Eccentric calcifications are seen in up to one-third of cases. Carcinoids tend to be highly vascular and, in a dynamic contrast-enhanced CT study, typical carcinoid tumors may demonstrate intense enhancement after contrast administration (Figure 15.24). This is particularly helpful for distinguishing the tumor from obstructive atelectasis or an adjacent mucus plug.

Foreign bodies and mucus plugs

Aspirated foreign bodies are by far the most common cause of intraluminal airway abnormality in childhood.[91,92] Clinically, most patients are children with varying degrees of cough and a recent history of foreign body aspiration. Most inhaled foreign bodies are food and broken fragments of teeth that frequently lodge in a main or lobar bronchus.[92] In most cases, radiological manifestations include obstructive lobar or segmental overinflation or atelectasis. Diagnosis requires careful integration of clinical data and radiographic findings, and a definitive diagnosis is usually made by conventional chest studies. CT is far more sensitive than chest radiography at demonstrating radiolucent foreign bodies.[93,94] In some instances, CT may provide additional diagnostic information showing subtle low-density intrabronchial material which is often the only finding that can help suggest the diagnosis.[93,94] Although in the

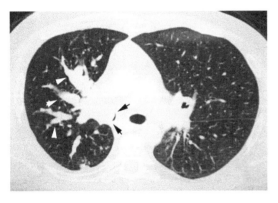

Figure 15.22
Bronchogenic carcinoma. HRCT scan (2-mm collimation) at the level of the carina shows an endobronchial nodule obstructing the right main bronchus (arrows). Note postobstructive multiple V-shaped mucoid impactions (white arrowheads).

(a)

(b)

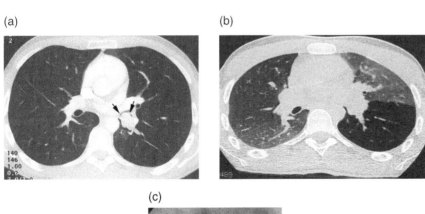

(c)

Figure 15.23
Bronchial carcinoid. (a) HRCT image (2.0-mm collimation) at the level of the intermediate bronchus shows a well defined, round, and partially endobronchial nodule (arrows) in the inferior bronchus of the left lower lobe. (b) Expiratory CT scan (lung windowing) shows overinflation and air trapping of the left lower lobe. (c) Photograph obtained during bronchoscopy shows a typical well defined 'reddy' nodule (arrows). The patient was an 18-year-old man with recurrent pneumonia and chronic cough.

(a)

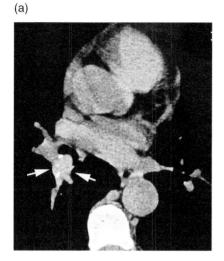

(b)

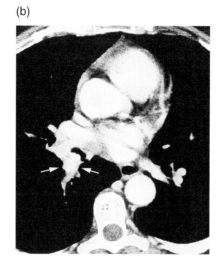

Figure 15.24
Bronchial carcinoid. (a) HRCT scan (2-mm collimation) shows a nodule with eccentric calcifications (arrows) obstructing partially the intermediate bronchus. Note the extraluminal component of tumor. (b) On contrast enhanced CT scan (mediastinal window) the nodule demonstrates marked contrast enhancement (arrows). The patient was a 45-year-old woman with a 3-year history of chronic cough and recurrent pneumonia.

majority of pediatric cases aspiration of a foreign body is diagnosed immediately or within 2–3 days of the event, exceptionally the diagnosis may not be made for weeks or sometimes even months. Once within the lung parenchyma, prolonged irritation with intermittent infections may result in massive hemoptysis.[92]

Intrabronchial retention of large plugs of inspissated mucus can occur in cases of disturbed bronchial secretion and/or impaired clearing mechanism.[95] Mucus plugs produce a variety of imaging appearances that are generally familiar, but sometimes can be difficult to differentiate from congenital, neoplastic, or infectious processes.[96] Based on radiological features or pathological states, mucus plugs have been described as gloved-finger, tooth-paste shadow, bronchial mucocele, and mucoid impaction.[96,97] Rod-like shadows are commonly seen in bronchial atresia, allergic bronchopulmonary aspergillosis, bronchiectasis, bronchial stenosis, bronchogenic carcinoma, and mucoviscidosis. Lobar collapse may result if a lobar bronchus is occluded by the excessive mucus and collateral ventilation does not permit air to enter the lung distal to the obstruction.[95]

The use of bronchoscopy for clearing retained secretions appears to be effective in patients who demonstrate lobar or segmental atelectasis[98] (Figure 15.25).

Parenchymal causes of cough

Pulmonary parenchymal causes of cough can be divided into diseases of the alveoli and of the interstitium. The distinction is somewhat arbitrary because these areas of the lung are intimately contiguous, and disease of one usually affects the other. There are, however, some diseases that appear radiographically distinct (i.e. either predominantly alveolar filling or interstitial).

Alveolar filling diseases

The radiographic hallmarks of alveolar disease include air bronchogram and ill-defined (fuzzy) margins. Distribution of disease can be focal or diffuse. Focal alveolar disease usually respects the anatomical barriers in the lungs, such as pleural fissures, demonstrating a lobar or segmental distribution. Diffuse alveolar disease may present with characteristic distributions (e.g. 'butterfly' or 'batwing' appearances) occupying central or peripheral regions. Finally, areas of alveolar disease may coalesce together to form larger areas of confluent alveolar disease.

Regarding alveolar disease, an important diagnostic key is to know whether it is acute or chronic. Acute alveolar disease is usually associated with infection, pulmonary hemorrhage, edema (cardiogenic or non-cardiogenic), and acute respiratory distress syndrome.

Any acute or chronic infection that involves the sinuses, upper airways, lower airways, and lungs may lead to acute or chronic cough. Tuberculosis should be considered early in the evaluation of patients with chronic cough when the likelihood of active tuberculosis is high.[99]

The chest radiograph represents an important initial examination in all patients suspected of having a pulmonary infection. In most cases the radiographic findings are suggestive or consistent with the diagnosis of pneumonia and sufficiently specific in the proper clinical context to preclude the need for additional imaging. However, there is wide disagreement among physicians on the presence or absence of pneumonia on chest radiographs, and a chest radiograph that shows 'no pneumonia' may not be sufficient to rule out the diagnosis.[100] In one large series, approximately 10% of patients with proven pulmonary infection had an apparently normal chest radiograph.

(a)

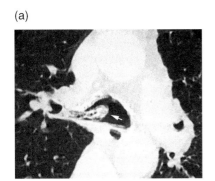

(b)

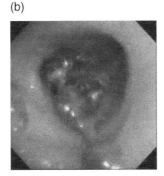

(c)

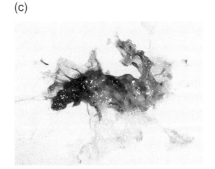

Figure 15.25

Mucus plug. (a) HRCT scan (2-mm collimation) at the level of the carina shows a 'tongue-like' material (arrow) filling the lumen of the main right bronchus and extending into the carina. Note the presence of tiny black lucencies (air bubbles) within the material. (b) Fiberoptic bronchoscopy demonstrated a tenacious mucous material that was subsequently removed. Note hematic content of mucus plug (c). The patient was a 55-year-old man with chronic bronchitis. (Courtesy of C Puzo, Barcelona)

Numerous reports have documented the usefulness of CT in the diagnosis and management of thoracic infections.

Non-resolving and recurrent pneumonia

Causes and patterns of non-resolving or recurrent pneumonia will depend on the nature of the underlying predisposition. Recurrent pneumonias may involve either a single or multiple areas of lung parenchyma. This anatomical distribution is extremely helpful in establishing a differential diagnosis. In infants, inhalational conditions (e.g. foreign body, lipid) and congenital malformations (congenital adenomatoid cystic malformation, bronchogenic cyst, and pulmonary sequestration) should be strongly considered when the recurrence appears in the same lobe; in pediatric patients, multilobar recurrent pneumonia could be associated with asthma, immunodeficiency syndromes, cystic fibrosis, or primary ciliary dyskinesias. In adults, bronchial obstruction secondary to bronchogenic carcinoma is the leading cause of recurrent pneumonia; other causes are foreign bodies, broncholithiasis, and aspiration. Multilobar recurrent pneumonia suggest a broader differential diagnosis. Aspiration is the most common cause of recurrent bilateral pneumonia. Other causes are structural abnormalities of the tracheobronchial tree and non-infectious illnesses such as cryptogenic organizing pneumonia and chronic eosinophilic pneumonia. Wegener's granulomatosis and other pulmonary vasculitis

may also present with recurrent pulmonary infiltrates. CT should be used in unresolved cases or when complications of pneumonia are suspected.

Diffuse parenchymal lung diseases

The most common clinical manifestations of patients with diffuse parenchymal lung diseases (DPLDs) are cough, dyspnea, fatigue, fever, and chest pain. HRCT scanning plays an integral role in the evaluation and diagnosis of DPLDs. The American Thoracic Society (ATS) and European Respiratory Society (ERS) have recommended an integrated clinical, radiological, and pathological approach to the diagnosis of DPLDs.[101] The differential diagnosis of DPLDs is extensive. Over 200 diseases can result in such a syndrome and the resulting clinical, physiological, and radiographical manifestations are often similar. A specific diagnostic cause of DPLDs can be established by combining a careful clinical history, physical examination, chest radiograph, HRCT, and, when indicated, bronchoscopic or surgical lung biopsy (Figure 15.26).

According to the ATS/ERS guidelines, DPLDs have been classified into four categories: DPLD of known cause (e.g. drugs, associated with a connective tissue disease, environmental exposure, etc.); granulomatous DPLD (e.g. sarcoidosis); rare DPLD with well-defined clinicopathological features (e.g. lymphangioleiomyomatosis, pulmonary Langerhans' cell histiocytosis, pulmonary alveolar

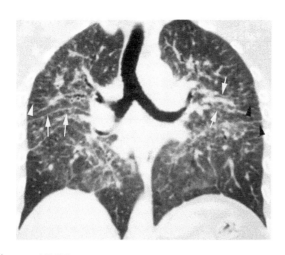

Figure 15.26
Sarcoidosis. Coronal inspiratory HRCT image acquired during a breath hold using a 16-row detector multislice CT scanner shows multiple small nodules in a predominantly peribronchoarterial and subpleural distribution (arrows) in association with thickening of the interlobular septa (arrowheads). Note bilateral upper lobes scarring. The patient was a 59-year-old woman with sarcoidosis.

proteinosis, and eosinophilic pneumonia); and the idiopathic interstitial pneumonias (IIPs), a heterogeneous group of non-neoplastic disorders resulting from damage to the lung parenchyma by varying patterns of inflammation and fibrosis.[101]

Connective tissue disorders

Chronic cough is a frequent respiratory manifestation in many autoimmune and collagen disorders. The connective tissue diseases are a heterogeneous group of immunologically mediated disorders in which the lungs are an important target organ because of their abundant connective tissue. Connective tissue disorders include rheumatoid arthritis, systemic lupus erythematosus (SLE), scleroderma, Sjögren syndrome, mixed connective tissue disease, relapsing polychondritis, and ankylosing spondylitis. Cough is observed in over 50% of patients with Sjögren syndrome and is the most common pulmonary symptom.[102] The most common form of diffuse pulmonary lung disease in patients with collagen vascular disorders is a chronic pulmonary fibrosis indistinguishable from other causes of usual interstitial pneumonia (UIP).[103] Rarely, the chronic pulmonary fibrosis may precede the extrapulmonary manifestations of the disease. Other complications of the connective tissue diseases include esophageal dysfunction leading to recurrent aspiration and secondary infection (in scleroderma and mixed connective tissue disease); respiratory muscle weakness contributing to atelectasis

and secondary infection (in SLE and polymyositis);[104] and drug-induced lung disease (methotrexate and gold treatment in rheumatoid arthritis). The approach to diagnosis of connective tissue disorders is discussed in the section on practical imaging in connective tissue disorders in Chapter 7.

Idiopathic interstitial pneumonias

A diagnosis of IIPs requires exclusion of other causes of pulmonary disease. HRCT features of IIPs are well recognized and several recent studies have shown that, in some cases, HRCT can help suggest a specific diagnosis with a degree of accuracy that approaches that of tissue biopsy.[105–110] The topic of IIPs and the value of imaging studies in its diagnosis are discussed in Chapter 6.

Smoking-related ILD

Smoking-related ILD is a term used to describe a heterogeneous group of diseases etiologically linked to cigarette smoking that can represent different degrees of severity of small airway and parenchymal reaction to cigarette smoke or other environmental exposures.[111,112] These diseases are desquamative interstitial pneumonia, respiratory bronchiolitis interstitial lung disease, and pulmonary Langerhans' cell histiocytosis.

Cough, which may be either non-productive or associated with non-purulent sputum, affects 75–80% of patients with smoking-related ILD.[113] Clinical context and knowledge of the appearance of smoking-related ILD on HRCT should allow the radiologist to make an appropriate differential diagnosis.

Langerhans' cell histiocytosis is one of these diseases that can be easily diagnosed by CT. In the early stage, HRCT demonstrates ill-defined nodular opacities (1–10 mm in diameter) mainly in a peribronchiolar distribution.[114] Cavitated nodules are seen in about 10% of the cases. In a later stage, cystic spaces ranging from a few millimeters to several centimeters in diameter are frequently seen. They may be round or irregular in shape, and their margins are smooth[114] (Figure 15.27). Sometimes, cystic changes can be difficult to differentiate from emphysema. Lack of visible walls in emphysema may be the only discriminating feature.

Cough and gastroesophageal reflux

Gastroesophageal reflux (GER), usually caused by transient relaxation of the low esophageal sphincter (LES), has been considered one of the commonest causes of chronic cough.

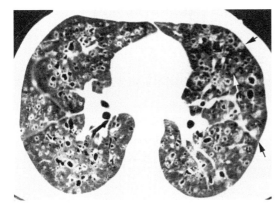

Figure 15.27
Langerhans' cell histiocytosis. HRCT scan (2-mm collimation) at the level of the right middle lobe bronchus shows numerous bilateral cystic lesions of various size. A few well marginated nodules are also visible (arrows). The patient was a 28-year-old male heavy smoker with chronic cough.

A significative number of patients with chronic bronchitis have gastrointestinal reflux,[115] and there is some evidence to suggest an association between reflux and asthma.[116] It would certainly be possible that intermittent microaspirative phenomena could produce mucosal injury of bronchioles and subsequent airflow obstruction. The best single test for diagnosing cough due to GER is 24-hour esophageal pH monitoring.[117] Barium swallow has low sensitivity and specificity, and is of little value in the initial evaluation of chronic cough due to GER.[118]

Thin-section CT findings that have been associated with obliterative bronchiolitis include bronchial dilatation, mosaic perfusion, bronchial wall thickening, and air trapping.[45]

Other causes of cough: idiopathic chronic cough

A proportion of cases, variously estimated at between 5 and 20%, remain unexplained after intensive investigations and trials. These patients are predominantly middle-age women with objective evidence of abnormality such as heightened cough reflex sensitivity and airway inflammation. Many patients with idiopathic chronic cough are labeled with a diagnosis of psychogenic cough but this is probably incorrect and it is perhaps more likely that any abnormal illness behavior is secondary to the adverse impact on psychosocial aspects of quality of life. Both chest radiograph and CT are normal.

Other imaging diagnostic studies

Many patients with cough will require other diagnostic studies than chest radiograph or CT. Plain sinus radiographs therefore are of little value in the evaluation of chronic cough, and sinus CT scanning should be reserved for refractory cases which may require surgical intervention.[119]

References

1. Widdicombe JG. Neurophysiology of the cough reflex. Eur Respir J 1995; 8: 1193–202.
2. Karlsson JA, Sant'Ambrogio G, Widdicombe J. Afferent neural pathways in cough and reflex bronchoconstriction. J Appl Physiol 1988; 65: 1007–23.
3. Shannon R, Baekey DM, Morris KF, Lindsey BG. Ventrolateral medullary respiratory network and a model of cough motor pattern generation. J Appl Physiol 1998; 84: 2020–35.
4. Irwin RS, Curley FJ, French CL. Chronic cough. The spectrum and frequency of causes, key components of the diagnostic evaluation, and outcome of specific therapy. Am Rev Respir Dis 1990; 141: 640–7.
5. Smyrnios NA, Irwin RS, Curley FJ. Chronic cough with a history of excessive sputum production. The spectrum and frequency of causes, key components of the diagnostic evaluation, and outcome of specific therapy. Chest 1995; 108: 991–7.
6. McGarvey LP, Heaney LG, Lawson JT et al. Evaluation and outcome of patients with chronic non-productive cough using a comprehensive diagnostic protocol. Thorax 1998; 53: 738–43.
7. Irwin RS, Rosen MJ, Braman SS. Cough. A comprehensive review. Arch Intern Med 1977; 137: 1186–91.
8. Braman SS. Chronic cough due to acute bronchitis: ACCP evidence-based clinical practice guidelines. Chest 2006; 129: 95S–103S.
9. Irwin RS, Corrao WM, Pratter MR. Chronic persistent cough in the adult: the spectrum and frequency of causes and successful outcome of specific therapy. Am Rev Respir Dis 1981; 123: 413–17.
10. Irwin RS, Madison JM. The diagnosis and treatment of cough. N Engl J Med 2000; 343: 1715–21.
11. Shah RM, Kaji AV, Ostrum BJ, Friedman AC. Interpretation of chest radiographs in AIDS patients: usefulness of CD4 lymphocyte counts. Radiographics 1997; 17: 47–58; discussion 59–61.
12. Brown MJ, Miller RR, Muller NL. Acute lung disease in the immunocompromised host: CT and pathologic examination findings. Radiology 1994; 190: 247–54.
13. Janzen DL, Padley SP, Adler BD, Muller NL. Acute pulmonary complications in immunocompromised non-AIDS patients: comparison of diagnostic accuracy of CT and chest radiography. Clin Radiol 1993; 47: 159–65.
14. Primack SL, Muller NL. High-resolution computed tomography in acute diffuse lung disease in the immunocompromised patient. Radiol Clin North Am 1994; 32: 731–44.
15. Tomiyama N, Muller NL, Johkoh T et al. Acute parenchymal lung disease in immunocompetent patients: diagnostic accuracy of high-resolution CT. AJR Am J Roentgenol 2000; 174: 1745–50.
16. Kauczor HU, Wolcke B, Fischer B et al. Three-dimensional helical CT of the tracheobronchial tree: evaluation of

imaging protocols and assessment of suspected stenoses with bronchoscopic correlation. AJR Am J Roentgenol 1996; 167: 419–24.

17. Boiselle PM, Ernst A. State-of-the-art imaging of the central airways. Respiration 2003; 70: 383–94.

18. LoCicero J 3rd, Costello P, Campos CT et al. Spiral CT with multiplanar and three-dimensional reconstructions accurately predicts tracheobronchial pathology. Ann Thorac Surg 1996; 62: 811–17.

19. Vining DJ, Liu K, Choplin RH, Haponik EF. Virtual bronchoscopy. Relationships of virtual reality endobronchial simulations to actual bronchoscopic findings. Chest 1996; 109: 549–53.

20. Remy-Jardin M, Remy J, Artaud D, Fribourg M, Duhamel A. Volume rendering of the tracheobronchial tree: clinical evaluation of bronchographic images. Radiology 1998; 208: 761–70.

21. Stark P. Imaging of tracheobronchial injuries. J Thorac Imaging 1995; 10: 206–19.

22. Webb EM, Elicker BM, Webb WR. Using CT to diagnose nonneoplastic tracheal abnormalities: appearance of the tracheal wall. AJR Am J Roentgenol 2000; 174: 1315–21.

23. Lee KS, Yoon JH, Kim TK et al. Evaluation of tracheobronchial disease with helical CT with multiplanar and three-dimensional reconstruction: correlation with bronchoscopy. Radiographics 1997; 17: 555–67; discussion 568–70.

24. Whyte RI, Quint LE, Kazerooni EA et al. Helical computed tomography for the evaluation of tracheal stenosis. Ann Thorac Surg 1995; 60: 27–30; discussion 30–21.

25. Gamsu G, Webb WR. Computed tomography of the trachea: normal and abnormal. AJR Am J Roentgenol 1982; 139: 321–6.

26. Greene R, Lechner GL. "Saber-sheath" trachea: a clinical and functional study of marked coronal narrowing of the intrathoracic trachea. Radiology 1975; 115: 265–8.

27. Restrepo S, Pandit M, Villamil MA et al. Tracheobronchopathia osteochondroplastica: helical CT findings in 4 cases. J Thorac Imaging 2004; 19: 112–6.

28. Boiselle PM, Dippolito G, Copeland J et al. Multiplanar and 3D imaging of the central airways: comparison of image quality and radiation dose of single-detector row CT and multi-detector row CT at differing tube currents in dogs. Radiology 2003; 228: 107–11.

29. Baroni RH, Feller-Kopman D, Nishino M et al. Tracheobronchomalacia: comparison between end-expiratory and dynamic expiratory CT for evaluation of central airway collapse. Radiology 2005; 235: 635–41.

30. Davis SD, Berkmen YM, King T. Peripheral bronchial involvement in relapsing polychondritis: demonstration by thin-section CT. AJR Am J Roentgenol 1989; 153: 953–4.

31. Im JG, Chung JW, Han SK, Han MC, Kim CW. CT manifestations of tracheobronchial involvement in relapsing polychondritis. J Comput Assist Tomogr 1988; 12: 792–3.

32. Lee KS, Ernst A, Trentham DE et al. Relapsing polychondritis: prevalence of expiratory CT airway abnormalities. Radiology 2006; 240: 565–73.

33. Hautmann H, Gamarra F, Pfeifer KJ, Huber RM. Fiberoptic bronchoscopic balloon dilatation in malignant tracheobronchial disease: indications and results. Chest 2001; 120: 43–9.

34. Mayse ML, Greenheck J, Friedman M, Kovitz KL. Successful bronchoscopic balloon dilation of nonmalignant tracheobronchial obstruction without fluoroscopy. Chest 2004; 126: 634–7.

35. Gudbjerg CE. Roentgenologic diagnosis of bronchiectasis; an analysis of 112 cases. Acta Radiol 1955; 43: 210–26.

36. Gudbjerg CE. Bronchiectasis; radiological diagnosis and prognosis after operative treatment. Acta Radiol 1957; 1–146.

37. Lee PH, Carr DH, Rubens MB, Cole P, Hansell DM. Accuracy of CT in predicting the cause of bronchiectasis. Clin Radiol 1995; 50: 839–41.

38. Bankier AA, Fleischmann D, Mallek R et al. Bronchial wall thickness: appropriate window settings for thin-section CT and radiologic-anatomic correlation. Radiology 1996; 199: 831–6.

39. Nelson SW, Christoforidis A. Reversible bronchiectasis. Radiology 1958; 71: 375–82.

40. Ricketti AJ, Greenberger PA, Mintzer RA, Pattersen R. Allergic bronchopulmonary aspergillosis. Chest 1984; 86: 773–8.

41. Mintzer RA, Rogers LF, Kruglik GD et al. The spectrum of radiologic findings in allergic bronchopulmonary aspergillosis. Radiology 1978; 127: 301–7.

42. McCarthy DS, Simon G, Hargreave FE. The radiological appearances in allergic broncho-pulmonary aspergillosis. Clin Radiol 1970; 21: 366–75.

43. Neeld DA, Goodman LR, Gurney JW, Greenberger PA, Fink JN. Computerized tomography in the evaluation of allergic bronchopulmonary aspergillosis. Am Rev Respir Dis 1990; 142: 1200–5.

44. Hansell DM, Strickland B. High-resolution computed tomography in pulmonary cystic fibrosis. Br J Radiol 1989; 62: 1–5.

45. Colby TV. Bronchiolitis. Pathologic considerations. Am J Clin Pathol 1998; 109: 101–9.

46. Ryu JH, Myers JL, Swensen SJ. Bronchiolar disorders. Am J Respir Crit Care Med 2003; 168: 1277–92.

47. Visscher DW, Myers JL. Bronchiolitis: the pathologist's perspective. Proc Am Thorac Soc 2006; 3: 41–7.

48. Pipavath SJ, Lynch DA, Cool C, Brown KK, Newell JD. Radiologic and pathologic features of bronchiolitis. AJR Am J Roentgenol 2005; 185: 354–63.

49. Lee KS, Im JG. CT in adults with tuberculosis of the chest: characteristic findings and role in management. AJR Am J Roentgenol 1995; 164: 1361–7.

50. Aquino SL, Gamsu G, Webb WR, Kee ST. Tree-in-bud pattern: frequency and significance on thin section CT. J Comput Assist Tomogr 1996; 20: 594–9.

51. Im JG, Itoh H, Han MC. CT of pulmonary tuberculosis. Semin Ultrasound CT MR 1995; 16: 420–34.

52. Im JG, Itoh H, Lee KS, Han MC. CT-pathology correlation of pulmonary tuberculosis. Crit Rev Diagn Imaging 1995; 36: 227–85.

53. Garg K, Lynch DA, Newell JD, King TE Jr. Proliferative and constrictive bronchiolitis: classification and radiologic features. AJR Am J Roentgenol 1994; 162: 803–8.

54. Muller NL, Miller RR. Diseases of the bronchioles: CT and histopathologic findings. Radiology 1995; 196: 3–12.

55. Franquet T, Muller NL. Disorders of the small airways: high-resolution computed tomographic features. Semin Respir Crit Care Med 2003; 24: 437–44.

56. Rossi SE, Franquet T, Volpacchio M, Gimenez A, Aguilar G. Tree-in-bud pattern at thin-section CT of the lungs: radiologic-pathologic overview. Radiographics 2005; 25: 789–801.

57. Lee KS, Hwang JW, Chung MP, Kim H, Kwon OJ. Utility of CT in the evaluation of pulmonary tuberculosis in patients without AIDS. Chest 1996; 110: 977–84.

58. Leung AN. Pulmonary tuberculosis: the essentials. Radiology 1999; 210: 307–22.

59. Leung AN, Brauner MW, Gamsu G et al. Pulmonary tuberculosis: comparison of CT findings in HIV-seropositive and HIV-seronegative patients. Radiology 1996; 198: 687–91.

60. Franquet T, Muller NL, Oikonomou A, Flint JD. Aspergillus infection of the airways: computed tomography and pathologic findings. J Comput Assist Tomogr 2004; 28: 10–16.

61. Franquet T, Serrano F, Gimenez A, Rodriguez-Arias JM, Puzo C. Necrotizing aspergillosis of large airways: CT findings in eight patients. J Comput Assist Tomogr 2002; 26: 342–5.

62. Gotway MB, Dawn SK, Caoili EM et al. The radiologic spectrum of pulmonary Aspergillus infections. J Comput Assist Tomogr 2002; 26: 159–73.

63. Aquino SL, Kee ST, Warnock ML, Gamsu G. Pulmonary aspergillosis: imaging findings with pathologic correlation. AJR Am J Roentgenol 1994; 163: 811–5.

64. Franquet T, Muller NL, Gimenez A et al. Spectrum of pulmonary aspergillosis: histologic, clinical, and radiologic findings. Radiographics 2001; 21: 825–37.

65. Marinelli DL, Albelda SM, Williams TM et al. Nontuberculous mycobacterial infection in AIDS: clinical, pathologic, and radiographic features. Radiology 1986; 160: 77–82.

66. Erasmus JJ, McAdams HP, Farrell MA, Patz EF Jr. Pulmonary nontuberculous mycobacterial infection: radiologic manifestations. Radiographics 1999; 19: 1487–505.

67. Miller WT Jr. Spectrum of pulmonary nontuberculous mycobacterial infection. Radiology 1994; 191: 343–50.

68. Nishimura K, Kitaichi M, Izumi T, Itoh H. Diffuse panbronchiolitis: correlation of high-resolution CT and pathologic findings. Radiology 1992; 184: 779–85.

69. Akira M, Kitatani F, Lee YS et al. Diffuse panbronchiolitis: evaluation with high-resolution CT. Radiology 1988; 168: 433–8.

70. Miller WT Jr, Sais GJ, Frank I et al. Pulmonary aspergillosis in patients with AIDS. Clinical and radiographic correlations. Chest 1994; 105: 37–44.

71. Mamelak AN, Obana WG, Flaherty JF, Rosenblum ML. Nocardial brain abscess: treatment strategies and factors influencing outcome. Neurosurgery 1994; 35: 622–31.

72. Sarosi GA, Johnson PC. Progressive disseminated histoplasmosis in the acquired immunodeficiency syndrome: a model for disseminated disease. Semin Respir Infect 1990; 5: 146–50.

73. Sarosi GA, Johnson PC. Disseminated histoplasmosis in patients infected with human immunodeficiency virus. Clin Infect Dis 1992; 14: S60–7.

74. Marti-Bonmati L, Ruiz Perales F, Catala F, Mata JM, Calonge E. CT findings in Swyer-James syndrome. Radiology 1989; 172: 477–80.

75. Moore AD, Godwin JD, Dietrich PA, Verschakelen JA, Henderson WR Jr. Swyer-James syndrome: CT findings in eight patients. AJR Am J Roentgenol 1992; 158: 1211–15.

76. King TE Jr. Overview of bronchiolitis. Clin Chest Med 1993; 14: 607–10.

77. Sherman S, Skoney JA, Ravikrishnan KP. Routine chest radiographs in exacerbations of chronic obstructive pulmonary disease. Diagnostic value. Arch Intern Med 1989; 149: 2493–6.

78. Barrios RJ, Kheradmand F, Batts L, Corry DB. Asthma: pathology and pathophysiology. Arch Pathol Lab Med 2006; 130: 447–51.

79. Hansell DM. Bronchiectasis. Radiol Clin North Am 1998; 36: 107–28.

80. Hansell DM, Wells AU, Rubens MB, Cole PJ. Bronchiectasis: functional significance of areas of decreased attenuation at expiratory CT. Radiology 1994; 193: 369–74.

81. Gurney JW, Jones KK, Robbins RA et al. Regional distribution of emphysema: correlation of high-resolution CT with pulmonary function tests in unselected smokers. Radiology 1992; 183: 457–63.

82. Matsuoka S, Kurihara Y, Yagihashi K, Nakajima Y. Morphological progression of emphysema on thin-section CT: Analysis of longitudinal change in the number and size of low-attenuation clusters. J Comput Assist Tomogr 2006; 30: 669–74.

83. Karlan MS, Livingston PA, Baker DC Jr. Diagnosis of tracheal tumors. Ann Otol Rhinol Laryngol 1973; 82: 790–9.

84. Pearson FG, Todd TR, Cooper JD. Experience with primary neoplasms of the trachea and carina. J Thorac Cardiovasc Surg 1984; 88: 511–8.

85. McCarthy MJ, Rosado-de-Christenson ML. Tumors of the trachea. J Thorac Imaging 1995; 10: 180–98.

86. Grillo HC, Mathisen DJ. Primary tracheal tumors: treatment and results. Ann Thorac Surg 1990; 49: 69–77.

87. Hajdu SI, Huvos AG, Goodner JT, Foote FW Jr, Beattie EJ Jr. Carcinoma of the trachea. Clinicopathologic study of 41 cases. Cancer 1970; 25: 1448–56.

88. Vaaler AK, Forrester JM, Lesar M et al. Obstructive atelectasis in patients with small cell lung cancer. Incidence and response to treatment. Chest 1997; 111: 115–20.

89. Shure D. Radiographically occult endobronchial obstruction in bronchogenic carcinoma. Am J Med 1991; 91: 19–22.

90. Kvale PA. Chronic cough due to lung tumors: ACCP evidence-based clinical practice guidelines. Chest 2006; 129: 147S–53S.

91. Marom EM, McAdams HP, Erasmus JJ, Goodman PC. The many faces of pulmonary aspiration. AJR Am J Roentgenol 1999; 172: 121–8.

92. Pattison CW, Leaming AJ, Townsend ER. Hidden foreign body as a cause of recurrent hemoptysis in a teenage girl. Ann Thorac Surg 1988; 45: 330–1.

93. Newton JP, Abel RW, Lloyd CH, Yemm R. The use of computed tomography in the detection of radiolucent denture base material in the chest. J Oral Rehabil 1987; 14: 193–202.

94. Bissonnette RT, Connell DG, Fitzpatrick DG. Preoperative localization of low-density foreign bodies under CT guidance. Can Assoc Radiol J 1988; 39: 286–7.

95. Glazer HS, Anderson DJ, Sagel SS. Bronchial impaction in lobar collapse: CT demonstration and pathologic correlation. AJR Am J Roentgenol 1989; 153: 485–8.

96. Felson B. Mucoid impaction (inspissated secretions) in segmental bronchial obstruction. Radiology 1979; 133: 9–16.

97. Proto AV. Evaluation of the bronchi with CT. Semin Roentgenol 1984; 19: 199–210.

98. Kreider ME, Lipson DA. Bronchoscopy for atelectasis in the ICU: a case report and review of the literature. Chest 2003; 124: 344–50.

99. Rosen MJ. Chronic cough due to tuberculosis and other infections: ACCP evidence-based clinical practice guidelines. Chest 2006; 129: 197S–201S.

100. Marrie TJ, Majumdar SR. Management of community-acquired pneumonia in the emergency room. Respir Care Clin N Am 2005; 11: 15–24.

101. American Thoracic Society/European Respiratory Society International Multidisciplinary Consensus Classification of the Idiopathic Interstitial Pneumonias. This joint statement of the American Thoracic Society (ATS), and the European Respiratory Society (ERS) was adopted by the ATS board of directors, June 2001 and by the ERS Executive Committee, June 2001. Am J Respir Crit Care Med 2002; 165: 277–304.

102. Strimlan CV, Rosenow EC 3rd, Divertie MB, Harrison EG Jr. Pulmonary manifestations of Sjogren's syndrome. Chest 1976; 70: 354–61.

103. Desai SR, Veeraraghavan S, Hansell DM et al. CT features of lung disease in patients with systemic sclerosis: comparison with idiopathic pulmonary fibrosis and nonspecific interstitial pneumonia. Radiology 2004; 232: 560–7.

104. Arakawa H, Yamada H, Kurihara Y et al. Nonspecific interstitial pneumonia associated with polymyositis and dermatomyositis: serial high-resolution CT findings and functional correlation. Chest 2003; 123: 1096–103.

105. Hunninghake GW, Lynch DA, Galvin JR et al. Radiologic findings are strongly associated with a pathologic diagnosis of usual interstitial pneumonia. Chest 2003; 124: 1215–23.

106. Lee KS, Chung MP. Idiopathic interstitial pneumonias: clinical findings, pathogenesis, pathology and radiologic findings. J Korean Med Sci 1999; 14: 113–27.

107. Lee KS, Chung MP. Diagnostic accuracy of thin-section CT in idiopathic interstitial pneumonia. Radiology 2000; 215: 918–9.

108. McAdams HP, Rosado-de-Christenson ML, Wehunt WD, Fishback NF. The alphabet soup revisited: the chronic interstitial pneumonias in the 1990s. Radiographics 1996; 16: 1009–33; discussion 1033–04.

109. Muller NL, Coiby TV. Idiopathic interstitial pneumonias: high-resolution CT and histologic findings. Radiographics 1997; 17: 1016–22.

110. Raghu G. Interstitial lung disease: a diagnostic approach. Are CT scan and lung biopsy indicated in every patient? Am J Respir Crit Care Med 1995; 151: 909–14.

111. Craig PJ, Wells AU, Doffman S et al. Desquamative interstitial pneumonia, respiratory bronchiolitis and their relationship to smoking. Histopathology 2004; 45: 275–82.

112. Vassallo R, Ryu JH, Colby TV, Harman T, Limper AH. Pulmonary Langerhans'-cell histiocytosis. N Engl J Med 2000; 342: 1969–78.

113. Caminati A, Harari S. Smoking-related interstitial pneumonias and pulmonary Langerhans cell histiocytosis. Proc Am Thorac Soc 2006; 3: 299–306.

114. Abbott GF, Rosado-de-Christenson ML, Franks TJ, Frazier AA, Galvin JR. From the archives of the AFIP: pulmonary Langerhans cell histiocytosis. Radiographics 2004; 24: 821–41.

115. David P, Denis P, Nouvet G et al. [Lung function and gastroesophageal reflux during chronic bronchitis. Bull Eur Physiopathol Respir 1982; 18: 81–6.

116. Ayres JG, Miles JF. Oesophageal reflux and asthma. Eur Respir J 1996; 9: 1073–8.

117. Kiljander TO, Salomaa ER, Hietanen EK, Terho EO. Chronic cough and gastro-oesophageal reflux: a double-blind placebo-controlled study with omeprazole. Eur Respir J 2000; 16: 633–8.

118. Richter JE, Castell DO. Gastroesophageal reflux. Pathogenesis, diagnosis, and therapy. Ann Intern Med 1982; 97: 93–103.

119. Pratter MR, Bartter T, Lotano R. The role of sinus imaging in the treatment of chronic cough in adults. Chest 1999; 116: 1287–91.

Index

Page numbers in *italics* refer to tables and figures.